Obstetric Evidence Based Guidelines

SERIES IN MATERNAL–FETAL MEDICINE

Available

Howard Carp, *Recurrent Pregnancy Loss: Causes, Controversies and Treatment*
ISBN 9780415421300

Vincenzo Berghella, *Maternal-Fetal Evidence Based Guidelines*
ISBN 9780415432818

Of related interest

Joseph J Apuzzio, Anthony M Vintzelos, Leslie Iffy, *Operative Obstetrics*
ISBN 9781842142844

Isaac Blickstein, Louis G Keith, *Prenatal Assessment of Multiple Pregnancy*
ISBN 9780415384247

Tom Bourne, George Condous, *Handbook of Early Pregnancy Care*
ISBN 9781842143230

Gian Carlo Di Renzo, Umberto Simeoni, *The Prenate and Neonate:*
The Transition to Extrauterine life
ISBN 9781842140444

Asim Kurjak, Guillermo Azumendi, *The Fetus in Three Dimensions:*
Imaging, Embryology and Fetoscopy
ISBN 9780415375238

Asim Kurjak, Frank A Chervenak, *Textbook of Perinatal Medicine,* second edition
ISBN 9781842143339

Catherine Nelson-Piercy, *Handbook of Obstetric Medicine,* third edition
ISBN 9781841845807

Dario Paladini, Paolo Volpe, *Ultrasound of Congenital Fetal Anomalies*
ISBN 9780415414449

Donald M Peebles, Leslie Myatt, *Inflammation and Pregnancy*
ISBN 9781842142721

Felice Petraglia, Jerome F Strauss, Gerson Weiss, Steven G Gabbe, *Preterm Birth:*
Mechanisms, Mediators, Prediction, Prevention and Interventions
ISBN 9780415392273

Ruben A Quintero, *Twin-Twin Transfusion Syndrome*
ISBN 9781842142981

Baskaran Thilaganathan, Shanthi Sairam, Aris T Papageorghiou,
Amor Bhide, *Problem Based Obstetric Ultrasound*
ISBN 9780415407281

Obstetric Evidence Based Guidelines

Edited by

Vincenzo Berghella MD FACOG
Director, Division of Maternal–Fetal Medicine
Professor, Department of Obstetrics and Gynecology
Jefferson Medical College of Thomas Jefferson University
Philadelphia, PA
USA

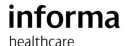

informa
healthcare

© 2007 Informa UK Ltd

First published in the United Kingdom in 2007 by Informa Healthcare, Telephone House, 69–77 Paul Street, London EC2A 4 LQ. Informa Healthcare is a trading division of Informa UK Ltd. Registered Office: 37/41 Mortimer Street, London W1T 3JH. Registered in England and Wales number 1072954.

Tel: +44 (0)20 7017 6000
Fax: +44 (0)20 7017 6699
Website: www.informahealthcare.com

Although every effort has been made to ensure that all owners of copyright material have been acknowledged in this publication, we would be glad to acknowledge in subsequent reprints or editions any omissions brought to our attention.

Although every effort has been made to ensure that drug doses and other information are presented accurately in this publication, the ultimate responsibility rests with the prescribing physician. Neither the publishers nor the authors can be held responsible for errors or for any consequences arising from the use of information contained herein. For detailed prescribing information or instructions on the use of any product or procedure discussed herein, please consult the prescribing information or instructional material issued by the manufacturer.

A CIP record for this book is available from the British Library.

Library of Congress Cataloging-in-Publication Data

Data available on application

ISBN-10: 0 415 70188 0
ISBN-13: 978 0 415 70188 4

Distributed in North and South America by
Taylor & Francis
6000 Broken Sound Parkway, NW, (Suite 300)
Boca Raton, FL 33487, USA
Within Continental USA
Tel: 1 (800) 272 7737; Fax: 1 (800) 374 3401
Outside Continental USA
Tel: (561) 994 0555; Fax: (561) 361 6018
Email: orders@crcpress.com

Distributed in the rest of the world by
Thomson Publishing Services
Cheriton House
North Way
Andover, Hampshire SP10 5BE, UK
Tel: +44 (0)1264 332424
Email: tps.tandfsalesorder@thomson.com

Composition by C&M Digitals (P) Ltd, Chennai, India
Printed and bound in India by Replika Press Pvt. Ltd
Cover image. Leonardo da Vinci, The babe in the Womb © 2007 The Royal Collection, Her Majesty Queen Elizabeth II

Contents

Contributors

Marianna Andreani MD
Department of Obstetrics and Gynecology
University of Milano-Bicocca
Monza
Italy

Valerie A Arkoosh MD
Department of Anesthesia
University of Pennsylvania School of Medicine
Philadelphia, PA
USA

Ariella Baylson MD BS
Jefferson Medical College of Thomas Jefferson University
Philadelphia, PA
USA

George Bega MD
Director of 3D Imaging Program
Research Assistant Professor
Jefferson Medical College of Thomas Jefferson University
Philadelphia, PA
USA

Michele Berghella MD
Department of Obstetrics and Gynecology
Ospedale Civile Santo Spirito
Pescara
Italy

Vincenzo Berghella MD
Director, Maternal–Fetal Medicine
Professor, Obstetrics and Gynecology
Jefferson Medical College of Thomas Jefferson University
Philadelphia, PA
USA

Sandra Patricia Bogota-Ángel MD
Department of Obstetrics and Gynecology
Crozer Chester Medical Center
Upland, PA
USA

Irina D Burd MD PHD
Department of Obstetrics and Gynecology
University of Pennsylvania
Philadelphia, PA
USA

Suneet P Chauhan MD
Director, Maternal–Fetal Medicine
Aurora Health Care
West Allis, WI
USA

Julie Takeuchi Crawford MD
Department of Obstetrics and Gynecology
Oregon Health and Science University
Portland, OR
USA

Jeff M Denney MD
Department of Obstetrics and Gynecology
Drexel University College of Medicine
Philadelphia, PA
USA

Gary Emmett MD
Director, General Pediatrics
Thomas Jefferson University
and
A I DuPont Hospital for Children
Philadelphia, PA
USA

Alessandro Ghidini MD
Perinatal Diagnostic Center
Inova Alexandria Hospital
Associate Professor, Obstetrics and Gynecology
Georgetown University
Alexandria, VA and Washington, DC
USA

Jay Goldberg MD MSCP
Director, General Obstetrics and Gynecology
Associate Professor, Obstetrics and Gynecology
Jefferson Medical College of Thomas Jefferson University
Philadelphia, PA
USA

Manish Gopal MD
Department of Obstetrics and Gynecology
University of Pennsylvania
Philadelphia, PA
USA

Marianne Greenberg BSN CRNP
Division of Maternal–Fetal Medicine
Department of Obstetrics and Gynecology
Jefferson Medical College of Thomas Jefferson University
Philadelphia, PA
USA

Jay S Greenspan MD MBA
Interim Chairman, Department of Pediatrics
Thomas Jefferson University and A I Dupont
    Hospital for Children
Philadelphia, PA and Wilmington, DE
USA

Colleen Horan MD
Department of Obstetrics and Gynecology
Jefferson Medical College of Thomas Jefferson University
Philadelphia, PA
USA

Thomas M Jenkins MD
Director of Prenatal Diagnosis
Legacy Center for Maternal–Fetal Medicine
Portland, OR
USA

Dawnette Lewis MD MPH
Assistant Clinical Professor
Division of Maternal–Fetal Medicine
Department of Obstetrics and Gynecology
North Shore University Hospital
New York University School of Medicine
Manhasset, NY
USA

Anna Locatelli MD
Department of Obstetrics and Gynecology
University of Milano-Bicocca
Monza
Italy

Mark C Molnar DO
Physician Health Alliance OB/GYN
Moses Taylor Hospital
Scranton, PA
USA

Victoria S Myers MD
Vincent Obstetrics and Gynecology Service
Massachusetts General Hospital
Harvard Medical School
Boston, MA
USA

Amen Ness MD
Clinical Assistant Professor
Stanford University Medical Center
Stanford, CA
USA

Sarah Poggi MD
Perinatal Diagnostic Center
Inova Alexandria Hospital
Assistant Clinical Professor
Georgetown University
Alexandria, VA and Washington, DC
USA

Normal G Rosenblum MD PHD
Director, Gynecologic Oncology
Professor, Obstetrics and Gynecology
Jefferson Medical College of Thomas Jefferson University
Philadelphia, PA
USA

Juan Carlos Sabogal MD
Department of Obstetrics and Gynecology
Jefferson Medical College of Thomas Jefferson University
Philadelphia, PA
USA

Rolf Alexander Schlichter MD
Department of Anesthesia
Hospital of the University of Pennsylvania
Philadelphia, PA
USA

Adele Schneider MD
Division of Genetics
Department of Pediatrics
Albert Einstein Medical Center
Philadelphia, PA
USA

Anthony C Sciscione MD
Director, Maternal–Fetal Medicine
Department of Obstetrics and Gynecology
Christiana Care Health Services
Wilmington, DE
USA

David F Silver MD
Women's Cancer Center of Nevada
Gynecologic Oncology
Las Vegas, NV
USA

Jorge E Tolosa MD
Associate Professor
Division of Maternal–Fetal Medicine
Department of Obstetrics and Gynecology
Oregon Health and Science University
Portland, OR
USA

Patrizia Vergani MD
Department of Obstetrics and Gynecology
University of Milano-Bicocca
Monza
Italy

John F Visintine MD
Division of Maternal–Fetal Medicine
Jefferson Medical College of Thomas Jefferson University
Philadelphia, PA
USA

Acknowledgments

Drs Jorge Tolosa, Suneet Chauhan, Jason Baxter, Lauren Plante, Bud Weiner, Leo Pereira, Regina Arvon, Alisa Modena, Amen Ness, Marie O'Neill, Jim Airoldi, Ted Hayes, John Visintine for reviewing and improving many of these guidelines.

My 'bosses' and mentors, for having given me a chance to practice the job I love, and showing me how to be an obstetrician: my father Andrea Berghella, Stanley Zinberg, Ron Wapner, Richard Depp, Ronald Bolognese, and Louis Weinstein. Finally, but perhaps most importantly, Lynn Stierle, for having been my trusted and patient assistant all these years.

Dedication

To Paola, Andrea, Pietro, mamma and papà, for giving me the serenity,
love, and strength at home now, then, and in the
future to fulfill my dreams and spend my talents as best as I could.

Abbreviations

Ab	antibody		CRL	crown–rump length
AC	abdominal circumference		CSE	combined spinal epidural
ACA	anticardiolipin antibody		CSF	cerebrospinal fluid
ACE	angiotensin-converting enzyme		CT	computed tomography
ACOG	American College of Obstetricians and Gynecologists		CVS	chorionic villus sampling
			DES	diethylstilbestrol
ACS	acute chest syndrome		DIC	disseminated intravascular coagulation
ADR	autosomic dysreflexia		DM	diabetes mellitus
AF	amniotic fluid		DNA	deoxyribonucleic acid
AFI	amniotic fluid index		DRVVT	dilute Russell's viper venom time
AFP	alpha fetoprotein		DV	ductus venosus
AFV	amniotic fluid volume		DVP	deepest vertical pocket
Ag	antigen		DVT	deep vein thrombosis
AIDS	acquired immunodeficiency syndrome		ECV	external cephalic version
ALT	alanine aminotransferase		EDC	estimated date of confinement
ANA	antinuclear antibodies		EDD	estimated date of delivery (synonym of EDC)
APA	antiphospholipid antibodies			
APS	antiphospholipid syndrome		EKG	electrocardiogram
aPT	activated prothrombin time		ERCD	elective repeat cesarean delivery
aPTT	activated partial thromboplastin time		FBS	fetal blood sampling
AROM	artificial rupture of membranes		FDA	Food and Drug Administration
ART	assisted reproductive technologies		fFN	fetal fibronectin
ARV	antiretroviral therapy		FGR	fetal growth restriction
ASA	aspirin		FHR	fetal heart rate
ASD	atrial septal defect		FISH	fluorescent in-situ hybridization
AST	aspartate aminotransferase		FLM	fetal lung maturity
AT III	antithrombin III		FM	femur length
AZT	ziduvidine		FOB	father of baby
bid	'bis in die', i.e. twice per day		FPO	fetal pulse oximetry
BMI	body mass index		FPR	false-positive rate
BP	blood pressure		FTS	first trimester screening
BPD	biparietal diameter		FVL	factor V Leiden
BPD	bronchopulmonary dysplasia		g	grams
BPP	biophysical profile		GA	gestational age
CAFS	conotruncal anomaly face syndrome		GBS	group B streptococcus
CAP	community-acquired pneumonia		GDM	gestational diabetes mellitus
CBC	complete blood count		GI	gastrointestinal
CD	cesarean delivery		HAART	highly active antiretroviral therapy
CDC	Center for Disease Control		HAV	hepatitis A virus
CF	cystic fibrosis		HBsAg	hepatitis B surface antigen
CHD	congenital heart defect		HBV	hepatitis B virus
CL	cervical length		HCG	human chorionic gonadotropin
CMV	cytomegalovirus		Hct	hematocrit
CNS	central nervous system		HCV	hepatitis C virus

HG	hyperemesis gravidarum	PC	protein C
Hgb	hemoglobin	PCEA	patient-controlled epidural analgesia
HIE	hypoxic-ischemic encephalopathy	PCI	placental cord insertion
HIV	human immunodeficiency virus	PCR	polymerase chain reaction
HR	heart rate	PE	pulmonary embolus
HSG	hysterosalpinogram	PFT	pulmonary function tests
HSV	herpes simplex virus	PGM	prothrombin gene mutation
HTN	hypertension	PID	pelvic inflammatory disease
IAI	intra-amniotic infection	PIH	pregnancy-induced hypertension
ICU	intensive care unit	PL	pregnancy loss
IM	intramuscular	PNC	prenatal care
IND	investigational new drug	po	'per os', i.e. by mouth
ITP	idiopathic thrombocytopenic purpura	PPH	postpartum hemorrhage
IUGR	intrauterine growth restriction (synonym of FGR)	PPHN	persistent pulmonary hypertension of the newborn
IUPC	intrauterine pressure catheter	PPROM	preterm premature rupture of membranes
IV	intravenous	pRBC	packed red blood cells
IVH	intraventricular hemorrhage	PROM	preterm rupture of membranes
IVIG	intravenous immune globulin	PS	protein S
L&D	Labor and Delivery (unit)	PT	prothrombin time
LA	lupus anticoagulant	PTB	preterm birth
Lab	laboratory	pTT	partial thromboplastin time
LBW	low birth weight (infants)	PSV	peak systolic velocity
LDP	luteal phase defect	PTL	preterm labor
LFT	liver function test	PTU	propylthiouracil
LMP	last menstrual period	PUBS	percutaneous umbilical blood sampling
LMW	low molecular weight	qd	once a day
LMWH	low molecular weight heparin	qid	four times per day
LR	likelihood ratio	qhs	before bedtime
LR	lactated Ringer's solution	QS	quadruple screen
MAS	meconium aspiration syndrome	RBC	red blood cell
MCA	middle cerebral artery	RCT	randomized controlled trial
MCV	mean corpuscular volume	RDS	respiratory distress syndrome
MOM	multiple of the median	REPL	recurrent early pregnancy loss
MRI	magnetic resonance imaging	RNA	ribonucleic acid
MTHFR	methylenetetrahydrofolate reductase	ROM	rupture of membranes
MVP	maximum vertical pocket	RPL	recurrent pregnancy loss
NA	not available	RPR	rapid plasma reagin
NAIT	neonatal alloimmune thrombocytopenia	RR	respiratory rate
NEC	necrotizing enterocolitis	Rx	treatment
NICU	neonatal intensive care unit	SAB	spontaneous abortion
NIH	National Institute of Health	SC	subcutaneous
NIH	non-immune hydrops	SCI	spinal cord injury
NRFHR	non-reassuring fetal heart rate	SDP	single deepest pocket
NRFHT	non-reassuring fetal heart testing	SIDS	sudden infant death syndrome
NRFS	non-reassuring fetal status	SLE	systemic lupus erythromatosus
NS	normal saline	SPTB	spontaneous preterm birth
NSAID	non-steroidal anti-inflammatory drug	STD	sexually transmitted disease (synonym of STI)
NST	non-stress test		
NT	nuchal translucency	STI	sexually transmitted infection
NTD	neural tube defect	STS	second trimester screening
n/v	nausea and/or vomiting	TB	tuberculosis
OR	operating room	TCD	transcerebellar diameter
PAPP-A	pregnancy-associated plasma protein-A	TG	*Toxoplasma gondii*

tid	three times per day	UFH	unfractionated heparin
TOL	trial of labor	U/S (or u/s)	ultrasound
TRAP	twin reversal arterial perfusion	VAS	visual analogue scale
TSH	thyroid-stimulating hormone	VBAC	vaginal birth after cesarean
TSI	thyroid-stimulating immune globulins	VDRL	venereal disease research laboratory
TTTS	twin–twin transfusion syndrome	VSD	ventricular septal defect
TVU	transvaginal ultrasound	VTE	venous thromboembolism
UA	umbilical artery	WHO	World Health Organization

Introduction

To me, pregnancy has always been the most fascinating and exciting area of interest, as care involves not one, but at least two persons – the mother and the fetus – and leads to the miracle of a new life. I was a third-year medical student, when, during a lecture, a resident said: 'I went into obstetrics because this is the easiest medical field. Pregnancy is a physiology process, and there isn't much to know. It's simple'. I knew from my 'classic' background that 'obstetrics' means to 'stand by, stay near', and that indeed pregnancy used to receive no medical support at all.

After almost 20 years practicing obstetrics, I know now that while physiologic and at times simple, obstetrics and maternal–fetal medicine can be the **most complex of the medical fields**: pregnancy is based on a different physiology than for non-pregnant women and can include any medical disease, require surgery, etc. It is not so simple. In fact, ignorance can kill, in this case with the health of the woman and her baby both at risk. Too often I have gone to a lecture, journal club, rounds, or other didactic event to hear presented only one or a few articles regarding the subject, without the presenter reviewing the pertinent best literature and data. It is increasingly difficult to read and acquire all the knowledge that is published, certainly in obstetrics, with over 20 journals publishing on this subject. Some residents or even authorities would state at times that 'there is no evidence' on a topic. Indeed, we used to be the field with the worst use of randomized trials.[1] As the best way to find something is to look for it, my co-authors and I searched for the best evidence. On careful investigation, we found data on almost everything we do in obstetrics, especially on our interventions. Indeed, **our field is now the pioneer for a number of meta-analyses and extension of work for evidence based reviews.**[2] Obstetricians are now blessed with lots of data, and should make the best use of it.

The **aims** of this book are to **summarize the best evidence available in the obstetrics and maternal–fetal medicine literature,** and make the results of randomized trials and meta-analyses **easily accessible to guide clinical care.** The intent is to bridge the gap between knowledge (the evidence) and its easy application. To reach these goals, we reviewed all trials on effectiveness of interventions in obstetrics. **Millions of pregnant women have participated in thousands of properly conducted randomized controlled trials (RCTs).** The efforts and sacrifice of mothers and their fetuses for science should be recognized at least

Table 1	*Obstetric evidence*
> 600 current Cochrane reviews	
Hundreds of other current meta-analyses	
Thousands of RCTs	
Millions of pregnant women randomized	

by the physicians' awareness and understanding of these studies. Some of the trials have been summarized in over 600 Cochrane reviews, with hundreds of other meta-analyses also published in obstetric topics (Table 1). All of the Cochrane Reviews, other meta-analyses and trials in obstetrics and maternal–fetal medicine were reviewed and referenced. The material presented in single trials or meta-analyses is too detailed to be readily translated to advice for the busy clinician who needs to make dozens of clinical decisions a day. Even the Cochrane Library, the undiscussed leader for evidence based medicine efforts, has been criticized for its lack of flexibility and relevance in failing to be more easily understandable and clinically readily usable.[3] It is the gap between research and clinicians that needed to be filled, making sure that proven **interventions** are clearly highlighted, and are included in today's care. All pilots fly planes under similar rules to maximize safety; by analogy, all obstetricians should manage all aspects of pregnancy with similar, evidence based rules. Indeed, **only interventions that have been proven to provide benefit should be used routinely.** On the other hand, *primum non nocere*: interventions that have clearly been shown to be not helpful or indeed harmful to mother and/or baby should be avoided. Another aim of the book is to make sure the pregnant woman and her unborn child are not penalized by the medical community. In most circumstances, medical disorders of pregnant women can be treated as in non-pregnant adults. Moreover, there are several effective interventions for preventing or treating specific pregnancy disorders.

Evidence based medicine is the concept of treating patients according to the best available evidence. While George Bernard Shaw said: 'I have my own opinion, do not confuse me with the facts', this can be a deadly approach, especially in medicine, and may compromise two or more lives at the same time in obstetrics and maternal–fetal medicine. What should be the basis for our interventions

Table 2	*Why did we write this book?*

Many aims:

- Improve the health of women and their children
- 'Make it easy to do it right'
- Clinical best care
- Research ideas
- Education
- Develop lectures
- Decrease disease, use of detrimental interventions, therefore costs
- Reduce medico-legal risks

Table 3	*Who is this book for?*

- Generalists
- Residents
- Nurses
- Medical students
- MFM attendings
- MFM fellows
- Other consultants on pregnancy
- Even lay public who wants to know 'the evidence'
- Politicians responsible for health care

in medicine? Meta-analyses allow summarizing of the best research data available. As such, they provide the best guidance for 'effective' clinical care.[4] It is unscientific and unethical to practice medicine or to teach or conduct research without first knowing all that has already been proven.[4] In the absence of trials or meta-analyses, lower-level evidence is reviewed. This book aims at providing a current systematic review of the evidence, **so that current practice and education, as well as future research, can be based on the full story from the best-conducted research, not just the latest data or someone's opinion** (Table 2). These evidence based guidelines cannot be used as a 'cookbook', or a document dictating the best care. The knowledge from the best evidence presented in the guidelines needs to be integrated with other knowledge gained from clinical judgment, individual patient circumstances, and patient preferences, to lead to best medical practice. These are guidelines, not rules. Even the best scientific studies are not always perfectly related to any given individual and clinical judgment must still be applied to allow the best 'particularizations' of the best knowledge for the individual, unique patient. Evidence based medicine informs clinical judgment, but does not substitute it. However, it is important to understand that greater clinical experience by the physician actually correlates with inferior quality of care, if not integrated with knowledge of the best evidence.[5] The appropriate treatment is given in only 50% of visits to general physicians.[5] At times, limitations in resources may also limit the physicians' knowledge. Guidelines and clinical pathways based on evidence not only point to the right management but also can decrease medico-legal risk.[6]

We aimed for brevity and clarity. Suggested management of the healthy or sick mother and child is stated as straightforwardly as possible, **for everyone to easily understand and implement** (Table 3). If you find the Cochrane Reviews, scientific manuscripts and books difficult to 'translate' into care of your patients, this book is for you. We wanted to prevent information overload. On the other hand, as remarked by Albert Einstein, 'everything should be made as simple as possible, but not simpler'. Key management points are highlighted at the beginning of each guideline, and in bold in the text. The chapters are divided into two volumes: one on obstetrics and one on maternal–fetal medicine. Please contact us (vincenzo.berghella@jefferson.edu or www.jefferson.edu/mfm) for any comments, criticisms, corrections, missing evidence, etc.

I have the most fun discovering the best ways to alleviate discomfort and disease. The search for the best evidence for these guidelines has been a wonderful, stimulating journey. Keeping up with evidence based medicine is exciting. The most rewarding part, as a teacher, is the dissemination of knowledge. I hope, truly, that this effort will be helpful to you, too.

References

1   Cochrane AL. 1931–1971: a critical review, with particular reference to the medical profession. In: Medicines for the Year 2000. Office to Health Economics; London: 1979: 1–11. [review]

2   Dickersin K, Manheimer E. The Cochrane Collaborations: evaluation of health care services using systematic reviews of the results of randomized controlled trials. Clin Obstet Gynecol 1998: 41: 315–31. [review]

3   Summerskill W. Cochrane Collaborations and the evolution of evidence. Lancet 2005; 366: 1760. [review]

4   Chalmers I Academia's failure to support systematic reviews. Lancet 2005; 365: 469. [III]

5   Arky RA. The family business – to educate. N Engl J Med 2006; 354: 1922–6. [review]

6   Ransom SB, Studdert DM, Dombrowski MP, Mello MM. Brennan TA. Reduced medico-legal risk by compliance with obstetric clinical pathways: a case-control study. Obstet Gynecol 2003; 101: 751–5. [II–2]

How to 'read' this book

The knowledge from all current available randomized controlled trials (RCTs) and meta-analyses in obstetrics is summarized and easily available for clinical implementation. Key management points are highlighted at the beginning of each guideline, and in bold in the text. Relative risks and 95% confidence intervals from studies are generally not quoted, unless trends were evident, to avoid crowding the text. Instead, the straight recommendation for care is made if one intervention is superior to the other, with the percent improvement often quoted to assess degree of benefit. If there is insufficient evidence to compare to interventions or managements, this is clearly stated.

An evidence based book must be based on adequate references, so to let "res ipsa loquitur" ('things speak for themselves'). Cochrane Reviews with 0 RCT are not referenced, and, instead of referencing a meta-analysis with only one RCT, the actual RCT is referenced. If meta-analysis includes >10 RCTs, not all RCTs are referenced, for brevity and because they can be easily accessed by reviewing the meta-analysis. If new RCTs are not included in meta-analysis, they are obviously referenced. Each reference was reviewed and evaluated for quality according to a modified method as outlined by the US Preventive Services Task Force (www.ahrq.gov):

I	Evidence obtained from at least one properly designed randomized controlled trial.
II-1	Evidence obtained from well-designed controlled trials without randomization.
II-2	Evidence obtained from well-designed cohort or case-control analytic studies, preferably from more than one center or research group.
II-3	Evidence obtained from multiple time series with or without the intervention. Dramatic results in uncontrolled experiments could also be regarded as this type of evidence.
III (review)	Opinions of respected authorities, based on clinical experience, descriptive studies, or reports of expert committees.

These levels were quoted after each reference. For RCTs and meta-analyses, the number of subjects studied was stated, and, sometimes, more details were provided to aid the reader to understand the study better.

Part I
Normal pregnancy

1

Prenatal care

Marianne Greenberg

KEY POINTS

- Prenatal care is probably of benefit to medically high-risk women, but there are insufficient data to recommend for or against prenatal care in low-risk women.
- A small reduction in the traditional number of prenatal visits in both developed and developing countries has not been associated with adverse biological maternal or perinatal outcomes, but women may feel less satisfied with fewer visits.
- There is no evidence that physicians need to be involved in the prenatal care of every woman experiencing an uncomplicated pregnancy, and some problems, in particular those involving social issues, may be better handled by midwives and other medical professionals such as general practitioners.
- Women should be allowed to carry their record.
- Continuity of care by midwives has been associated with less need for pain relief in labor, decreased incidence of cesarean delivery, less need for neonatal resuscitation, as well as improved patient satisfaction.
- Regular exercise during low-risk pregnancies is beneficial to overall maternal fitness and sense of well-being, with insufficient data to assess impact on maternal or fetal outcomes.
- Folic acid supplementation is recommended for neural tube defects (NTD) prevention, with 400 μg/day for all women, and 4 mg/day for women with prior children with NTD. All reproductive-age women should be on folic acid supplementation. Otherwise, supplementation should start at least 1 month before conception and continue until at least 28 days after conception.
- Most studies report that sexual activity is associated with better pregnancy outcomes, probably because women that are sexually active are healthier to begin with compared to women with less sexual activity.
- Breastfeeding is the best feeding method for most infants, and should be strongly encouraged. Counseling and education may facilitate breastfeeding success.
- Unsensitized RhD-negative women should be offered anti-D immunoglobin phophylaxis.

- Sweeping or 'stripping' of membranes during cervical examination at ≥ 38 weeks reduces the rate of post-term delivery.
- In women with late (> 32 weeks) pregnancy itching not associated with liver disease and a rash, chlorpheniramine 4 mg three times per day (tid) decreases itching.
- Massage with Trofolastin cream (*Centella asiatica* extract, α-tocopherol, and collagen elastin hydrolases) applied daily decreases the development of stretch marks. Massage with Verum ointment (tocopherol, panthenol, hyaluronic acid, elastin, and menthol) also decreases the development of stretch marks. These products are not widely available.
- Magnesium lactate or citrate chewable tablets 122 mg in the morning and twice this amount in the evening for 3 weeks for women with leg cramps are associated with significant improvement in persistent leg cramps.
- Water gymnastics for 1 hour weekly starting at <19 weeks reduces back pain in pregnancy, and allows more women to continue to work, with no adverse effects. A specially shaped pillow used for 1 week when laying in a lateral position reduces back pain in late pregnancy and improves sleep compared with a regular pillow. Both physiotherapy and acupuncture starting <32 weeks for 10 sessions might reduce back and pelvic pain.
- Dietary fiber supplements (such as 10 mg/day of either corn-based biscuits – Fibermed – or 23 g of wheat bran) increase the frequency of defecation and are associated with softer stools. Stimulant laxatives (such as senna 14 mg, or dioctyl sodium succinate 120 mg and dihyroxyanthroquinone 100 mg – Normax) resolve constipation compared with bulk-forming laxatives, but are more likely to be associated with diarrhea and abdominal pain. All these products are not widely available. Docusate sodium is a similar product and widely available.
- Rutoside capsules 300 mg tid for 8 weeks in the last 3 months of pregnancy improve leg edema symptoms, accompanied by a decrease in ankle circumference. Rutoside safety in pregnancy has not been sufficiently studied, and this product is not widely available.
- Oral hydroxyethyl rutosides decrease symptoms in women with hemorrhoids, and reduce the signs identified by the healthcare provider, but the safety data in pregnancy is still insufficient.

Introduction

Definition

Prenatal care (PNC) is the care provided to pregnant women to prevent complications and decrease the incidence of perinatal and maternal morbidity/mortality.[1]

Purpose

Prenatal care identifies pregnancies with maternal or fetal conditions associated with maternal or perinatal morbidity/mortality, and provides interventions to prevent such complications. Care should be systematic, evidence based, and provide both medical and psychological support as well as ongoing risk assessment. It should result in informed shared decision making between the patient and provider.

Prenatal care vs no prenatal care

The value of prenatal care (PNC) is controversial, as there is no definite evidence that it improves birth outcomes. **There are no randomized controlled trials (RCTs) of prenatal care vs no prenatal care.** Most studies are observational, comparing outcomes in women who have had prenatal care vs those without prenatal care. While some results show benefit, others do not. Selection bias (women who self-select to PNC are usually more inclined to have better outcomes) leads to confounding bias (e.g. risk factors associated with low birth weight [LBW] and neonatal death are also risk factors for inadequate PNC). Specific interventions for specific risks may reduce morbidity and mortality. Nonetheless, **prenatal care is probably of benefit to medically high-risk women,** while there are insufficient data to recommend for or against prenatal care in low-risk women.[2]

Frequency (and content) of prenatal care

PNC usually consists of 7–11 visits/pregnancy in developed countries, with an initial prenatal visit (PNV), followed by visits every 4–6 weeks to 28 weeks, every 3 weeks to 34 to 36 weeks, then weekly until delivery. Uncomplicated multiparous women may need fewer visits than uncomplicated nulliparous ones. Individual patient needs and risk factors should be assessed at the first prenatal visit, and reassessed at each appointment thereafter. Usual practice incorporates:

- routine visits for **prenatal education and reassurance**[3]
- provision of evidence-based screening tests at appropriate intervals
- problem-oriented visits as needed
- condition-specific care for high-risk patients.

A small reduction in the traditional number of prenatal visits in both developed and developing countries **has not** been associated with adverse maternal or perinatal outcomes, but women may feel less satisfied with fewer visits.[4] The schedule of visits should be determined by the purpose of the appointment. **A minimum of 4 PNC visits is recommended even for low-risk women.**[4] There is insufficient evidence to assess the effectiveness of prenatal education. Women can be offered the opportunity to attend prenatal classes, but there is no trial to assess their benefit. Individualized prenatal education directed toward avoidance of a cesarean delivery does not increase the rate of vaginal birth after cesarean section.[3]

Organizational issues

There is no evidence that physicians need to be involved in the prenatal care of every woman experiencing an uncomplicated pregnancy, and some problems, in particular those involving social issues, may be **better handled by midwives and other medical professionals such as general practitioners.**[4]

A formal, structured record should be used for documenting care during the pregnancy. Structured records with reminder aids help ensure that providers incorporate evidence-based guidelines into clinical practice. There is no trial comparing different records. **Women should be allowed to carry their record.**[5] Carrying the record is **associated with increased maternal control and satisfaction during pregnancy, increased availability of antenatal records during hospital attendance, but also with more operative deliveries.** More women in the case-notes-carrying group would prefer to hold their antenatal records in another pregnancy.[5]

Continuity of care by midwives during prenatal care and delivery is associated with decreased need for pain relief in labor, decreased (by 21%) incidence of cesarean delivery, less need for neonatal resuscitation, as well as improved patient satisfaction compared with care by a combination of midwives and physicians. It is not clear whether these associations are due to greater continuity of care, or to midwifery care.[6]

Initial visit

Ideally, this visit should occur prior to 12 weeks of gestation. Women should receive *written* information regarding their pregnancy care services, the proposed schedule of visits, screening tests that will be offered, and lifestyle issues, such as nutrition and exercise. Major parts of the visit include history, counseling, physical examination, and laboratory testing.

History and counseling

- A comprehensive history should be performed (Table 1.1), possibly using standardized record forms (e.g. www.acog.org). In particular, the woman who may require additional care or referral should be identified.

Table 1.1 *History and counseling*

Initial visit ≤ 12 weeks	Visits occurring 16–27 weeks	Visit at 28 weeks	Visits occurring 28–33 weeks	Visits occurring 34–41 weeks
Comprehensive history: 　Genetic screening 　Screening and counseling 　for lifestyle/workplace issues Directed physical exam 　(includes weight, BMI, BP, 　and urine dipstick) First trimester ultrasound Calculate EDC Lab screening: 　Hgb/Hct 　Blood type, Rh, antibody screen 　Rubella titer 　RPR 　HBsAg 　HIV 　Urine culture 　Gonorrhea/*Chlamydia* (if risk factors) 　Pap 　Offer aneuploidy screening 　(e.g. first trimester 　or sequential screening) Identify women who may need 　additional care Additional laboratory screening 　as needed	Review, discuss, and record results of screening tests: BP, FH, urine dipstick Offer second trimester quadruple screen if first trimester screen missed 18–22 week ultrasound Discuss quickening, lifestyle, physiology of pregnancy	Review, discuss, and record results of screening tests: BP, FH, urine dipstick Lab screening: 　GDM screening 　Repeat Hgb/Hct 　Repeat antibody screen Administer RhD immunoglobulin 　to appropriate women Reassess infectious disease 　risk and test accordingly	Review, discuss, and record results of screening tests: BP, FH, urine dipstick Consider third trimester ultrasound	Review, discuss, and record results of screening tests: BP, FH, urine dipstick Pre-eclampsia precautions Screening for GBS at 35–37 weeks Assess fetal presentation ≥ 34 weeks: 　offer ECV if breech Offer membrane sweeping 　at ≥ 38 weeks

BMI, body mass index; BP, blood pressure; EDC, estimated date of confinement; Hgb/Hct, hemoglobin/hematocrit; RPR, rapid plasma reagin; HBsAg, hepatitis B surface antigen; HIV, human immunodeficiency virus; FH, fetal heart; GDM, gestational diabetes mellitus; GBS, group B streptococcus; ECV, external cephalic version; Pap, Papanicolaou smear (cervical cytologic screening).

- The estimated date of confinement (EDC) is calculated based on last menstrual period (LMP). **Early ultrasonography should be used to determine the EDC.** Accuracy of EDC is critical for timing of screening tests and appropriate interventions, managing complications, and consideration of post-dates induction. It also provides early identification of multiple pregnancies (see Chapter 3 for further details).
- Genetic screening – all couples should be screened for family history of genetic disorders, history of recurrent spontaneous pregnancy loss, and history of a previous fetus or child who was affected by a genetic disorder. Cystic fibrosis (CF) screening should be offered to women with a family history of CF, reproductive partners of individuals with CF, couples in whom one or both partners are Caucasian and are planning a pregnancy or are seeking prenatal care (see Chapter 5).
- Those patients belonging to an ethnic group at increased risk for a recessive condition (e.g. sickle cell anemia, Tay–Sachs disease, α- or β-thalassemia, etc.) should be offered specific screening. Women with a specific indication for genetic testing should be referred for genetic counseling and a discussion of options available for prenatal diagnosis (see Chapters 4 and 5 for further details).
- Assessment of risk factors related to lifestyle and workplace, and recommendations for modification in pregnancy – nutrition and nutritional supplements, and recommended weight gain.

Nutrition and nutritional supplements

Folic acid

Folic acid supplementation is recommended, with a minimum 400 μg/day for all women: [93% decrease in neural tube defects (NTD)] and 4 mg/day for women with prior children with NTD (69% decrease in NTD).[7] Supplementation should start at least 1 month before conception and continue until at least 28 days after conception (time of neural tube closure). Given the unpredictability of planned conception and that 50% of pregnancies are unplanned, all reproductive-age women should be on folic acid supplementation. Given that in several countries (e.g. Western countries) the baseline serum folate level is only 5 ng/ml, and that increases in this level are directly proportional with a decrease in the incidence of NTD, some experts have advocated 5 mg of folic acid per day as optimal supplementation.[8] **No increase in ectopic pregnancy, miscarriage, or stillbirth has been associated with folate supplementation, but it might increase (non-significant trend) the incidence of multiple gestations by 40%.**[7] The overall benefits or risks of fortifying basic foods such as grains with added folate have been insufficiently studied, but have been associated with an increase in supplementation of only 140–200 μg/day, and with only a 20–50% decrease in incidence of NTD.[9] Women taking anti-seizure medications, other drugs which might interfere with folic acid metabolism, those with homozygous MTHFR enzyme mutations, multiple gestations or those who are obese may need higher doses of folate supplementation. Women with first trimester diabetes mellitus, or exposure to valproic acid or high temperatures, might not experience decrease in NTD risk with folate supplementation due to these risks.

Vitamin A

Excess vitamin A intake can cause birth defects and miscarriages at doses >25 000 IU per day. Vitamin A supplements should be avoided, with maximum intake prior to and during pregnancy probably 5000 IU, certainly ≤10 000 IU. **Vitamin A supplementation may be beneficial to women with vitamin A deficiency, especially in prevention of night blindness, in developing countries.**[10] Optimal duration of supplement use cannot be evaluated. One large population-based trial in Nepal showed a possible beneficial effect on maternal mortality after weekly vitamin A supplements. Night blindness, associated with vitamin A deficiency, was assessed in a nested case-control study within this trial and found to be reduced but not eliminated. There is insufficient evidence to support vitamin A supplementation as intervention for anemia.[10]

Vitamin B₆ (pyridoxine)

There is insufficient evidence to evaluate pyridoxine supplementation during pregnancy. **For the aim of decreasing dental decay or missing/filled teeth, pyridoxine supplementation 20 μg/day (either as oral capsules or even better with lozenges) is associated with decreased incidence of these outcomes in pregnant women.**[11]

Vitamin C

The data are insufficient to assess if vitamin C supplementation either alone or in combination with other supplements is beneficial during pregnancy for either low- or high-risk women. There are **no trials** available to assess whether vitamin C supplementation may be useful for **all pregnant women.** All of the women involved in the trials were either at high risk of pre-eclampsia or preterm birth, or the women had established severe early onset pre-eclampsia (see also *Maternal–Fetal Evidence Based Guidelines*, Chapter 7). No difference is seen between women supplemented with vitamin C alone or in combination with other supplements compared with placebo for the risk of stillbirth, neonatal death, birth weight, or intrauterine growth restriction.[12] **Women supplemented with vitamin C compared with placebo are at** increased risk of giving birth preterm.[12] Women supplemented with vitamin C have a trend for decreased risk of pre-eclampsia. Only one study evaluated vitamin C supplementation alone; the remaining trials used either a combination of vitamin C and vitamin E, or vitamin C, vitamin E, aspirin, and fish oil. The data are too few to allow meaningful comparisons assessing the impact of vitamin C given alone compared with vitamin C given with other supplements; hence, any treatment effects found cannot be attributed directly to vitamin C.[12]

Vitamin D

There is insufficient evidence to evaluate the effects of vitamin D supplementation during pregnancy. Vitamin D 1000 IU/day in the third trimester is associated with no consistent effect on incidence of lower birth weight.[13] **Neonatal hypocalcemia is less common** with vitamin D supplementation compared to placebo.[13] There are limited data to assess any benefit of vitamin D supplements for complete vegetarians and women with extremely limited exposure to sunlight.

Vitamin E

There is insufficient evidence to assess if vitamin E supplementation either alone or in combination with other supplements is beneficial during pregnancy. There are **no trials** available to assess whether vitamin E supplementation may be useful for **all pregnant women**, or if vitamin E may be beneficial when used alone. All evidence tested women at high risk of pre-eclampsia or with established pre-eclampsia, and assessed vitamin E in combination with other supplements (usually vitamin C). Compared with placebo, vitamin E in combination with other supplements during pregnancy is associated with similar risk of stillbirth, neonatal death, perinatal death, preterm birth, intrauterine growth restriction, or birth weight.[14] Vitamin E in combination with other supplements compared with placebo is associated with a non-significant trend for decreased risk of developing clinical pre-eclampsia. There are no differences between women supplemented with vitamin E compared with placebo for any other outcomes.[14]

Multivitamin supplementation

There is insufficient evidence to recommend routine multivitamin supplementation for all women, or even only for women who are underweight, have poor diets, smokers, substance abusers, vegetarians, multiple gestations, or others. **Excess (>1) prenatal vitamin intake/day should be avoided. No prenatal multivitamin supplement has been shown to be superior to another.** Use of multivitamin supplements not specific for pregnancy should be discouraged, as often excess doses can pose risks to the pregnancy.

Table 1.2	*Usual content of multivitamin supplements*
Vitamin A 4000 IU (100% as beta-carotene): 50% RDA	
Vitamin C 120 mg: 200% RDA	
Vitamin D 400 IU: 100% RDA	
Vitamin E 30 IU: 100% RDA	
Vitamin B_6 2.6 mg: 104% RDA	
Vitamin B_{12} 8 µg: 100% RDA	
Thiamin 1.8 mg: 106% RDA	
Riboflavin 1.7 mg: 85% RDA	
Niacin 20 mg: 100% RDA	
Calcium 200 mg: 15% RDA	
Iron 28 mg: 156% RDA	
Folic acid 800 µg: 100% RDA	

RDA, recommended daily allowance.

Prenatal vitamins commonly contain supplements, as shown in Table 1.2.

Magnesium

There is insufficient high-quality evidence to show that dietary magnesium supplementation during pregnancy is beneficial. Including high- and low-quality trials, oral magnesium treatment from before the 25th week of gestation is associated with a lower frequency of preterm birth, a lower frequency of low birth weight, and fewer small for gestational age infants compared with placebo.[15] In addition, magnesium-treated women have less hospitalizations during pregnancy and fewer cases of antepartum hemorrhage than placebo-treated women. Incidences of pre-eclampsia and all other outcomes are similar. In the analysis of the one high-quality trial, no differences between magnesium and placebo groups are seen. Poor-quality trials are likely to have resulted in a bias favoring magnesium supplementation.[15]

Calcium

Calcium supplementation is associated with a **reduction in the incidence of pre-eclampsia in pregnancy in all women, particularly for women at high risk of hypertension and in women with low-dietary-calcium intake** (e.g. <600 mg/day)[16] (see also Chapter 1 in the *Maternal–Fetal Evidence Based Guidelines*). There is insufficient evidence to determine optimum dosage and the effect on other important maternal and fetal outcomes. There is no overall effect on the risk of preterm delivery, although there is a **reduction in preterm birth risk among women at high risk of developing**

hypertension. There is no evidence of any effect of calcium supplementation on stillbirth or death before discharge from hospital. In women at high risk of hypertension, calcium supplementation is associated with fewer babies with birth weight < 2500 g. In one study, childhood systolic blood pressure > 95th percentile was reduced[16] (see also Chapter 1 in the *Maternal–Fetal Evidence Based Guidelines*).

Iron

There is no evidence to advise against a policy of routine iron and folate supplementation in pregnancy. Routine (universal) iron supplementation is associated with **prevention of low hemoglobin at birth or at 6 weeks postpartum**.[17,18] Iron supplementation, however, has no detectable effect on any substantive measures of either maternal or fetal outcome. One trial, with the largest number of participants of selective vs routine supplementation, shows an increased likelihood of cesarean section and postpartum blood transfusion, but a lower perinatal mortality rate (up to 7 days after birth) associated with selective iron supplementation. There are few data derived from communities where iron deficiency is common and anemia is a serious health problem.[17] For iron supplementation only for women with anemia, see Chapter 11 in *Maternal–Fetal Evidence Based Guidelines*.

Zinc

There is insufficient evidence to evaluate fully the effect of zinc supplementation during pregnancy. Zinc supplementation is associated with **significant reduction in preterm birth (PTB)**.[19] The reductions in induction of labor and cesarean delivery are from small studies, with no other differences detected between groups of women who had zinc supplementation and those who had either placebo or no zinc during pregnancy. There is insufficient evidence to assess the best dose, gestational age and duration, and population for zinc supplementation in pregnancy.[19]

Iodine

Iodine supplementation **in populations with low iodine intake and high levels of endemic cretinism** results in an important reduction in the incidence of the condition, with no apparent adverse effects. Iodine supplementation in these populations is associated with **a reduction in deaths during infancy and early childhood, with decreased endemic cretinism at the age of 4 years, and better psychomotor development scores between 4 and 25 months of age**.[20]

Cholesterol-lowering diet

A cholesterol-lowering diet with omega-3 fatty acids and dietary counseling does not affect cord or neonatal lipids

Table 1.3	*Food safety in pregnancy*
Food-borne illness to avoid	Preventive strategy
Listeriosis	Cook all foods (especially meats); avoid raw meats; avoid unpasteurized cheese; wash fruits and vegetables throughly
Toxoplasmosis	Avoid unpasteurized cheese; avoid litter of outdoor cats
Salmonella	Cook all seafood, avoid uncooked shellfish/seafood
Mercury	Avoid excessive consumption of large, mercury-containing fish (see also Chapter 15)

but is associated with a **90% reduction in preterm delivery** <37 weeks in one trial.[21] Diet and weight gain in general have been insufficiently studied in pregnancy, not allowing for strong recommendations.

Food safety

Food safety and prevention of food-borne illness and infection is suggested in Table 1.3.

Antigen-avoidance diet

Antigen-avoidance diet (e.g. **avoiding chocolate, nuts, etc.) in pregnancy is unlikely to reduce substantially the incidence of the child's atopic diseases in high-risk women, and such a diet decreases birth weight, and might increase LBW and PTB**.[22]

Drugs and environment

Substance abuse

Screening for use and counseling for cessation of tobacco, alcohol, and recreational or illicit drug use is recommended. Counseling is effective in reducing substance abuse in pregnancy, although women who use illicit drugs may need specialized interventions (see Chapter 20 in the *Maternal–Fetal Evidence Based Guidelines*).

Over-the-counter, alternative/complementary, and prescription medications

Because of the possibility of teratogenicity, medication use, including alternative remedies, should be limited to circumstances where benefit outweighs risk. Beneficial medications should be continued in pregnancy when safe for both mother and fetus (see specific disease guidelines).

Enviromental/occupational risks and exposures

In general, working is not associated with poor pregnancy outcome. Some workplace exposures, such as toxic chemicals (e.g. lead and magnesium), radiation (>5 rad), heavy repeated lifting, prolonged standing (>8 hours), excessive work hours (>80 hours/week), and high fatigue score may be associated with pregnancy complications, but there is insufficient evidence on the effect of avoidance of these risks. There are insufficient safety data for paint, solvents, hair dyes, fumes, and anesthetic drugs, with no absolute evidence of harm. Hot tubs and saunas should avoid temperatures >102°F, especially in the first trimester, and prolonged exposure to avoid risk of dehydration. After 14 weeks, probably all these exposures are not harmful.

Domestic violence

Domestic violence against pregnant women is associated with increased risk of PTB, LBW, second and third trimester bleeding, and fetal injury. Domestic violence may escalate during pregnancy. Providers therefore need to enquire and be alert regarding signs and symptoms of abuse and provide opportunities for private disclosure.

Exercise

Regular exercise during low-risk pregnancies is beneficial to overall maternal fitness and sense of well-being, with insufficient data to assess the impact on maternal or fetal outcomes or assess effect in high-risk pregnancies.[23] Twenty minutes of light exercise about 3 times a week has not been associated with detrimental effects. Exercise in pregnancy should still increase heart rate (up to 140 bpm is safe with normal cardiac function). Walking, swimming, and other sports with a low chance of loss of balance are recommended. Avoid contact sports and sports with high chance of loss of balance. Avoid hypoglycemia and dehydration.

Travel

Counseling should include the proper use of passenger restraint systems in automobiles, reduction of risk of venous thromboembolism during long distance air travel by walking and exercises, and provision of care and prevention of illness during travel abroad.

Sex and sexuality

Intercourse has not been associated with adverse outcomes in pregnancy. Many women and some men are concerned that intercourse may harm the pregnancy, and women have a progressive decrease in sexual desire during the pregnancy. This in turn is associated with progressively decreasing frequency of sexual intercourse in pregnancy. Most women desire more communication regarding sex in pregnancy by their care providers. Healthcare provider counseling should be reassuring, in the absence of pregnancy complications. Semen may be detrimental to membranes in women with cervical dilatation and/or shortening, and orgasms do increase contractions. Preterm birth and other complications of pregnancy do not seem increased in most studies of sex in pregnancy. **Most studies report that sexual activity is associated with better pregnancy outcomes**, probably because women that are sexually active are healthier to begin with compared to women with less sexual activity.[24]

Labor and delivery

Women should be provided with written information and instruction regarding what to expect during labor and delivery, how to obtain care when labor begins, and the value of a support person during the labor process (see Chapters 6–8).

Breastfeeding

Breastfeeding is considered to be the best feeding method for most infants, and should be strongly encouraged. Counseling and education may facilitate breastfeeding success. Antigen-avoidance diet during lactation may reduce the risk of developing atopic eczema of the child of high-risk women, and may reduce atopic eczema in children already with atopic eczema during the first 12–18 months.[22]

Physical examination

The physical examination (see Table 1.1) should be both general and directed by any risks identified in the history.

Weight and height

Weight and height should be determined at the initial prenatal visit, so as to determine the body mass index (**BMI = weight [kg]/height squared [m²]**). Categories of BMI are given in Table 1.4.

Women with obesity are at increased risk for diabetes, shoulder dystocia, and primary cesarean section, and have better outcomes with a lower (or none) total weight gain. Women who are underweight (<50 kg or <120 lbs) are at

Table 1.4 *Body mass index (BMI) categories*	
Weight category	BMI
Underweight	<18.5
Normal weight	18.5–24.9
Overweight	25–29.9
Obesity (class I)	30–34.9
Obesity (class II)	35–39.9
Extreme obesity (class III)	≥ 40

increased risk for low birth weight and preterm birth, and have better outcomes with a higher total weight gain.

Blood pressure

Blood pressure measurement is recommended at each prenatal visit. Initial blood pressure evaluation may help to identify women with chronic hypertension, while third trimester blood pressure readings aid in pre-eclampsia screening. A blood pressure of ≥ 120/80 mmHg in the first or second trimester is not normal, and associated with later risk of pre-eclampsia. There are significant risks associated with hypertension and pre-eclampsia in pregnancy. This simple, inexpensive, and widely accepted screening tool may help to identify abnormal trends in blood pressure over time. Blood pressure should be taken in the sitting position using an appropriately sized cuff and correct technique (see Chapter 7 in *Maternal–Fetal Evidence Based Guidelines*).

Pelvic exam

A routine pelvic exam is not accurate for assessment of gestational age and is not a reliable predictive test of preterm birth or cephalopelvic disproportion. It is not recommended for these assessments. Abdominal and pelvic examination to detect gynecologic pathology can be included in the initial examination.

Laboratory screening

Recommended initial universal laboratory screening – serum for ABO/Rh(D) type and antibody screen, hemoglobin and hematocrit, rubella titer, rapid plasma reagin (RPR), hepatitis B surface antigen (HBsAg), human immunodeficiency virus (HIV). Urine dipstick for glucose, protein, and culture for asymptomatic bacteriuria. If indicated, cervical screening for gonorrhea and *Chlamydia*

polymerase chain reaction (PCR) tests, and Papanicolaou (Pap) smear (see below). Other laboratory testing may be ordered if other risks/conditions are present.

Universal (all pregnant women)
Serum

ABO/Rh (D) type and antibody screen: Testing for blood group, Rh status, and atypical red cell antibodies at the initial visit is recommended, repeating antibody testing at 26–28 weeks of pregnancy. **Unsensitized RhD-negative women should be offered anti-D immunoglobin at 28 weeks.** Anti-D immunoglobin should also be offered for any **invasive procedure** (amniocentesis, chorionic villus sampling [CVS], percutaneous umbilical sampling [PUBS]), for second or third trimester **bleeding,** for partial **molar pregnancies, spontaneous abortion, elective termination, and for any condition that might be associated with fetal–maternal hemorrhage, such as abdominal trauma, external cephalic version, or placental abruption.** It may also be offered for any first trimester threatened abortion, and for ectopic pregnancy, although the evidence is not as strong, and it is probably not cost-effective or necessary unless the bleeding is significant. As anti-D immunoglobin is a blood product, informed consent should be obtained before its administration. For the Rh-negative woman, offering blood group and Rh status testing of the father of the pregnancy, if he is certain, can be considered to determine if anti-D immunoglobin is necessary. Du-positive women do not need anti-D immunoglobulin (see Chapter 47 in *Maternal–Fetal Evidence Based Guidelines*).

Hemoglobin/hematocrit: Recommended at the first prenatal visit and repeated in the early third trimester for asymptomatic women. Prophylactic iron supplementation in all women is recommended to prevent anemia (see above). Pregnant women identified with anemia (hemoglobin <11.0 g/dl) should be treated as per anemia guideline (see Chapter 11 in *Maternal–Fetal Evidence Based Guidelines*).

Platelets: Initial determination of platelet count (optimally also before pregnancy) may help with later diagnosis of HELLP syndrome, gestational thrombocytopenia, or neonatal alloimmune thrombocytopenia, and with screening for idiopathic thrombocytopenic purpura (ITP).

Rubella immunity: Screen all women at first encounter. Non-immune pregnant women should be counseled to avoid exposure, and seek immunization postpartum. Rubella vaccine is a live attenuated vaccine, and therefore is contradicted in pregnancy (see Chapter 37 in *Maternal–Fetal Evidence Based Guidelines*).

Syphilis screening (RPR):   Screen all women at the initial prenatal visit with RPR or venereal disease research laboratory (VDRL) tests. Repeat screening in the early third trimester and at delivery can be considered for high-risk populations (see Chapter 34 in *Maternal–Fetal Evidence Based Guidelines*).

HBSAg: Screen at initial encounter, and rescreen high-risk populations in third trimester. Postnatal intervention is recommended in all HBsAg-positive women to reduce the risk of viral transmission to the neonate. Pregnancy and breastfeeding are not contraindications to immunization in women who are at risk for acquisition of the hepatitis B virus (see Chapters 28–30 in *Maternal–Fetal Evidence Based Guidelines*).

HIV serology: Screening is recommended for all pregnant women. Those at increased risk for infection and from communities with an increased prevalence of seropositive newborns should be retested in the third trimester. Women should be offered HIV screening as routine, and decliners should be encouraged to sign 'opt-out' consent. Providers should continue to strongly encourage testing to those women who decline screening, and to address concerns that pose obstacles to testing. It should be emphasized that testing not only provides the opportunity to maintain maternal health but also that interventions can be offered to dramatically reduce the risk of viral transmission to the fetus (see Chapter 31 in *Maternal–Fetal Evidence Based Guidelines*).

Urine

Dipstick for protein: Urine dipsticks for protein do not reliably detect the variable elevations in albumin that may occur in pre-eclampsia. The 24-hour urine collection provides optimal assessment of proteinuria. In women at high risk for pre-eclampsia, this collection is a reasonable screen for proteinuria as a baseline at the first prenatal visit, and when other signs/symptoms of pre-eclampsia are present (see Chapter 1 in *Maternal–Fetal Evidence Based Guidelines*).

Dipstick for glucose: Glycosuria ≥ 250 mg/dl on urine dipstick in the first or second trimester is associated with abnormal gestational diabetes screening later in pregnancy. Presence of significant glycosuria before 24–28 weeks is an indicator for earlier gestational glucose screening (see Chapter 4 in *Maternal–Fetal Evidence Based Guidelines*).

Culture for asymptomatic bacteriuria: Screening with urine culture is recommended prior to 16 weeks of gestation or at the first prenatal visit for all women. Pregnant women with asymptomatic bacteriuria are at increased risk for symptomatic infection and pyelonephritis. There is also a positive relationship between untreated bacteriuria and LBW/PTB. Treatment of asymptomatic bacteriuria prevents these complications (see Chapter 15).

Selective (only women with risk factors) laboratory screening

Infectious diseases

Hepatitis C serology: A test for hepatitis C antibodies should be performed in pregnant women at increased risk for exposure, such as those with a history of intravenous (IV) drug abuse, exposure to blood products or transfusion, organ transplants, and kidney dialysis (see Chapters 28–30 in *Maternal–Fetal Evidence Based Guidelines*).

Chlamydia* screening:**   All women under age 26 should be screened for ***Chlamydia, as well as those women in high-risk populations (multiple sex partners, new partner within past 3 months, single marital status, inconsistent use of barrier contraception, previous or concurrent sexually transmitted infection [STI], vaginal discharge, mucopurulent cervicitis, friable cervix, or signs of cervicitis on physical examination). Some agencies advocate universal *Chlamydia* screening. Rescreen in the third trimester if at increased risk for infection. Screening using PCR technology is most accurate (see Chapter 33 in *Maternal–Fetal Evidence Based Guidelines*).

Gonorrhea screening: All women under age 26 should be screened for gonorrhea, as well as those women in high-risk populations (prior STI, multiple sexual partners, having a partner with a past history of any STI, sex work, drug use, inconsistent condom use). Some agencies advocate universal gonorrhea screening. Rescreen in the third trimester if at increased risk for infection. Screening using PCR technology is most accurate (see Chapter 32 in *Maternal–Fetal Evidence Based Guidelines*).

Bacterial vaginosis (BV):   There is **no benefit** to routine screening and treatment for asymptomatic bacterial vaginosis. Consideration can be given to screening and treating women with a prior PTB and BV, and those women who are symptomatic (see Chapter 15).

Genital herpes: Routine serologic screening for herpes simplex virus (HSV) in asymptomatic pregnant women is not recommended. In the absence of lesions during the third trimester, routine serial cultures are not indicated for women with a history of recurrent genital herpes (see Chapter 44 in *Maternal–Fetal Evidence Based Guidelines*).

Varicella: Determine immunity at the first session by history. Over 90% of women reporting a history of chickenpox are serologically immune. Varicella vaccine (live attenuated) is not recommended during pregnancy, but seronegative women should be advised to take appropriate precautions (see Chapter 37 in *Maternal–Fetal Evidence Based Guidelines*).

Tuberculosis: PPD (purified protein derivative; tuberculin) screening can be offered to high-risk women at any gestational age in pregnancy, and follow-up chest X-ray is recommended for recent converters. High-risk factors included HIV disease, homeless or impoverished women, prisoners, and recent immigrants from areas where tuberculosis is prevalent (see Chapter 22 in *Maternal–Fetal Evidence Based Guidelines*).

Cytomegalovirus (CMV): CMV testing can be considered for day care workers, ICN nurses, adolescents with multiple partners or a history of sexually transmitted diseases (STDs), women with HIV infection, and those who are or care for patients on immunosuppressive medications. Good handwashing and practicing universal precautions are recommended to prevent transmission (see Chapter 41 in *Maternal–Fetal Evidence Based Guidelines*).

Parvovirus: Routine screening not recommended. Consider screening high-risk groups (see Chapter 43 in *Maternal–Fetal Evidence Based Guidelines*).

Toxoplasmosis: Universal screening is not recommended. Education regarding prevention of disease should be addressed (see Table 1.3) (see Chapter 42 in *Maternal–Fetal Evidence Based Guidelines*).

Pap screening

A Pap test should be obtained at the first prenatal visit if none has been documented during the preceding 12 months. A Pap test might also be avoided if three consecutive normal Pap tests have been documented in the last 3 years before pregnancy (see Chapter 30).

At the end of the initial visit, make plans for care in remainder of pregnancy, arranging follow-up appointments and/or testing.

Follow-up visits should provide

- Ongoing assessment of risk factors and anticipatory guidance.
- Opportunity for discussion and questions.
- Communication and review of test results.
- Follow-up physical examination and laboratory screening and testing.

Follow-up visit physical examination

- **Weight** – repeated weighing is controversial and can be confined to circumstances where it will affect clinical management. Weight gain is rarely the only sign of pre-eclampsia.
- **Blood pressure** measurement should be performed and recorded at each visit (see above).
- **Fetal heart tones** – identify at each visit. Whereas at <12 weeks ultrasound may be necessary, beginning at about 12 weeks of gestation Doppler portable devices may be sufficient. Fetal heart tone testing provides reassurance to the pregnant woman. It permits an earlier diagnosis of pregnancy loss.
- **Fundal height measurement** can be performed at each visit during the second and third trimester. Fundal height measurement may help to detect fetal growth restriction (FGR) and macrosomia, but there is poor reliability both with same and different raters. There is probably some value in evaluating trends. Although it will not impact on the underlying condition, it may affect decision making on fetal surveillance. **There is insufficient evidence to show whether this measurement has any impact, beneficial or not, on pregnancy outcomes, with no effect in the only trial.**[25]
- **Cervical examination** – routine digital examination of the cervix is not recommended as a screening measure for prevention of preterm birth (see Chapter 15). **Sweeping or 'stripping' of membranes during cervical examination at ≥ 38 weeks reduces the rate of post-term delivery** (see also Chapter 23). Cervical examination may assist in the identification of abnormal presentation, and therefore the opportunity to offer appropriate intervention (i.e. version).
- **Fetal movement** – there is no evidence that formalized kick counts reduce the incidence of fetal death (*see Chapter 51 in Maternal–Fetal Evidence Based Guidelines*). Nonetheless, women should be instructed to identify daily fetal movements after about 28 weeks.
- **Abdominal examination for fetal presentation** – start to perform at each visit from 34 weeks to allow possibility of external version of breech fetus. Ultrasound can be used to confirm fetal presentation and position.
- **Clinical pelvimetry** – Measurement of the bony birth canal is of no value in predicting CPD at delivery (see Chapter 6).
- **Routine evaluation for edema** has traditionally been a part of the evaluation for pre-eclampsia, but by itself, it is neither specific nor sensitive.

Follow-up visit laboratory screening

- See initial laboratory screening and Table 1.1.
- Each visit: urine dipstick for protein and glucose.
- **11–13 6/7 weeks (best at 11 weeks): first trimester screening**, which includes nuchal translucency (NT), pregnancy associated plasma protein A (PAPP-A), and β-human chorionic gonadotropin (β-HCG), should be

offered to all pregnant women interested in prenatal diagnosis of Down's syndrome (see Chapter 4).

- **15–21 weeks (best at 16–18 weeks): serum marker screening for neural tube defect, trisomy 18 (T18) and trisomy 21 (T21)** – screening of maternal serum using the measurement of HCG, α-fetoprotein (AFP), estriol, and dimeric inhibin A identifies approximately 80% of pregnancies with T21, >80% of T18, and >95% (by maternal serum AFP [MSAFP]) of open abdominal wall defects and NTD. This 'quadruple' test can be offered to all interested patients, especially those women presenting after 14 weeks, with pretest counseling emphasizing the nature, risks, and benefits of the test. Counseling regarding the variety of screening options and the limitations of testing should be made available to all pregnant women (see Chapter 4).
- **24–28 weeks: screening for gestational diabetes mellitus (GDM)** – women with risk factors for GDM should be screened with either one-step or two-step tests, since intervention (diet, exercise, glucose monitoring, and, as necessary, medical therapy) prevents maternal and perinatal morbidities (see Chapter 4 in *Maternal–Fetal Evidence Based Guidelines*). Universal glucose challenge screening for GDM is the most sensitive approach, but the following women are at low risk and are less likely to benefit from testing:

  - *age younger than 25 years*
  - *not a member of a racial or ethnic group with high prevalence of diabetes (e.g. Hispanic, African, Native American, South or East Asian, or Pacific Islands ancestry)*
  - *BMI ≤ 25*
  - *no history of abnormal glucose tolerance*
  - *no previous history of adverse pregnancy outcomes usually associated with GDM*
  - *no known diabetes in first-degree relative.*

- **35–37 weeks: screening for group B streptococcus** – Group B streptococcus (GBS) is a significant cause of morbidity and mortality in neonates. Approximately 10–30% of pregnant women are asymptomatically colonized with GBS in the vagina or rectum. Vertical transmission of this organism from mother to fetus occurs most commonly after onset of labor or rupture of membranes. All women should be screened for GBS colonization by rectovaginal culture at 35–37 weeks of gestation. Colonized women should be treated with intravenous antibiotics (penicillin is first choice if not allergic) in labor or with rupture of membranes (see Chapter 36 in *Maternal–Fetal Evidence Based Guidelines*).

Ultrasonography (see Chapter 3)

- Ultrasound has not been proven harmful to mother or fetus.
- **First trimester 'dating' ultrasonography (before 14 weeks of gestation)** is more accurate than LMP to determine gestational age. It should be considered in all women. Ultrasound examination at first prenatal visit (usually first trimester) vs at 18–20 weeks provides **more precise estimate of gestational age** (crown–rump length is associated with the most accurate estimation), **is associated with less women feeling worried about their pregnancy, and less women not feeling relaxed about their pregnancy.** First trimester ultrasound also allows earlier detection of multiple pregnancies, screening for Down's syndrome with NT, and diagnosis of non-viable pregnancies.
- **Second trimester 'anatomy' ultrasound:** generally, women are offered an ultrasound at 18–22 weeks gestation to screen for structural anomalies. **Routine use of ultrasound reduces the incidence of post-term pregnancies and rates of induction of labor for post-term pregnancy, increases early detection of multiple pregnancies, increases earlier detection of major fetal anomalies when termination of pregnancy is possible, increases detection rates of fetal malformations, decreased admission to special care nursery, and decreased poor spelling at school compared to selective ultrasound. Given the benefits mentioned, all pregnant women should be offered a second trimester ultrasound.** No significant differences are detected for substantive clinical outcomes such as perinatal mortality, possibly because of insufficient data.
- **Third trimester 'growth' ultrasound:** in low-risk or unselected populations, routine third trimester (>24 weeks) pregnancy ultrasound has not been associated with improvements in perinatal mortality. Selective ultrasound in later pregnancy is of benefit in specific situations, such as calculation of interval growth for suspected FGR, assessment of amniotic fluid index for suspect oligo- or polyhydramnios, assessment of malpresentation, etc.
- Routine umbilical artery or other Doppler, or uterine artery ultrasound in low-risk or unselected patients, has not been shown to be of benefit.

Preventive care

Influenza immunizations

Influenza vaccination is recommended to **all pregnant women** during flu season (usually October–March in the USA). Pregnant women should only be vaccinated with the inactivated influenza vaccine. There is no evidence that influenza vaccine is unsafe (see Chapter 37 in *Maternal–Fetal Evidence Based Guidelines*).

Abdominal decompression

Abdominal decompression consists of a rigid dome placed about the abdomen and covered with an airtight suit, with the space around the abdomen decompressed to −50 to −100 mmHg for 15–30 seconds out of each minute for 30 minutes once to three times daily, or with uterine contractions during labor. This is thought to 'pump' blood through the intervillous space. There is no evidence to support the use of abdominal decompression in normal pregnancies. There is no difference between the abdominal decompression groups and the control groups for low birth weight, admission for pre-eclampsia, Apgar score, perinatal mortality, and childhood development.[26]

Antibiotic for preterm birth or infection prevention

Antibiotic prophylaxis within unselected pregnant women (no specific risk factor or infection) is associated with similar incidence of premature preterm rupture of membranes (PPROM), PTB, and postpartum endometritis.[27,28]

Postpartum depression prevention
(see also Chapter 21 in Maternal–Fetal Evidence Based Guidelines)

Overall, women who receive a **psychosocial intervention are equally likely to develop postpartum depression as those receiving standard care**. The provision of **intensive postpartum support provided by public health nurses or midwives (professional support)** is associated with 32% less postpartum depression.[29] **Identifying mothers 'at-risk'** assisted the prevention of postpartum depression compared to intervening on the general population. Interventions with **only a postnatal component** appeared to be more beneficial than interventions that also incorporated an antenatal component. **Individually based interventions** may be more effective than those that are group-based. Women who received multiple-contact intervention are just as likely to experience postpartum depression as those who received a single-contact intervention.[29]

There is insufficient evidence to assess the effectiveness of **antidepressants** given immediately postpartum in preventing postnatal depression in all women or just in high-risk women. **Sertraline** (Zoloft – a selective serotonin reuptake inhibitor [SSRI]) **reduced the recurrence of postnatal depression and the time to recurrence** when compared with placebo in a very small trial.[30] Nortriptyline (a tricyclic antidepressant) did not show any benefit over placebo.[30]

Norethisterone enanthate, a synthetic **progestogen**, 200 mg intramuscularly administered once within 48 hours of delivery to unselected women, is associated with a significantly **higher risk of developing postpartum depression** at 6 weeks.[31]

Audit and feedback systems

In the developing world, **participatory intervention with women's groups** is associated with **decreased maternal and** neonatal mortality in one large cluster-randomized trial.[32] It is important to record and review the number and causes of death and morbidities for both mother and babies, to identify problems and possible interventions to improve outcomes. There is insufficient evidence on assessing audit and feedback systems regarding mortalities and morbidities.

Interventions for common pregnancy complaints

Itching in late pregnancy (>32 weeks) not due to liver disease

If there is no rash, aspirin (600 mg qid) has been reported to decrease itching,[33] but because of potential detrimental fetal effects (closure of ductus arteriosus and oligohydramnios), it should not be used after 32 weeks. As regards to both itching and a rash, chlorpheniramine 4 mg tid decreased itching in a small trial.[33]

Stretch marks

Some stretch marks (striae gravidarum) develop in about 50% of women by the end of pregnancy. **Massage with trofolastin cream (*Centella asiatica* extract, α-tocopherol and collagen elastin hydrolases) applied daily decreases the development of stretch marks by 59% compared to massage with placebo.**[34] **Massage with Verum ointment (tocopherol, panthenol, hyaluronic acid, elastin, and menthol) decreases the development of stretch marks by 74% compared to no treatment, so it is unclear in the study if the massage or the Verum ointment were beneficial.**[34] In women with stretch marks from a previous pregnancy, there is no benefit.[34] It is unclear which one of the ingredients (or combination) is beneficial, and if massage itself has any effect. These products are not widely available. There is no proven treatment for stretch marks once they have developed.

Leg cramps

If a woman reports uncomfortable leg cramps in pregnancy, **magnesium (lactate or citrate) chewable tablets 5 mmol (122 mg) in the morning and 10 mmol (244 mg) in the evening for 3 weeks are associated with one-third of women not having persistent leg cramps, compared with 94% of** placebo controls having persistent cramps.[35] Magnesium lactate 84 mg (MagTabSR) is available in the US. Multivitamins with mineral supplement have been understudied; they might decrease leg cramps, but it is unclear which one of the

12 ingredients (or combination) is beneficial (e.g. magnesium?). Sodium chloride has been understudied, and can be considered only in areas of low daily intake, with precautions regarding blood pressure effects. **Calcium supplements do not decrease leg cramps compared with placebo.**[35]

Back pain

Back pain is common in pregnancy, given weight gain and its uneven distribution. **Water gymnastics for 1 hour weekly, starting at < 19 weeks, reduces back pain in pregnancy, and allows more women to continue to work, with no adverse effects.**[36] **A specially shaped pillow (Ozzlo) used for 1 week when laying in a lateral position reduces back pain in late pregnancy and improves sleep compared with a regular pillow,** but this pillow is no longer commercially available.[36] **Both physiotherapy and acupuncture starting < 32 weeks for 10 sessions might reduce back and pelvic pain; individual acupuncture sessions are more beneficial than group physiotherapy sessions.**[36] Education, other exercises, massage, heat therapy, support belts, and analgesic therapy have not been studied in a trial in pregnancy for back pain relief.

Constipation

Constipation is common in pregnancy, given decreased bowel peristalsis (possibly related to increased progesterone). **Dietary fiber supplements (such as 10 mg/day of either corn-based biscuits – Fibermed – or 23 g of wheat bran) increase the frequency of defecation and are associated with softer stools.**[37] **Stimulant laxatives (such as senna 14 mg, or dioctyl sodium succinate 120 mg and dihydroxyanthroquinone 100 mg – Normax) resolve constipation, compared with bulk-forming laxatives (such as 10 ml of 60% sterculia and 40% frangula – Normacol standard, or 10 ml of 60% sterculia – Normacol special), but these stimulant laxatives are also more likely to be associated with diarrhea and abdominal pain.**[37] Docusate Sodium is a similar product and widely availble. These findings in pregnant women are consistent with non-pregnant evidence. In non-pregnant adults, exercise, increase in water intake, dietary counseling, and certain foods (e.g. prunes) have shown relief in constipation. Bran or wheat fiber supplements daily should be used for women who complain of constipation in pregnancy; women who do not have sufficient benefit from fiber should receive stimulant laxatives, but should be warned of side effects.

Varicosities and leg edema (venous insufficiency)

Rutoside capsules 300 mg tid for 8 weeks in the last 3 months of pregnancy improve leg edema symptoms compared with women taking a placebo, accompanied by a decrease in ankle circumference.[38] There are insufficient data to absolutely confirm rutoside safety in pregnancy. This product is not widely availble, except for combination compounded products. In small studies, external pneumatic compression for 30 minutes is associated with a non-significant reduction in lower leg volume compared with simple resting, and immersion in water at 32°C for 50 minutes is associated with greater diuresis and fall in blood pressure than 50 minutes of bed rest.[38] External pneumatic compression and immersion in water cannot be recommended for leg edema/varicosities, since there is no evidence they lessen symptoms. Moreover, outcomes for these two interventions were short term, right after the intervention, and it is unknown for how long these changes are sustained. It is also unknown whether they are of any benefit in maternal or fetal outcomes. Leg elevation, compression hosiery, and swimming have not been studied for leg edema/varicosities relief.

Hemorrhoids

Hemorrhoidal disease is common during pregnancy, given obstruction of normal venous return from the growing uterus. **Oral hydroxyethyl rutosides decrease symptoms compared with a placebo group in women with hemorrhoids, and reduce the signs identified by the healthcare provider.**[39] Rutosides are associated with mild side effects such as gastrointestinal discomfort, and **their safety data in pregnancy are still insufficient.** They are also not widely available. Constipation is a predisposing factor for hemorrhoids, and should be treated. Sitz baths, ice, or ointments have been insufficiently studied for treatment of hemorrhoids in pregnancy.

Pelvic girdle pain

Pelvic girdle pain may be related to poor muscle function in the back and pelvis, and is common. Acupuncture and stabilizing exercises are effective in the management of pelvic girdle pain during pregnancy, with acupuncture superior to exercises.[40]

REFERENCES

1. American Academy of Pediatrics, American College of Obstetricians and Gynecologists. Guidelines for Perinatal Care, 5th edn. American Academy of Pediatrics: Elk Grove Village, IL, and American College of Obstetricians and Gynecologists: Washington, DC: 2002. [review]
2. Vintzileos AM. The impact of prenatal care on neonatal deaths in the presence and absence of antenatal high-risk conditions. Am J Obstet Gynecol 2002; 186: 1011–16. [II–2]
3. Gagnon AJ. Individual or group antenatal education for childbirth/parenthood. Cochrane Database Syst Rev 2007; 1. [meta-analysis: 6 RCTs, n = 1443 women]
4. Villar J, Carroli G, Khan-Neelofur D, Piaggio G, Gulmezoglu M. Patterns of routine antenatal care for low risk pregnancy. Cochrane Database Syst Rev 2007; 1. [meta-analysis: 10 RCTs; n > 60 000]

5. Brown HC, Smith HJ. Giving women their own case notes to carry during pregnancy. Cochrane Database Syst Rev 2007; 1. [meta-analysis: 3 RCTs, n=675]

6. Hodnett ED. Continuity of caregivers for care during pregnancy and childbirth. Cochrane Database Syst Rev, 2007; 1. [meta-analysis: 2 RCTs, n=1815]

7. Lumley L, Watson L, Watson M, Bower C. Periconceptional supplementation with folate and/or multivitamins for preventing neural tube defects. Cochrane Database Syst Rev 2007; 1. [meta-analysis; 4 RCTs, n=6425]

8. Wald NJ. Folic acid and the prevention of neural-tube defects. N Engl J Med 2004; 350: 101–3. [editorial]

9. Honein MA, Paulozzi LJ, Mathews TJ, Erickson JD, Wong LY. Impact of folic acid fortification of the US food supply on the occurrence of neural tube defects. JAMA 2001; 285: 2981–6. [observational]

10. van den Broek N, Kulier R, Gulmezoglu AM, Villar J. Vitamin A supplementation during pregnancy. Cochrane Database Syst Rev 2007; 1. [meta-analysis: 5 RCTs, n=23 426]

11. Hillman RW, Cabaud PG, Schenone RA. The effects of pyridoxine supplements on the dental caries experience of pregnant women. Am J Clin Nutr 1962; 10: 512–15. [1 RCT, n=371]

12. Rumbold A, Crowther CA. Vitamin C supplementation in pregnancy. Cochrane Database Syst Rev 2007; 1. [meta-analysis: 5 RCTs, n=766]

13. Mahomed K, Gulmezoglu AM. Vitamin D supplementation in pregnancy. Cochrane Database Syst Rev 2007; 1. [2 RCTs, n=232]

14. Rumbold A, Crowther CA. Vitamin E supplementation in pregnancy. Cochrane Database Syst Rev 2007; 1. [meta-analysis: 4 RCTs, n=566]

15. Makrides M, Crowther CA. Magnesium supplementation in pregnancy. Cochrane Database Syst Rev 2007; 1. [7 RCTs, n=2,689]

16. Atallah AN, Hofmeyr GJ, Duley L. Calcium supplementation during pregnancy for preventing hypertensive disorders and related problems. Cochrane Database Syst Rev 2007; 1. [meta-analysis: 11 RCTs, n≥6600]

17. Mahomed K. Iron supplementation in pregnancy. Cochrane Database Syst Rev 2007; 1. [meta-analysis: 20 RCTs, n=>6000]

18. Mahomed K. Iron and folate supplementation in pregnancy. Cochrane Database Syst Rev 2007; 1. [meta-analysis: 8 RCTs, n=5449]

19. Mahomed K. Zinc supplementation in pregnancy. Cochrane Database Syst Rev 2007; 1. [7 RCTs, n=>2500, most studies included all women presenting for PNC]

20. Mahomed K, Gulmezoglu AM. Maternal iodine supplements in areas of deficiency. Cochrane Database Syst Rev 2007; 1. [3 RCTs, n=1551]

21. Khoury J, Henriksen T, Christophersen B, Tonstad S. Effect of a cholesterol-lowering diet on maternal, cord, and neonatal lipids, and pregnancy outcome: a randomized clinical trial. Am J Obstet Gynecol 2005; 193: 1292–301. [RCT, n=290]

22. Kramer MS, Kakuma R. Maternal dietary antigen avoidance during pregnancy and/or lactation for preventing or treating atopic disease in child. Cochrane Database Syst Rev 2007, 1. [meta-analysis: 4 RCTs, n=451]

23. Kramer MS. Aerobic exercise for women during pregnancy. Cochrane Database Syst Rev 2007; 1. [meta-analysis: 10 RCTs, n=688]

24. Berghella V, Klebanoff M, McPherson C et al. Sexual intercourse association with asymptomatic bacterial vaginosis and trichomonas vaginalis treatment in relationship to preterm birth. Am J Obstet Gynecol 2002; 187: 1277–82. [II-2]

25. Lindhard A, Nielsen PV, Mouritsen LA et al. The implications of introducing the symphyseal-fundal height-measurement. A prospective randomized controlled trial. Br J Obstet Gynecol 1990; 97: 675–80. [RCT; n=1639]

26. Hofmeyr GJ, Kulier R. Abdominal decompression in normal pregnancy. Cochrane Database Syst Rev 2007; 1. [meta-analysis: 3 RCTs, n=>700]

27. Thinkhamrop J, Hofmeyr GJ, Adetoro O, Lumbiganon P. Prophylactic antibiotic administration in pregnancy to prevent infectious morbidity and mortality. Cochrane Database Syst Rev 2007; 1. [meta-analysis: 6 RCTs, n=2189, both low- and high-risk women; see also Chapter 15 for high-risk women, such as those with prior PTB]

28. McGregor JA, French JI, Richter R et al. Cervicovaginal microflora and pregnancy outcome: results of a double-blind, placebo-controlled trial of erythromycin treatment. Am J Obstet and Gynecol 1990; 163: 1580–91. [RCT, n=229]

29. Dennis C-L, Creedy D. Psychosocial and psychological interventions for preventing postpartum depression. Cochrane Database Syst Rev 2007; 1. [meta-analysis: 15 RCTs, n=>7600]

30. Howard LM, Hoffbrand S, Henshaw C, Boath L, Bradley E. Antidepressant prevention of postnatal depression. Cochrane Database of Syst Rev 2007; 1. [meta-analysis: 2 RCTs, n=73; intention to treat analyses were not carried out in either trial]

31. Lawrie TA, Hofmeyr GJ, de Jager M et al. A double-blind randomised placebo controlled trial of postnatal norethisterone enanthate: the effect on postnatal depression and serum hormones. Br J Obstet Gynaecol 1998; 105: 1082–90. [RCT, n=180]

32. Manandhar DS, Osrin D, Shrestha BP et al. Effect of participatory intervention with women's groups on birth outcomes in Nepal: cluster-randomized controlled trial. Lancet 2004; 364: 970–9 [RCT, n=6212]

33. Read MD. A new hypothesis of itching in pregnancy. Practitioner 1977; 218: 845–7. [RCT; n=36]

34. Young GL, Jewell D. Creams for preventing stretch marks in pregnancy. Cochrane Database Syst Rev 2007; 1. [meta-analysis: 2 RCTs, n=130]

35. Young GL, Jewell D. Interventions for leg cramps in pregnancy. Cochrane Database Syst Rev 2007; 1. [meta-analysis: 5 RCTs, n=352]

36. Young G, Jewell D. Interventions for preventing and treating pelvic and back pain in pregnancy. Cochrane Database Syst Rev 2007; 1. [meta-analysis: 3 RCTs, n=376]

37. Jewell DJ, Young G. Interventions for treating constipation in pregnancy. Cochrane Database Syst Rev 2007; 1. [meta-analysis: 2 RCTs, n=185]

38. Young GL, Jewell D. Interventions for varicosities and leg oedema in pregnancy. Cochrane Database Syst Rev 2007; 1. [meta-analysis: 3 RCTs, n=115]

39. Quijano CE, Abalos E. Conservative management of symptomatic and/or complicated haemorrhoids in pregnancy and the puerperium. Cochrane Database Syst Rev 2007; 1. [meta-analysis: 2 RCTs; n=150 women]

40. Elden H, Ladsfors L, Fagevik M, Ostgaard H-C, Hagberg H. Effects of acupuncture and stabilizing exercises as adjunct to standard treatment in pregnant women with pelvic girdle pain: randomized single blind controlled trial. BMJ 2005; 330: 761–6 [RCT, n=386]

2

Physiological changes in pregnancy

Colleen Horan

Tables 2.1–2.6 are intended to provide a summary of expected physiological changes that are found in normal pregnancy.[1] It is important to keep these changes in mind when evaluating a pregnant women's review of systems, physical examination findings, and laboratory values. Findings which might indicate a diseased state in the non-pregnant female or male patient may reflect normal adaptations in pregnancy, and conversely, failure of these adaptations may represent pathology in the pregnant patient. Expected changes reported are averages, at times with wide variations.

Reference

1. Lind T. Maternal Physiology: CREOG Basic Science Monograph in Obstetrics and Gynecology. American College of Obstetricians and Gynecologists, Washington DC: 1985. [review]

Table 2.1 *Cardiovascular system*

Parameter	Expected change	Comments
Heart size	Increases 12%	Increased diastolic filling and muscle hypertrophy
Murmurs	Physiological systolic and diastolic	Ejection murmurs attributable to increased stroke volume usually occur in early or mid-systole and are best heard along the left sternal edge
ECG	Positional heart changes result in changes that resemble ischemia	Heart is pushed upward and forward, deviating electrical axis to the left by 15–20 degrees, causing flattened or inverted T in lead III
Cardiac output	Increases 1.5 l/min	Greatest increase occurs immediately after delivery with redistribution of blood flow from uterus
Rhythm	Increase in atrial and ventricular extrasystole	SVT not infrequent
Heart rate	Increases from 70 to 85 beats per minute	
Stroke volume	Increases from 63 to 70 ml	
Systolic and diastolic BP	Decreases soon after beginning of pregnancy and mid-pregnancy (100–110/60–70 mean levels); then returns to pre-pregnant values by third trimester and term	**Supine hypotension** – decreased venous return due to compression from gravid uterus Increased blood flow through alternative pathways such as paravertebral-azygous veins

(Continued)

Table 2.1 *(Continued)*		
Parameter	Expected change	Comments
Pulse pressure	Increases	
Venous pressure	Increases in femoral system Unchanged in arms	
Peripheral resistance	Decreases	
Pulmonary BP	Unchanged	
Blood flow to uterus	Increases by 500 ml/min	No autoregulation
Blood flow to kidneys	Increases by 400 ml/min	
Blood flow to skin	Increases by 300–400 ml/min	
Blood flow to breasts	Increases by 200 ml/min	

ECG, electrocardiogram; BP, blood pressure; SVT, supraventricular tachycardia.

Table 2.2 *Respiratory system*		
Parameter	Expected change	Comments
Anatomy	Increase of subcostal angle from 68° to 103° → 3 cm increase in transthoracic diameter	Increased upper respiratory capillary engorgement can cause increased congestion, epistaxis, and intubation trauma
Tidal volume	Increases by 300 ml or 40%	
Expiratory reserve volume	Decreases by 200 ml	Cephalad displacement of diaphragm
Residual volume	Decreases by 300 ml or 20 %	
Inspiratory capacity	Increases by 300 ml	
Functional residual volume	Decreases by 500 ml	
Minute volume	Increases by 40% or 3 L/min beginning in first trimester	Increased rate of induction of, and emergency from, inhaled anesthetics
Maximum breathing capacity	Unchanged	
Forced expiratory volume	Unchanged	
Peak expiratory flow rate	Unchanged	
Closing volume	May increase	
Pulmonary diffusing capacity	Decreases by 4 ml/min/mmHg	
Oxygen requirement	Increases by 30–40 ml/min	
Carbon dioxide output	Increases; expressed as respiratory quotient	
Carbon dioxide pressure	Decreases from 35–40 mmHg to 28–30 mmHg	
Oxygen pressure	Increases	
pH	Mild increase (7.40–7.44 is normal)	Compensated respiratory alkalosis
pO_2	Mild increase (100–104 is normal)	
pCO_2	Decreases (30–31 mmHg is normal)	

Table 2.3 *Renal system and homeostasis*		
Parameter	Expected change	Comments
Glomerular filtration rate	Increases from 97 ml/min to 128 ml/min by 10 weeks	
Glucose excretion	Increases	Random glycosuria
Protein excretion	Increases (up to 300 mg/24 hours is normal)	
Renin, angiotensins I and II	Increases	Diminished vascular response causes less pressor effect from angiotensin
Anatomic changes	Dilation of renal calyces and ureters to pelvic brim; 'physiological' hydronephrosis, right > left	Increased risk of pyelonephritis; screen for asymptomatic bacteruria
Potassium	Increased retention	
Sodium	Increased retention	
Urine output	No significant change	
Vitamin excretion	Increased loss of folate, vitamin B_{12}, and ascorbic acid	
Osmolality	Decreases 10 mOsm/kg in first trimester, then stable	
Sodium	Decreases 3 mEq/L in first trimester, then stable	
Potassium	Decreases 0.5 mEq/L	
Calcium	Decreases (total and ionized)	Increased intestinal absorption of calcium and increased bone turnover
Magnesium	Decreases 10–20% in first half of pregnancy	
Zinc	Decreases	
Copper	Increases from 1.14 mg/L to 2.03 mg/L by term	
Chloride	Unchanged	
Bicarbonate	Decreases markedly (18–22 mEq/L is normal)	Compensates for decrease in pCO_2
Total protein	Decreases from 72 g/L to 62 g/L	
Albumin	Decreases from 47 g/L to 36 g/L	
Urea, creatinine, and uric acid	Decrease first trimester; stabilize second trimester; increase toward term	
Vitamin B_6	Decreases	
Blood glucose	Fasting levels **decrease** in first trimester, then unchanged	Postprandial levels remain elevated longer, prolonging return to fasting state Increased glucose levels allow passive diffusion across placenta to fetus
Folate	Decreases 50% toward term	
Vitamin B_{12}	Decreases 50% or more	Vitamin B_{12} levels in folate-deficient women will increase with folate supplementation alone

Table 2.4 *Endocrine system*		
Parameter	Expected change	Comments
Pituitary gland	Increases to 50% greater weight than adult male	Attributable to increase of prolactin-secreting cells in anterior lobe
Prolactin	Increases from 300 to 5000 mIU/L	
FSH/LH	Decrease to nearly undetectable	
ACTH	Increases	
Human growth hormone	Decreases	
Melanocyte-stimulating hormone	Increases	May be responsible for linea nigra, chloasma, and increased areolae pigmentation
Vasopressin	Unchanged	Stimulation of nerve endings in breast causes reflex increase in oxytocin and vasopressin
Oxytocin	Unchanged	
Thyroid anatomy	Unchanged	
TSH	**Unchanged**	May be suppressed during late first to early second trimester due to HCG-mediated increase in thyroid hormone production – subtle effect may be exacerbated by conditions that increase HCG levels, such as hyperemesis, molar pregnancies, and multiples
Thyroid-binding globulin	Increases – doubles by end of first trimester; triples by term	Due to estrogen effect on liver
Thyroxine (T_4)	Increased total circulating level; **unchanged free fraction**	Fetal thyroid hormone production commences at about 18 weeks
Triiodothyronine (T_3)	Increased total circulating level; **unchanged free fraction**	
Reverse T_3	Unchanged in maternal circulation; increased in cord blood	
Adrenal anatomy	Unchanged	
CBG	Increases – doubles by second trimester	
Cortisol	Increases to 3 times nonpregnant values	Episodic pattern of release is maintained
Aldosterone	Increases 2-fold by term	
Deoxycorticosterone	Increases by 20–100 times	
Testosterone	Increased total amount; decreased free fraction	
Androstenedione	Increases by 50%	10-fold increased rate of transformation to estradiol and estrone
DHEA	Unchanged or small decrease	
Catecholamines	Unchanged	
Pancreas	Hypertrophy of islets due to hyperplasia of B cells	

(Continued)

Table 2.4   *(Continued)*

Parameter	Expected change	Comments
Insulin	Increased fasting levels toward term Hyperplasia of pancreatic B cells	Proportionally less increase of glucagons compared to insulin; so insulin:glucagon ratio is increased
Glucagon	Increased fasting levels	
Glucose	Slight decrease	Especially fasting levels (see Table 2.3)
Parathyroid hormone	Increased during end of pregnancy	Maintains calcium levels in face of increased renal absorption and transfer to fetus
25-Hydroxyvitamin D	Unchanged	
1,25-Dihydroxyvitamin D	Increases	
Calcitonin	No change to slight increase	
Progesterone	Increases from 0.2 µg/ml to 139 µg/ml (up to 1000-fold)	Production originates in corpus luteum over first 7–8 weeks; then placenta takes over
Estradiol	Increases about 500-fold from 0.05 µg/ml to 18 µg/ml	
17-Hydroxyprogesterone	Increases to maximum level by week 8	
Relaxin	Increases	Corpus luteum
Estriol	Increases	
Human placental lactogen (hPL)	Increases about 5000-fold from 0.002 µU/ml to 10 µU/ml	
HCG	Increases to maximum values by 8–10 weeks	Peak 93 U/ml Term 14 U/ml

FSH, follicle-stimulating hormone; LH, luteinizing hormone; ACTH, adrenocorticotropic hormone; TSH, thyroid-stimulating hormone; CBG, corticosteroid-binding globulin; DHEA, dehydroepiandrosterone; HCG, human chorionic gonadotropin.

Table 2.5   *Gastrointestinal system*

Parameter	Expected change	Comments
Appetite	Increases	
Gastric reflux	Increases	Cardiac sphincter laxity and anatomic displacement Treated during labor and delivery/anesthetic procedures with non-particulate oral antacids
Gastric secretion	Decreased acidity; increased volume	'Full stomach' effect increases risk of aspiration Intubation requires cuffed endotracheal tube
Gastric motility	Decreases	
Intestinal absorption	Increases	
Intestinal transit time	Delayed	
Large intestine	Greater absorption; slower transit time	
Liver	Unchanged	
Gallbladder	Larger due to passive dilation	

Table 2.6 *Hematologic system*

Parameter	Expected change	Comments
Plasma volume	40–60% **increase** from 12 to 36 weeks; 70–100% increase in multiple gestations	Offsets blood loss at delivery
Total erythrocyte volume	Increases 15–30%	Greater increase with iron supplementation
Hematocrit	**Decreases** 3–5% by 36 weeks	Physiological anemia due to greater proportionate increase in plasma volume compared to erythrocyte volume; less change with iron supplementation
Hemoglobin	**Decreases** 2–10% by third trimester	
Mean corpuscular volume	Unchanged	Good indicator of iron status Slight increase with iron supplementation
Erythrocyte sedimentation rate	Significantly **increased**	Provides little diagnostic value; combined with physiologic increase in WBCs can cause false suspicion for infection
WBCs	**Increase** 8% by term and may increase further postpartum	Predominantly due to increase in neutrophils
Serum iron	**Decreases** 35% by term	
Serum transferrin	**Increases** by 100% or more by second trimester	TIBC markedly increased
TIBC	**Increases** by 25–100%	
Serum ferritin	**Decreases** markedly (even with iron supplementation)	Nadir 30% or less of normal values Best test to assess iron deficiency anemia in pregnancy
Erythropoietin	**Increases** 4-fold	
Alpha-fetoprotein	Increases	Larger increase in neural tube defects, abdominal wall defects, and fetal death
Glutamatic–oxalacetic transaminase and glutamatic–pyruvic transaminase	Unchanged	
Creatinine kinase	Decreases first half of pregnancy	
Lipase	Decreases	
Alkaline phosphatase	Increases	Heat-stable fraction formed by placenta
Lipids	Increase	Triglycerides, cholesterol, phospholipids, and free fatty acids all increase progressively
Fibrinogen	Increases 2 g/L by term	Overall increased tendency towards thrombosis
Factors VII, VIII, and X	Increase	
Factors XI and XIII	Decrease by about 30%	
Antithrombin III	Decreases	
Fibrin, FDP	Increase progressively	
Protein S	Decreases	
Protein C	Unchanged	

WBCs, white blood cells; TIBC, total iron-binding capacity; FDP, fibrin degradation products.

3

Ultrasound in pregnancy: if, when, what

Sandra Patricia Bogota-Ángel and George Bega

KEY POINTS

- There is **no** clear **evidence** that **ultrasound** examination during pregnancy **is harmful.** Prenatal exposure to ultrasound is not associated with adverse influence on school performance or neurobehavioral function. There is no evidence of an adverse effect on speech, vision, or hearing. There is no clear effect on non-right-handedness.
- Ultrasound should be performed by **trained and experienced professionals**, with continuing education and ongoing quality-monitoring programs.
- Before the examination **every pregnant woman** should be **informed on expectations** about the obstetric ultrasound, as well as its benefits and risks.
- Routine use of ultrasound reduces the incidence of post-term pregnancies and rates of induction of labor for post-term pregnancy, increases early detection of multiple pregnancies, increases earlier detection of major fetal anomalies when termination of pregnancy is possible, increases detection rates of fetal malformations, decreases admission to special care nursery, and decreases poor spelling at school compared with selective ultrasound. No significant differences are detected for substantive clinical outcomes such as perinatal mortality, possibly because of insufficient data.
- Ultrasound examination is the best method to estimate gestational age dating in pregnancy. Ultrasound-based gestational age estimates are lower than last menstrual period (LMP)-based gestational age estimates, and generate a higher rate of preterm birth and lower rate of post-term birth. The crown–rump length (CRL) is associated with the most accurate estimation, with an error of around 2.1 days, and is most accurate in assessing gestational age at about 8–12.5 weeks [CRL about 15–60 mm]. CRL should be used for dating < 14 weeks, and biparietal diameter (BPD) and femur length at 14 weeks and after.
- Ultrasound examination at first prenatal visit (usually first trimester) vs at 18–20 weeks **provides more precise** estimate of gestational age, is associated with less women feeling worried about their pregnancy, and less women not feeling relaxed about their pregnancy. First trimester ultrasound **also allows earlier detection of multiple pregnancies, screening for Down's syndrome with nuchal translucency, and diagnosis of non-viable pregnancies.**
- Given the benefits mentioned above, **all pregnant women should be offered a first trimester (11–14 weeks) as well as a second trimester (18–24 weeks) ultrasound.**
- In low-risk or unselected populations, **routine third trimester (> 24 weeks) pregnancy ultrasound** has **not** been associated with improvements in perinatal mortality.
- In low-risk or unselected populations, **routine umbilical artery Doppler ultrasound examination,** usually around 28–34 weeks, does **not result in reduced perinatal mortality.**

Background

Since the late 1970s ultrasound evaluation of the embryo and fetus has been a tool for prenatal care around the world. Its range of clinical application in obstetrics has expanded since then. Nevertheless, the related controversies around this screening and diagnostic technique have been growing as well. This guideline presents evidence about some topics related to its safety, as well as if this test should be used at all, when/how often it should be used, and what should be looked for on the ultrasound.

Safety of ultrasonography

The temperature elevation and its possible effect of cavitations, or the formation of microbubbles in the tissues exposed to ultrasound waves, are known mechanical effects and the main concerns about ultrasound. Effects of ultrasound on tissues have been studied with animal experimentation. In humans, however, the information comes from epidemiologic data and population studies. No epidemiologic studies have shown harmful effects in humans, so far. **There is no clear evidence that ultrasound** examination during pregnancy is harmful.[1] Prenatal exposure to ultrasound is not associated with an adverse influence on school performance or neurobehavioral function. There is no evidence of an adverse effect on speech, vision, on hearing. There is no clear effect on non-right-handedness.[1,2]

As ultrasound is a form of energy and may produce secondary effects in the tissues it traverses, it should be performed only with valid medical indications and with the shortest duration possible and at the lowest settings to avoid unnecessary exposure to ultrasonic waves. Exposing the fetus to ultrasonography with no anticipation of medical benefit is not justified. It is best to keep the thermal index and mechanical index on the ultrasound (usually appear on screen automatically) both at <1.[3,4]

About quality

Ultrasound scanning in pregnancy should always be considered as a medical procedure, with the examination of the fetus as its goal. Levels of expertise vary between the different healthcare centers. Since ultrasound screening efficiency is operator-dependent, **continuing education and ongoing quality-monitoring programs** are important strategies in each center offering ultrasound diagnosis. The ongoing risks of false-negative tests and/or misinterpretation of the images obtained (either false positives or wrong diagnoses) can be minimized if those examinations are carried out and interpreted by **trained and experienced professionals**. Sensitivity of ultrasound screening for pregnancy varies widely. Appropriate accreditation, documentation, and continuous careful quality control are essential.[3,4]

About informed consent and patient's expectations

Even though a formal written informed consent is not always needed, **before the examination every pregnant woman should be informed on expectations about the obstetric ultrasound, as well as its benefits and risks.** The patients should know that ultrasound evaluation is a screening test with wide variations in detection rates for fetal anomalies, and that all ultrasound diagnoses, especially false-positive and false-negative results, can put both mother and fetus at risk.

Whether the sex of the fetus should be revealed or not to the patient with a singleton gestation should be addressed. It may be harmful for the physician–patient relationship to withhold this information, especially if the patient previously requested it. Although a moral conflict may exist in some cultures around the world where this information is used by the patient for elective abortions based on sex selection and sex preferences, in general disclosing fetal gender

during ultrasound can benefit not only the doctor–patient relationship but also the parent–child relationship.[5]

Should an obstetric ultrasound be done, and if yes, when?
Routine vs selective use of ultrasound (if)

Routine (i.e. performed on every pregnant woman) ultrasound examination is associated with the following effects compared with selective ultrasound examination (i.e. performed only on women with specific indications):[1]

1. **Reduces by 39% the incidence of post-term pregnancies and rates of induction of labor for post-term pregnancy** by allowing a more precise estimation of exact gestational age.
2. **Increases by 92% the early detection of multiple pregnancies.** Although all trials have shown twin pregnancies are diagnosed earlier, there is insufficient evidence to assess differences in perinatal mortality.
3. **Increases earlier detection of major fetal anomalies when termination of pregnancy is possible.**
4. **Increases detection rates of fetal malformations.** 90% of congenital malformations occur in patients without risk factors and in which clinical signs may be absent. Detection rates by ultrasound for fetal malformations in the general population show a range of sensitivity from 17 to 74%. This wide variation is in part the result of the difference in ascertainment, type of patient recruitment (can alter the frequency and severity of malformations), and variation in the skills of the individual performing the ultrasound. These aspects make it difficult to obtain a single estimate of the sensitivity of routine ultrasonographic screening for fetal malformations.
5. **No significant differences are detected for substantive clinical outcomes such as perinatal mortality,** with a trend (14% decrease) for benefit but insufficient size to assess perinatal mortality accurately. There is insufficient evidence to support or refute the benefit of routine ultrasound in reducing the mortality overall as well as in infants with life-threatening anomalies. This latter result may be attributed in part to the small sample size in terms of numbers of anomalies. Improvement of perinatal morbidity and mortality rates could theoretically be achieved through more accurate gestational age estimation and earlier detection of special conditions such as multiple gestation and major malformations. A lowering mortality rate as a consequence of early and selective termination of fetal malformations can be reached, but not improvement in the proportion of live births.

6. **Reduces by 14% admission to special care nursery**. It has not been controlled if this is related to more prenatal care in general.
7. **Reduces by 27% poor spelling at school**. There are also trends for improvements in other school-age activities and sensory skills.
8. **No differences in handedness, with a trend towards more left-handedness and more ambidexterity**.

If only one routine ultrasound examination is done, it is usually performed at 18–22 weeks (<24 weeks). Earlier examination provides more accurate assessment of gestational age; later examination (e.g. between 18 and 22 weeks) allows more full inspection of fetal anatomy, but is more complex and time-consuming (see later in this chapter).

Gestational age dating in pregnancy

Precise estimation of gestational age is extremely important for optimal obstetric care, including evaluation of fetal growth, interpretation of maternal screening markers, choosing the appropriate gestational age to perform interventions, and management of preterm and post-term pregnancies.

For gestational age estimation, cardinal numbers should be preferred to ordinal numbers to avoid confusion. So week 0 is 1–7 days after last menstrual period (LMP), week 2 is 8–14 days, etc. Six weeks of gestation is then 1 month (lay person estimation), and 38 weeks = 9 months. Some other definitions (not uniformly accepted, with variation in literature): first trimester: 0–13 6/7 weeks; second trimester: 14–27 6/7 weeks; third trimester: 28 weeks to delivery; term 37–41 6/7 week; preterm: 20–36 6/7 weeks; post-term: ≥42 weeks.

Ultrasound examination is the best method to estimate gestational age dating in pregnancy.[6] The first day of the LMP should be asked of all pregnant women for calculating the approximate date when the dating ultrasound should be booked. Compared with LMP, ultrasound-based gestational age is more precise. The error, even with certain LMP, is often due to late ovulation (>14 days after LMP). Some have stated that there is no reason to use LMP for dating when adequate ultrasound data are available by 24 weeks.[7] **Ultrasound-based gestational age estimates are lower than LMP-based gestational age estimates, and generate a higher rate of preterm birth and a lower rate of post-term birth**. Naegele's rule (add 7 – some suggest 10 – days to first day of LMP, add 1 year, take back 3 months), manual assessment of uterine size, quickening, etc., should not be used unless ultrasound dating is unavailable. In general, the earlier the ultrasound is obtained in the pregnancy, the more accurate the dating will be. Multiple parameters and equations have been evaluated to estimate gestational age. **The crown–rump length (CRL) is associated with the most accurate estimation, with an error of around 2.1 days, and is most accurate in assessing gestational age at about 8–12.5 weeks** (CRL

about 15–60 mm). For biparietal diameter (BPD), the error is around 2.8 days, and is most accurate between 12 and 14 weeks (second-best ultrasound parameter for estimation of gestational age after CRL). **CRL should be used for dating <14 weeks, and BPD and femur length (FL) at 14 weeks and after**. Combining three or more parameters can slightly increase, rather than decrease, the error, but a combination of BPD, AC (abdominal circumference), and FL is commonly used for dating by ultrasound in the second and third trimesters.[7] Repeated examinations improve the prediction only marginally, and the estimated date of confinement (EDC) should always be set by the earliest ultrasound, as the earlier the examination is made, the smaller is the prediction error. Whereas prediction of gestational age by ultrasound can be very accurate, prediction of date of delivery remains less accurate, with an error of usually ≥7–8 days, given other biological factors.

Gestational age determination can generally follow simple suggestions[7] (Table 3.1).

The transcerebellar diameter (TCD) is an accurate predictor of gestational age, and can be used between 14 and 28 weeks reliably with the use of normograms.[8] There is some reliability in gestational age prediction even up to 35 weeks, and TCD is spared effects from fetal growth restriction (FGR), and so can be used to assess pregnancies at risk for this complication. The presence of epiphyses in lower extremities usually signifies a gestational age of >32 weeks.

Table 3.1   *Gestational age determination*
• The first day of the LMP should be asked of all pregnant women. They should be asked if they have regular menses, have taken oral contraceptive pills within the last 2 months, or have had any unusual bleeding in the first trimester. The woman should be asked if she is certain of her LMP (but this is still not precise)
• IVF pregnancies should be dated by the date of embryo transfer minus 14 days to obtain LMP, and then EDC by Naegele's rule. There is no need to ever change dating in these pregnancies
• First trimester (0–13 6/7 weeks): if LMP- and ultrasound-based dating differ by ≥7 days, preference should be given to the ultrasound-based date
• Early second trimester (14–20 6/7 weeks): if LMP- and ultrasound-based dating differ by ≥10 days, preference should be given to the ultrasound-based date
• Late second trimester (21–27 6/7 weeks): if LMP- and ultrasound-based dating differ by ≥14 days, preference should be given to the ultrasound-based date
• Third trimester (28–42+ weeks): if LMP- and ultrasound-based dating differ by ≥21 days, preference should be given to the ultrasound-based date

LMP, last menstrual period; IVF, in-vitro fertilization; EDC, estimated date of confinement.

Ultrasound examinations (when and what)

First trimester

Ultrasonographic evaluation in the first trimester (0–13 6/7 weeks) is the most accurate method to determine exact gestational age. For gestational age determination, it is best performed at 8–12.5 weeks with the CRL used to determine gestational age. **Ultrasound examination at first prenatal visit vs at 18–20 weeks provides more precise estimate of gestational age, is associated with 20% less women feeling worried about their pregnancy, and 27% less women not feeling relaxed about their pregnancy.**[1,4] First trimester ultrasound also allows **earlier detection of multiple pregnancies, screening for Down's syndrome with nuchal translucency (NT), and diagnosis of non-viable pregnancies.** No other important maternal or perinatal outcome differences are detected, with insufficient data to accurately assess some rare outcomes such as perinatal mortality. Transvaginal scanning is preferred in cases of a pregnancy resulting from ovulation induction or other assisted reproductive technologies, first trimester bleeding, abdominal pain, or increased risk of aneuploidy, and should be used if transabdominal examination is inconclusive for diagnosis. First trimester screening for congenital defects by transvaginal ultrasound is an option for pregnant women who meet certain criteria, and should be done by experienced sonographers and confirmed at 18–22 weeks.

Nuchal translucency is measured at the area of the back of the fetal neck and is to be reassured between weeks 10 and 14 of gestation. It has been associated with chromosomal and anatomical abnormalities in the fetus according to recent studies of high-risk or selected populations. Screening permits choosing the earliest definitive diagnostic procedures, e.g. chorionic villus sampling (CVS), allowing women to prepare for a child with health problems and also providing the option to terminate the pregnancy earlier (see Chapter 4).

If not performed routinely (best at 11–12 weeks), indications by experts (no trials) for first trimester ultrasound are shown in Table 3.2, and essential elements in Table 3.3.

Ultrasound diagnosis of missed abortion/embryonic demise

<u>Missed abortion:</u>   Mean gestational sac size of ≥20 mm and no heart beat by transvaginal ultrasound.

<u>Embryonic demise:</u>   CRL of ≥5 mm and no heart beat by transvaginal ultrasound. With a mean gestational sac size of >10 mm, a yolk sac should be seen to help discriminate a true gestational sac from a pseudosac (associated with abnormal pregnancy).

Table 3.2   *Indications for first trimester ultrasound*[3,4]
• To confirm the presence of an intrauterine pregnancy
• To evaluate suspected ectopic pregnancy
• To define the cause of vaginal bleeding
• To evaluate pelvic pain
• To estimate gestational age
• To diagnose or evaluate multiple gestations
• To confirm cardiac activity and identify non-viable pregnancies
• As an adjunct to chorionic villus sampling, embryo transfer, and localization and removal of an intrauterine device
• To evaluate maternal pelvic masses and/or uterine anomalies
• To evaluate suspected hydatiform mole

Table 3.3   *Essential elements for first trimester ultrasound*[3,4]
• Gestational sac (location, mean diameter)
• Yolk sac (diameter)
• Fetal biometry, e.g. crown–rump length (CRL)[a]
• Development of fetal anatomy in early pregnancy, including recognition of anomalies such as cystic hygroma
• Fetal viability (cardiac activity)
• Fetal number (amnionicity and chorionicity have to be reported for multiples)
• Ultrasound features of early pregnancy failure, e.g. ectopic pregnancy, hydatidiform mole
• Uterus, adnexa, and cul-de-sac
• Any other abnormalities (e.g. leiomyomata)

[a]CRL is a more accurate indicator of gestational age than gestational sac size.

If the β-human chorionic gonadotropin (β-HCG) is >1500 mIU/ml, a gestational sac should be visualized by transvaginal ultrasound; if the gestational sac is not seen in the uterus, suspect ectopic pregnancy.

Prognostic ability: The presence of normal embryonic cardiac activity in the uterine cavity in the first trimester has a >90% prediction for a live birth in both symptomatic and asymptomatic pregnancies.

Precautions and pitfalls

Physiologic midgut herniation at 7–11 weeks (resolve ≥12 weeks); do not confound with omphalocele. The rhombencephalon can look as a cystic mass up to 8–10 weeks, and should not be confused with a central nervous system (CNS) anomaly; ventriculomegaly cannot be assessed well in the first trimester. The amnion and chorion are expected to be fused by 14 weeks.

Second trimester (aka 'anatomy', or 'standard' ultrasound)

The best timing for just one ultrasound screening of the fetal anatomy and dating is the early to mid second trimester (18–22 weeks),[1] not only to obtain an accurate estimation of gestational age or a satisfactory inspection of the fetal anatomy but also as a tool to detect anomalies so as to allow patients to choose about whether or not to proceed with their pregnancies. This is therefore usually called the anatomy, or standard ultrasound examination (nomenclature such as Level I, II, etc., ultrasound is controversial and less descriptive). Given the benefits highlighted above, **all pregnant women should be offered a second trimester ultrasound**. At least two aspects are important about early fetal anomalies detection with ultrasound: first, the estimated sensitivity to detect anomalies varies widely, with higher rates of detection for major anomalies than for the minor anomalies, and some organs (e.g. neural tube defects) vs others (e.g. heart). The best moment for detection of most malformations is around 20–24 weeks even in specialized centers. Secondly, it is important for the woman to obtain this information as early as possible. In some circumstances more than one second trimester ultrasound is necessary, especially if the initial second trimester ultrasound is performed at 18–19 weeks. Experts have suggested (no trials) indications (Table 3.4) and essential elements (Table 3.5) for ultrasound.

Third trimester

The potential benefit of a third trimester ultrasound examination greatly depends on how many and how accurate the prior (if any) ultrasounds have been. If the first and only ultrasound is in the third trimester, it probably has similar benefits to the routine second trimester ultrasound, except early detection and accurate dating are not possible. Assuming prior accurate second trimester ultrasound(s) have been done, ultrasound evaluations in the third trimester involve assessments of fetal growth, amniotic fluid volume, and placenta, trying to identify a compromised or malformed fetus, etc. **In low-risk or unselected populations, routine late (>24 weeks) pregnancy ultrasound has not been associated with improvements in perinatal morbidity or mortality.[9,10] Placental grading, as an adjunct to third trimester ultrasound examination, was associated with a significant reduction in the stillbirth rate in one trial,[11] with more research needed in placental grading for prediction of poor perinatal outcome for routine recommendation.** Third trimester ultrasound may decrease the incidence of a growth-restricted infant, but increase the rate of iatrogenic interventions.[9,10] There are no data on the potential psychological effects of routine ultrasound in late pregnancy, and the effects on both short- and long-term neonatal and childhood outcome.

Table 3.4 *Indications for second (and third) trimester ultrasound*[3,4]
• Estimation of gestational age (if uncertain dates, scheduled cesarean delivery, induction of labor, or other elective termination of pregnancy)
• Evaluation of fetal growth
• Vaginal bleeding
• Abdominal and pelvic pain
• Insufficient cervix
• Determination of fetal presentation
• Suspected multiple gestation
• Adjunct to amniocentesis
• Significant discrepancy between uterine size and clinical dates
• Pelvic mass
• Suspected hydatidiform mole
• Adjunct to cervical cerclage placement
• Suspected ectopic pregnancy
• Suspected fetal death
• Suspected uterine abnormality
• Evaluation of fetal well-being (e.g. biophysical profile [BPP], Doppler)
• Suspected amniotic abnormalities
• Suspected placental abruption
• Adjunct to external cephalic version
• Premature rupture of membranes or premature labor (for estimation of fetal weight)
• Abnormal biochemical markers during screening
• Follow-up evaluation of placental location for suspected placenta previa
• History of previous congenital anomaly
• Evaluation of fetal condition in late registrants for prenatal care

Doppler

Umbilical artery: In low-risk or unselected populations, **routine Doppler ultrasound examination, usually of the umbilical artery at around 28–34 weeks, does not result in increased antenatal, obstetric, and neonatal interventions, and no overall differences are detected for substantive short-term clinical outcomes such as perinatal mortality.**[12] There was a strong non-significant trend towards less perinatal mortality for late ultrasound with umbilical artery Doppler in one trial.[13] There is no available evidence to assess the effect on substantive long-term outcomes such as childhood neurodevelopment. There is no available evidence to assess maternal outcomes, particularly psychological effects. Further evaluation regarding the safety of Doppler ultrasound is required.[12]

Uterine artery: There is insufficient evidence to assess the effect of routine mid-pregnancy uterine Doppler ultrasound for prediction and prevention of pre-eclampsia, intrauterine growth restriction, or adverse pregnancy

Table 3.5   *Essential elements for second (and third) trimester ultrasound[3,4]*

- Fetal cardiac activity (abnormal heart rate or rhythm should be reported)
- Number (multiple pregnancies require additional information: chorionicity, amnionicity, comparison of fetal sizes, estimation of amniotic fluid volume at each side of the membranes, and fetal gender)
- Presentation
- A qualitative or semiquantitative (e.g. AFI, SDP, two-diameter pocket) estimate of the amniotic liquid volume (see Chapter 50 in *Maternal–Fetal Evidence Based Guidelines*)
- The placental location, appearance, and relationship to the internal cervical os should be recorded. (The apparent position early in pregnancy may not correlate well with its location at the time of delivery. Therefore, if low-lying placenta or placenta previa are suspected early in gestation, verification in the third trimester by ultrasound is indicated. Transabdominal, transperineal, or transvaginal (best modality) views may be helpful in visualizing the internal cervical os and its relation to the placenta. Transvaginal ultrasound may be considered if the cervix appears shortened or if the patient complains of regular uterine contractions)
- The umbilical cord and the number of vessels in the cord should be evaluated when possible
- Gestational age assessment. Fetal trimester CRL measurement is the most accurate means for sonographic dating. After this period, a variety of sonographic parameters such as the biparietal diameter, head circumference, abdominal circumference, and femoral diaphysis length can be used to estimate gestational age. The variability of gestational age estimations, however, increases with advancing pregnancy (see Table 3.1)
- Fetal weight estimation can be calculated by obtaining measurements, such as biparietal diameter, head circumference, abdominal circumference, and femoral length. None of the several equations for estimating fetal weight based on such fetal biometric measurements is superior to others; ideally, the equations should be derived by actual fetal weights of the local or institutional population. Results can be compared to fetal weight percentiles from published nomograms. Consecutive ultrasound examinations for growth evaluation should typically be performed no less than 2–3 weeks apart.
- Evaluation of the maternal uterus and adnexal structures should be performed
- Fetal anatomy survey: fetal anatomy is best assessed by ultrasound ≥ 18 weeks. Essential elements of a standard examination:
  - Head and neck: cerebellum, choroids plexus, cisterna magna, lateral cerebral ventricles, midline falx, cavum septi pellucidi
  - Chest: the basic cardiac inspection includes a four-chamber view of fetal heart (outflow tracts can be added if technically feasible)
  - Abdomen: stomach (presence, size, situs), kidneys, bladder, umbilical cord (insertion site into fetal abdomen and vessel number)
  - Spine: cervical, thoracic, lumbar, and sacral spine
  - Extremities: legs and arms (presence or absence)
  - Gender: for evaluation of multiple gestations

AFI, amniotic fluid index; SDP, single deepest pocket; CRL, crown–rump length.

outcome (see also Chapters 1 and 39 in *Maternal–Fetal Evidence Based Guidelines*).

There is insufficient evidence to assess the benefit of Doppler screening of any other fetal or maternal vessel.

Other types of obstetric ultrasound

Limited ultrasound examination is performed when a specific question requires investigation: for example, to assess amniotic fluid volume, to verify fetal life or death, to evaluate fetal biophysical profile, to guide amniocentesis, to localize the placenta in antepartum bleeding, to evaluate fetal position, etc. It is appropriate generally only if a prior complete standard ultrasound examination has been done. A **specialized** (aka detailed or targeted) **ultrasound examination** should be considered for a patient who, by history, clinical evaluation, or prior scanning evaluation, is suspected of having an anatomic or physiological abnormality in the fetus. This ultrasound

examination must be done by a person with expertise in obstetric ultrasonography and maternal and fetal disease. Other specialized examinations might include fetal Doppler, biophysical profile, fetal echocardiography, or other biometric studies. A '**genetic**' **ultrasound** can be performed with the aim of detecting anomalies or markers associated with fetal aneuploidy (no trials on its efficacy). **Three-dimensional ultrasound examination** is not considered a required modality for all pregnant women at this time,[4] but it can add accuracy in the assessment of the fetus identified to have anomalies (especially CNS) on two-dimensional examination.

References

1. Neilson JP. Ultrasound for fetal assessment in early pregnancy. Cochrane Database Syst Rev 2007; 1. [meta-analysis: 9 RCTs, n=>24 000]
2. Newnham JP, Doherty DA, Kendall GE et al. Effects of repeated prenatal ultrasound examinations on childhood outcome up to 8 years

of age: follow-up of a randomized trial. Lancet 2004; 364: 2038–44. [follow-up at 8 years of RCT of 5 vs 1 ultrasounds in pregnancy]

3. American Institute of Ultrasound in Medicine. AIUM practice guideline for the performance of antepartum obstetric ultrasound examination. J Ultrasound Med 2003; 22: 1116–25. [review]

4. American College of Obstetricians and Gynecologists. Ultrasonography in pregnancy. ACOG Practice Bulletin No. 58. American College of Obstetricians and Gynecologists; Washington, DC: 2004. [review]

5. Raphael T. Disclosing the sex of the fetus: a view from the UK. Ultrasound Obstet Gynecol 2002; 20: 421–4. [review]

6. Gardosi J. Dating of pregnancy: time to forget the last menstrual period. Ultrasound Obstet Gynecol 1997; 9(6): 367–8. [review]

7. Taipale P, Hiilesmaa V. Predicting delivery date by ultrasound and last menstrual period in early gestation. Obstet Gynecol 2001; 97: 189–94. [II–3]

8. Chavez MR, Ananth CV, Smulian JC et al. Fetal transcerebellar measurement with particular emphasis on the third trimester: a reliable predictor of gestational age. Am J Obstet Gynecol 2004; 191: 979–84. [II–2]

9. Bricker L, Neilson J. Routine ultrasound in late pregnancy (after 24 weeks gestation). Cochrane Database Syst Rev 2007; 1. [meta-analysis: 7 RCTs, n = 25 036]

10. McKenna D, Tharmaratnam S, Mahsud S et al. A randomized trial using ultrasound to identify the high-risk fetus in a low-risk population. Obstet Gynecol 2003; 101: 626–32. [RCT, n = 1998]

11. Proud J, Grant AM. Third trimester placental grading by ultrasonography as a test of fetal wellbeing. BMJ 1987; 294: 1641–4. [RCT, n = 2000]

12. Bricker L, Neilson JP. Routine Doppler ultrasound in pregnancy. Cochrane Database Syst Rev 2007; 1. [meta-analysis: 5 RCTs; n = 14 338]

13. Newnham JP, Evans SF, Michael CA, Stanley FJ, Landau LI. Effects of frequent ultrasound during pregnancy: a randomised controlled trial. Lancet 1993; 342: 887–91. [RCT, n = 2834]

4

Screening for aneuploidy and prenatal diagnosis

Thomas M Jenkins and Dawnette Lewis

KEY POINTS

- Population screening for women in a high-risk category should have **genetic counseling services available** to discuss the different modalities, advantages and disadvantages, and the time frame for each test prior to screening. All women should have counseling available if desired or if an 'abnormal' result occurs.
- Issues of **sensitivity, specificity, and positive and negative predictive values** are vital to the interpretation of a screening test. Positive predictive value of a screening test is greatly influenced by **prevalence** rates in the population tested.
- **The performance of a screening test depends on** the **age of the women** screened (which determines prevalence of trisomies), **women's preference** of screening methods, their **choice of invasive testing**, and their **attitudes towards pregnancy termination**. There is, as of now, **no definitive non-invasive prenatal diagnostic test. The only diagnostic tests are invasive, i.e. chorionic villus sampling (CVS) and amniocentesis.**
- Compared to a Down's syndrome screening policy of amniocentesis for age ≥35 years of age and universal ultrasound at 18 weeks, a policy of **nuchal translucency (NT) screening is associated with similar numbers of Down's syndrome neonates born and a decrease in invasive tests.**
- First trimester screening (FTS) – NT, pregnancy-associated plasma protein-A (PAPP-A), and β-human chorionic gonadotropin (β-HCG) – **can be performed at 10 3/7 to 13 6/7 weeks, with the best detection rate achieved at 11 weeks.** The overall detection rate (sensitivity) for Down's Syndrome is about 84–87% (false-positive rate [FPR] = 5%). First trimester screening should be offered only if: appropriate training and ongoing quality monitoring programs are in place for both ultrasound (NT) and laboratory assays of analytes; sufficient information and resources are available to provide comprehensive counseling to women regarding the different options and limitations of these tests; and access to an appropriate diagnostic test (i.e. CVS) is available when screening results are positive. **Compared to management** using second trimester screening (STS), management using FTS is also associated with a significant reduction in induction for post-term pregnancy because of better dating with first trimester ultrasound.

- Analyte screening (**quadruple marker screen**) can **detect approximately 70–81%** of Down's pregnancies (FPR = 5%).
- **Integrative screening** has the **best detection rate for Down's syndrome (95%), with a low (1–4%) FPR, but** results are available **only in the second trimester. Step-wise or contigent sequential screening** offers **the same 95% detection rate, a reasonable 5% FPR, and availability of results in the first trimester.**
- **Second-trimester 'genetic' ultrasound** has an impact, among other things, on dating, induction rates, and anatomic evaluation of the fetus. As a modality for genetic screening, the data are more limited compared with other available tests. Major anomalies (e.g. congenital cardiac defects and duodenal atresia), and some markers (especially nuchal thickening, short humerus or femur, and echogenic bowel), are associated with a significantly higher risk for Down's syndrome.
- **Second trimester amniocentesis is safer than transcervical CVS or early amniocentesis (< 15 weeks). Early amniocentesis should never be performed. With expert operators (> 400 CVS), CVS by any route may be as safe as second trimester amniocentesis.**
- If **earlier diagnosis is required, transabdominal CVS is preferable to early amniocentesis or transcervical CVS.** In circumstances where transabdominal CVS may be technically difficult, the preferred options are transcervical CVS in the first trimester with expert operator, or second trimester amniocentesis, per patient preference.

Definition

Prenatal diagnosis: what once was only rudimentary ultrasound and invasive karyotype analysis by amniocentesis, prenatal diagnosis now incorporates screening for aneuploidies and fetal anomalies with many different modalities, including population screening, individual risk assessment, genetic counseling, and diagnostic testing.

Table 4.1 *Ideal fetal screening test*

Identify common or important fetal disorder

Be cost-effective

High detection rate; low false-positive rate

Be reliable and reproducible

Diagnostic test exists

Be positive early in pregnancy

Possible intervention if screening test is positive

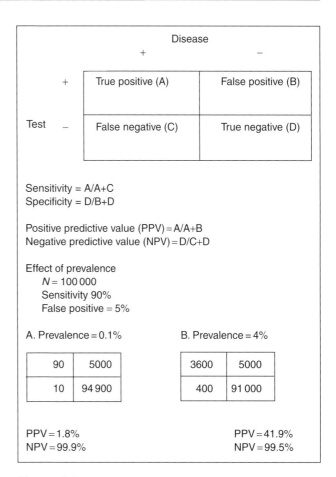

Figure 4.1
Screening test concepts and effect of prevalence

Screening vs diagnostic tests

Prior to screening a population with an available test, test specifics should be assessed. **Issues of prevalence, sensitivity, specificity, and positive and negative predictive values are vital to the interpretation of a screening test** and are a large part of the problem that exists in interpreting the value of a test by either practitioners or the public. Sensitivity of a screening test can also be called detection rate. Table 4.1 lists the characteristics of an ideal perinatal screening test. High sensitivity and specificity are preferable; however, the prevalence of a condition (based upon the population tested) will ultimately determine the value of a positive or negative result (Figure 4.1). With lower prevalence, the chance of a particular 'positive' test to be a true finding is much less. For example, based upon the numbers from Figure 4.1, if all the women with a positive test from group 'A' had a chorionic villus sampling (CVS), there would be one positive result for every 55 CVS performed. If all the women in group 'B' had a CVS, one out of every 2.4 tests would yield a positive result. **The performance of a screening test depends on the age of the woman screened** (which determines the prevalence of trisomies), **the woman's preference** for screening method, her **choice of invasive testing,** and her **attitude towards pregnancy termination. There is currently no definitive non-invasive prenatal diagnostic test. The only diagnostic tests are invasive, i.e. CVS and amniocentesis.**

Antenatal screening for Down's syndrome (Table 4.2)

History

Langdon Down, in 1866, reported that the skin of individuals with trisomy 21 appeared enlarged. In the 1970s data became available on the relationship between maternal age and increased risk for aneuploidy. A statistically relevant difference was seen between the 30–34-year-old group, and the 35–39-year-old group, so that this difference led to the offering of women 35 years of age or older diagnostic evaluation for karyotype. Maternal serum α-fetoprotein (MSAFP) was originally found to be elevated in women carrying fetuses with neural tube defects (NTDs); then in 1984 a low MSAFP was associated with a higher risk of Down's syndrome. Nuchal translucency (NT) first trimester ultrasound screening was introduced in the early 1990s. While livebirths to women > 35 years of age continue to increase, due to better, more diffuse screening, the number of Down's syndrome neonates is decreasing.

Principles

There is presently a general consensus in the USA that invasive testing for Down's syndrome be offered to those with a second-trimester risk of 1: 270 or higher (liveborn risk of 1: 380). The cut-off level and subsequent public policy was determined over 25 years ago and was based on a maternal age risk of 35 years at delivery. Factors considered in determining this value included the prevalence of disease, a

Table 4.2 *Screening tests for Down's syndrome*		
Test	FPR (%)	Sensitivity (%)
Age	5	25–30
First trimester (11–14 weeks)		
NT	5	70–80
PAPP-A and β-HCG	5	60–80
Age, NT, PAPP-A, and β-HCG (FTS)	5	85
Age, NT, PAPP-A, and HCG (FTS)	5	80–85
Second trimester (15–21 weeks)		
Age, MSAFP, HCG, uE$_3$ (TS)	5	60–70
Age, MSAFP, HCG, uE$_3$, inhibin (QS)	5	70–81
Integrative (non-disclosure of FTS)		
Integrated (NT, PAPP-A, QS)	4	95
Serum integrated (PAPP-A, QS)	5	85–90
Sequential (disclosure of FTS)		
Independent	11	95
Step-wise	5	95
Contigent	5	NA
Genetic ultrasound	5	50–70
Extended ultrasound[a]	5	80–85

FPR, false-positive rate; NT, nuchal translucency; PAPP-A, pregnancy-associated plasma protein-A; HCG, human chorionic gonadotropin; MSAFP, maternal serum α-fetoprotein; uE$_3$, unconjugated estriol; FTS, first trimester screening; TS, triple screen; QS, quadruple screen; NA, not available.
[a]genetic ultrasound and serum screening (QS).

perceived significant increase in the trisomy 21 risk after this age, the risk of invasive testing, the availability of resources, and a cost–benefit analysis. Since that time, a number of additional screening tests for Down's syndrome have become available that challenge the validity of maternal age as a single indication for invasive testing. There are a limited amount of randomized control trials for the evaluation of different tests. Most data come from cohort studies or cross-sectional analysis.

Age

The risk of fetal trisomy 21 increases with maternal age, but decreases with the gestational age at assessment in determining the risk, secondary to in-utero death rates (Table 4.3).[1]

Women > 35 years of age have a higher individual risk than younger women; however, the vast majority of Down's syndrome pregnancies are born to the < 35-year-old age group. Screening programs have been developed to try to detect affected pregnancies in both the 'higher' and 'lower' risk groups.

First trimester screening: nuchal translucency

Nuchal translucency is elevated in fetuses with Down's syndrome at **10 3/7 to 13 6/7 weeks** (crown–rump length [CRL] about 36–86 mm). The NT measurement is obtained in a mid-sagittal plane with the neck of the fetus in a neutral position. The amnion should be seen separately from the neck. The image should be enlarged > 75% of the screen. The measurement is obtained from the inner to inner aspects of the NT, and multiples of the medians are used to calculate the Down's syndrome risk via computer software. An increased NT is > 70% sensitive for trisomy 21, trisomy 18, and trisomy 13. Rigorous training, certification, and ongoing quality control are necessary to achieve the detection rates published in the literature (www.fetalmedicine.com;

Table 4.3 *Risk for Down's syndrome based upon maternal and gestational age*

Maternal age	Gestational age (weeks)			
	12	16	20	Liveborn
20	1/1068	1/1200	1/1295	1/1527
25	1/946	1/1062	1/1147	1/1352
30	1/626	1/703	1/759	1/895
31	1/543	1/610	1/658	1/776
32	1/461	1/518	1/559	1/659
33	1/383	1/430	1/464	1/547
34	1/312	1/350	1/378	1/446
35	1/249	1/280	1/302	1/356
36	1/196	1/220	1/238	1/280
37	1/152	1/171	1/185	1/218
38	1/117	1/131	1/142	1/167
39	1/89	1/100	1/108	1/128
40	1/68	1/76	1/82	1/97
42	1/38	1/43	1/46	1/55
44	1/21	1/24	1/26	1/30
45	1/16	1/18	1/19	1/23

www.ntqr.org). The optimal time to perform NT for Down's syndrome screening is about 11 weeks.

Compared to a Down's syndrome screening policy of amniocentesis for age ≥ 35 years old and ultrasound at 18 weeks, a policy of NT screening is associated with similar numbers of Down's syndrome neonates born (a non-significant 37.5% decrease) and **a significant 82% decrease in invasive tests.**[2] One explanation for the small non-significant difference in Down's syndrome neonates born alive may be that NT screening certainly identifies better Down's syndrome fetuses, but the majority of these identified Down's syndrome fetuses are those that would have miscarried without intervention.

Biochemistry

The maternal serum analytes measured are β-human chorionic gonadotropin (β-HCG) and pregnancy-associated plasma protein-A (PAPP-A). β-HCG normally decreases in pregnancy, but is increased in fetuses affected with trisomy 21. **Free** β-HCG performs better than **total HCG** as an independent marker, but there does not appear to be a clinically significant difference in sensitivity when either is combined with NT and PAPP-A for first trimester screening (FTS).[3] **PAPP-A** normally increases in pregnancy, but is decreased in fetuses affected with trisomy 21. HCG discrimination is greatest at 13 weeks, whereas PAPP-A's is greatest at 10 weeks, making 11 weeks the optimal time for first trimester analyte screening.

First trimester screening

First trimester screening consists of measurement of the NT combined with maternal serum screening (**PAPP-A** and β-**HCG**). Over 18 studies in over 200 000 women have been performed to assess the sensitivity of this screening test, making this the best studied screening test in pregnancy.[3–6] The gestational age for FTS is about **10 3/7 to 13 6/7 weeks** (about 73–98 days; CRL about 36–86 mm). The usual cut-off risk is 1: 270. The detection rate (sensitivity) is about **84–87%** (95% CI 80–90%). **The best detection rate is achieved at 11 weeks.**

First trimester screening should be offered only if the following criteria can be met: [3–6]

1. Appropriate training and ongoing quality monitoring programs are in place for both ultrasound (NT) and laboratory assays of analytes.
2. Sufficient information and resources are available to provide comprehensive counseling to women regarding the different options and limitations of these tests.
3. Access to an appropriate diagnostic test (i.e. CVS) is available when screening results are positive.

The Maternal Fetal Medicine Foundation (www.mfmf.org) and the Fetal Medicine Foundation (www.fetalmedicine.com) both provide nuchal translucency education and quality review programs. There is sufficient evidence to support implementing FTS for Down's syndrome provided the above three requirements are met. Almost 85% of women in the USA present for care within 12 weeks and can be offered FTS, which can provide high detection, early reassurance, more time/diagnostic options, and earlier completion of aneuploidy screening.

Compared to management using second trimester screening (STS), management using FTS is associated also with a significant reduction in induction for post-term pregnancy because of better dating with first trimester ultrasound.[7]

Nasal bone

Over 12 studies in over 18 000 women demonstrated that nasal bone when imaged at 11–14 weeks is absent in approximately 70% of Down's syndrome fetuses, and in only 1.5% of unaffected fetuses. When added to FTS (NT, PAPP-A, and β-HCG), it can increase the detection rate to about 95%, decreasing the false-positive rate (FPR) to 2%. Possibly owing to the difficulty of this examination, these data have not been confirmed in all studies. Most recently, abnormal ductus venosus Doppler flow and tricuspid regurgitation have also been found to be > 70% sensitive for trisomy 21, but there is insufficient prospective data for any increase in accuracy over FTS.

Second trimester screening

Maternal analyte screening had the first reported association with Down's syndrome with low **MSAFP** (multiples of the median [MoM] 0.75), followed by the association of high **HCG** (MoM 2.3) and a low **unconjugated estriol** (MoM 0.7), to form the 'triple screen'. The detection rate for women under 35 with a triple screen ranges between 57 and 74%, with a constant 5% FPR.[2,4] For women above 35 (using similar cut-off values), the sensitivity increases to 87%, but the FPR also balloons to 25%.[8] **Inhibin** was added to analyte screening (**quadruple screen**), but, since levels correlate somewhat with HCG, it is not an independent predictor like the other markers, and the increase in detection is more limited (7–11 percentage points). Approximately 70–81% of cases are detected in the majority of studies, holding the FPR at 5%.[3,5] This screening test can be performed between 15 and 22 weeks, with best results obtained at 16–18 weeks.

Other combinations of markers have been assessed since the advent of the 'triple screen'; however, with the addition of extra markers, the potential benefit versus the cost must be balanced. With each additional marker, costs to society reach into the millions secondary to the numbers of pregnancies tested each year. The relative cost and value of raising the sensitivity or lowering the FPR a few percentage points is an ongoing debate.

Combining both first and second trimester tests

Combined screening programs in the first trimester (using both ultrasound assessments of the NT as well as maternal analytes) and the second trimester (using maternal analytes) have been described. Patterns of testing include sequential testing (results given after each test) and integrated testing (delaying reporting until both tests have been completed).

Integrative screening

Integrative screening is performance of screening tests at different times during pregnancy with a single result provided to the patient only after all tests have been completed. A protocol for integrated screening for Down's syndrome is based upon tests performed during the first and second trimester (NT, PAPP-A, MSAFP, HCG, estriol, and inhibin). Mathematical models calculated that >85% of affected pregnancies would be detected with an FPR of only 0.9%. The FASTER trial (First- And Second-Trimester Evaluation of Risk) performed integrated screening in 33 557 women (84 with Down's syndrome).[5] Cut-off values for the different tests varied (first trimester combined test cut-off, 1: 150; second trimester 'quad screen', 1: 300). The authors report a sensitivity of 86% with first trimester screening (FPR = 5%), 85% with second trimester screening (FPR high at 8.5%), and, when combined, a 94% detection of Down's syndrome cases. If results are revealed after STS, the FPR is only 4.9%, with the **best sensitivity**. If NT is not available, an 'integrated serum screening test' has a detection rate of 85% with 3.9% FPR.[3] Disadvantages of integrative screening include the lack of early diagnosis, the physical and psychological ramifications created if an abnormality is found and the woman opts for termination (compared with the FTS), the increase in costs (compared with either FTS or STS), the perception of 'hiding' abnormal results, as well as the limitations it places on multiple gestations if discordant karyotypes are found.

Sequential screening

Sequential screening involves performance of different screening tests at different times during pregnancy with results provided to the patient after each test. There are three approaches to sequential testing: independent, stepwise, and contingent.

Independent: This approach involves the independent interpretation of FTS and STS. While the sensitivity is as exemplary with this approach as with integrative screening (94–95%), combining screening tests and revealing the results after each increases the chance for false-positive results. The FASTER trial[5] FPR was 10.8% with sequential independent screening, far too high for population-based usage. As a high FPR means higher loss rates due to more invasive testing, independent sequential screening is the least-efficient risk assessment strategy, and should NOT be used.

Step-wise: Both FTS and STS (usually quadruple screen [QS]) are performed, with results revealed after FTS: if FTS risk is above a certain cut-off, invasive testing (i.e. CVS) is offered; if FTS is below a certain cut-off, STS is recommended with a final risk revealed at that point. In the FASTER trial, such an approach (low cut-off, 1:150; high-cutoff, 1:300) had a detection rate of 95% with an FPR of 4.9%.[5] The advantages of this approach are a very high detection rate (as with integrative screening), with the option of early results in first trimester for the highest-risk women.

Contingent: Both FTS and STS (usually QS) are performed, with results revealed after FTS: if FTS risk is above a certain cut-off (e.g. 1/150), invasive testing (i.e. CVS) is offered; if FTS is below a certain cut-off (e.g. 1/300), no further screening is necessary; if FTS is in between, STS is recommended with a final risk revealed at that point. Careful determination of risk cut-offs is necessary. This strategy has not been studied prospectively.

'Genetic' ultrasound screening for Down's syndrome

An ultrasound of the fetus performed at **18–24 weeks** is associated with several important benefits (see Chapter 3). One of the benefits is the antenatal detection of anomalies. The identification of a fetus with an issue allows for directed counseling and optimization of antepartum, intrapartum, and postpartum care. Whether routine or targeted anatomic assessment is being performed, it should be done by experienced centers with ongoing quality assessment to increase detection of anomalies and limit false-positive results.

The in-utero diagnosis of Down's syndrome can be suspected when anomalies or physical features that occur more frequently in Down's syndrome than in the general population are noted on an ultrasound examination. Some of these major structural congenital anomalies, such as atrioventricular canal or duodenal atresia, strongly suggest the possibility of Down's syndrome and are independent indications to offer invasive testing. Although, when present, there is a high risk of trisomy 21, these anomalies have low sensitivity and, thus, are not useful in screening. For example, when **duodenal atresia** is identified, there is approximately a 40% risk of Down's syndrome, yet it is seen in only 8% of affected fetuses. About 50% of Down's syndrome fetuses have **congenital heart defects.**

Physical characteristics that are not structural anomalies but occur more commonly in fetuses with Down's syndrome are called **markers.** By comparing the prevalence of markers in Down's syndrome fetuses to their prevalence in the normal population, a likelihood ratio (LR) can be calculated which can be used to modify risk. This is the basis for ultrasound screening for Down's syndrome. In order for a marker to be useful for Down's syndrome screening, it should be sensitive (i.e. present in a high proportion of Down's syndrome pregnancies), specific (i.e. not commonly seen in normal fetuses), easily imaged in standard sonographic examination, and present early enough in the second trimester that diagnostic testing can be performed

Table 4.4 *Ultrasound changes associated with Down's syndrome*

Major anomalies
Congenital heart defects
Duodenal atresia

Major markers
Increased nuchal thickness
Hyperechoic bowel
Shortened humerus
Shortened femur
Echogenic intracardiac focus
Renal pyelectasis

Minor markers
Shortened or absent nasal bone
Foot length
'Sandal gap' of the foot
Widened ischial spine angle
Hypoplasia of the mid-phalynx of the fifth digit
Brachycephaly

so that results are available when pregnancy termination remains an option. A list of currently available markers and LRs are seen in Tables 4.4 and 4.5, respectively.[9–11] Markers commonly sought to assess the risk of Down's syndrome include the following:

Increased nuchal thickness: About 35% of Down's syndrome fetuses, but only 0.7% of normal fetuses, have a nuchal skin fold measurement ≥ 6 mm (some studies use ≥ 5 mm). When an increased nuchal fold is an isolated finding, the LR is strong at 10–17. Thus, the presence of an increased nuchal fold alone is usually an indication to offer invasive testing.

Increased echogenicity of the fetal bowel: When brighter than the surrounding bone, this factor has a Down's syndrome LR of 3.0–6.7, a finding that can also be seen with

Table 4.5 *Likelihood ratios and 95% confidence limits for isolated ultrasound markers*

Isolated sonographic marker	Nyberg et al[9] LR (95% CI)	Smith-Bindman et al[10] LR (95% CI)	Nicolaides[11] LR
Nuchal fold/thickening	11 (5.2–22)	17 (8–38)	9.8
Hyperechoic bowel	6.7 (2.7–16.8)	6.1 (3–12.6)	3.0
Short humerus	5.1 (1.6–16.5)	7.5 (4.7–12)	4.1
Short femur	1.5 (0.8–2.8)	2.7 (1.2–6)	1.6
EIF	1.8 (1.0–3)	2.8 (1.5–5.5)	1.1
Pyelectasis	1.5 (0.6–3.6)	1.9 (0.7–5.1)	1.0

LR, likelihood ratio; CI, confidence interval; EIF, echogenic intracardiac foci.

fetal cystic fibrosis, congenital cytomegalovirus (CMV) infection, swallowed bloody amniotic fluid, and severe fetal growth restriction (FGR).

Short humerus, and to a lesser degree, short femur: In the second trimester, these factors are associated with Down's syndrome, relative to the length expected from their biparietal diameter (BPD). This can be used to identify at-risk pregnancies by calculating a ratio of observed to expected (O/E) femur/humerus length based on the fetus' BPD. An O/E ratio for femur length of < 0.91 has a reported LR of 1.5–2.7 when present as an isolated finding. A short humerus is more strongly related to Down's syndrome, with reported LRs ranging from 4.1 to 7.5.

Pyelectasis: A renal AP diameter of ≥ 4–5 mm has an LR that ranges from 1.1 to 1.9 as an isolated marker. This has been found by some not to be significantly more frequent in Down's syndrome pregnancies than in normals (low specificity).[11]

Echogenic intracardiac foci: They occur in up to 5% of normal pregnancies and in approximately 13–18% of Down's syndrome gestations. The LR for Down's syndrome when an echogenic focus is present as an isolated marker has ranged from 1.0 to 2.8. This has been found by most investigators not to be significantly more frequent in Down's syndrome pregnancies than in normals (low specificity).[11] The risk does not seem to vary if the focus is in the right or left ventricle or if it is unilateral or bilateral, but may be affected by ethnicity.

Other markers described include a hypoplastic fifth middle phalanx of the hand, short ears, a sandal gap between the first and second toes, an abnormal iliac wing angle, an altered foot to femur ratio, and a short or absent nasal bone. These markers are inconsistently used because of the time and expertise required to obtain them. Mild ventriculomegaly (10–15 mm) can be an indication for invasive prenatal diagnosis, since it is associated with a 1–2% risk of aneuploidy if isolated. If the karyotype is normal, mild ventriculomegaly is still associated with about 8% structural anomalies, 3% perinatal death, and 10–20% abnormal neurodevelopment.

Except for major anomalies and increased nuchal thickness, isolated 'genetic ultrasound' markers should in general not be used as the sole indication for invasive testing. As with other screening modalities, 'genetic' ultrasound can be used to alter the a priori risk in either direction. A positive LR can be used to increase estimated risk. The magnitude of the increase depends upon the marker(s) or anomalies seen. While most of the clinical prospective data justifying this approach have come from a baseline age-related risk, some have advocated using these LRs to adjust whichever baseline risk, even that derived by other screening tests (e.g. FTS and/or QS, or even integrative or consecutive approaches). A benign second trimester scan having none of the known markers and no anomalies has been suggested to have an LR of 0.4–0.5, assuming the image quality is satisfactory when the 'genetic ultrasound' is normal. It is doubtful that the same sensitivity can be achieved in every center.

Ultrasound screening for other chromosomal abnormalities

Fetal aneuploidy other than Down's syndrome can be suspected based on ultrasound findings.[12] The rates reported are usually in high-risk populations and may overestimate the strength of the association when such findings are noted on a screening examination.

Trisomy 18

Choroid plexus cysts (CPCs) have a very weak association with trisomy 18, and should not be the sole indication for invasive testing if isolated. The presence of CPCs should be an indication for a detailed second trimester ultrasound for trisomy 18 major anomalies, such as cardiac, central nervous system (CNS), hand defects, etc.

FTS and STS with MSAFP, HCG, unconjugated estriol, and inhibin (QS) have a high detection rate for trisomy 18.

Second trimester ultrasound also has a high detection rate for trisomy 18.

Positive screening for aneuploidy but normal karyotype

Nuchal translucency

An NT above the 95% percentile for gestational age, and especially ≥ 3.5 mm at 10 3/7 to 13 6/7 weeks is associated with an increased risk of other anomalies and syndromes, with the risk directly proportional to the increase in NT[13] (Table 4.6).

The list of anomalies is long,[13] and a detailed second trimester ultrasound is recommended, as is the list of genetic syndromes. The incidence of cardiac anomalies is ≥ 3.7% for NT ≥ 3.5 mm, so that a fetal cardiac ultrasound by an experienced operator is recommended.

First trimester PAPP-A and β-HCG

A low PAPP-A in FTS in the presence of a normal karyotype is associated with several adverse pregnancy outcomes,

Table 4.6 *Risks of chromosome abnormalities and (if normal karyotype) of fetal death or anomalies according to nuchal translucency measurement*

| NT | Chromosomal defects (%) | Normal karyotype | | | |
		Fetal death (%)	Major fetal anomalies (%)	Alive and well (%)	Cardiac defects (%)
<95th centile	0.2	1.3	1.6	97	0.6
95–99th centiles	3.7	1.3	2.5	93	0.6
3.5–4.4	21.1	2.7	10.0	70	3.7
4.5–5.4	33	3.4	18.5	50	6.7
5.5–6.4	50	10	24	30	13
≥6.5	65	19	46	15	20

NT, nuchal translucency.

including fetal loss, preterm birth (PTB), and FGR. Low free HCG is associated with fetal loss.

Second trimester screening

High MSAFP is associated with NTDs, as well as abdominal wall defects and several other fetal abnormalities. High MSAFP, negative amniotic fluid acetylcholinesterase (AChE), and normal ultrasound can be associated with congenital nephrosis or other syndromes, or normal pregnancy. Unexplained high MSAFP is associated with mild increases in the incidence of pre-eclampsia, abruption, placental ischemia, PTB, fetal demise, low birth weight, and sudden infant death syndrome (SIDS). No trials have assessed the specific management needed to prevent these complications.

Low unconjugated estriol is associated with steroid sulfatase deficiency, Smith–Lemli–Opitz syndrome, or other conditions when very low, usually <0.3 MoM.

MSAFP screening for NTD

Elevated (usually ≥2.5 MoM) MSAFP between 14 and 21 weeks is associated with a ≥90–95% sensitivity for NTDs (false-negative rate 5%). Given that ultrasound is also ≥95% sensitive for NTDs, the routine use of MSAFP screening may be most important for pregnancies that will not have a detailed second trimester ultrasound.

Screening for aneuploidies in twins

NT is accurate in estimating Down's risk in dizygotic twins, using each NT separately for each fetus. In monochorionic twins, the average NT is the most effective screening method. Detection rates comparable to singletons can be achieved (see also Chapter 38 in *Maternal–Fetal Evidence Based Guidelines*).

Detection rates of FTS or STS tests are usually lower than in singletons, with higher rates of false-positive and false-negative results. Chorionicity does not seem to affect serum analytes in FTS or STS.

Pre-test general counseling

There is no treatment for aneuploidy, so the woman must be aware that the **main aims of screening for aneuploidy** are the **possibility of termination**, and the **knowledge of the diagnosis**, with no definite proof that this knowledge will improve outcome. Similarly, there are usually minimal, experimental, and often no treatments for fetal anomalies, so the woman must be aware that the main aims of screening for anomalies are (similarly) the possibility of termination, and the knowledge of the diagnosis, with no definite proof that this knowledge will improve outcome. Down's syndrome is the most frequent chromosomal disorder among liveborn infants, with an expected prevalence of about 1/600–1/800 live births, and the most common identifiable cause of mental retardation, with a life expectancy of almost 50 years (see Chapter 5).

Although complicated, discussion of sensitivity (detection rates) at 5% FPR of main screening tests (highlighted in Table 4.2) is necessary. Specific resources (time, expertise, plus the availability of genetic counseling) are paramount. Continuing education of healthcare providers is necessary. Some couples might prefer a screening approach with earliest detection even with a higher, for example 5%, FPR (e.g. FTS), some might prefer highest detection with lowest FPR (e.g. integrative screening), but most might opt in the near future for sequential screening, such as step-wise or contingent screening, as these become available commercially.

No matter the sensitivity of available tests, for women undergoing screening, particularly those in a higher-risk group, detailed discussions regarding the advantages and disadvantages of screening vs diagnostic testing should occur. After such counseling, each woman can make the most informed and best choice for her situation. Since screening tests will never detect 100% of diseases, the option of diagnostic testing in higher-risk populations can be offered. Several studies have shown that most pregnant women prefer early (vs later) screening for Down's syndrome.

Too great a portion of the population believes that the whole purpose behind screening for aneuploidy is so that a couple can terminate a pregnancy prior to viability. While it is true that couples faced with the reality of an aneuploid pregnancy may opt for termination, the purpose of prenatal diagnosis and screening is to provide information. If an abnormality is found, depending on the specifics, couples can be provided with specific information regarding their situation. When a couple decides to carry an abnormal pregnancy to term, the antenatal, intrapartum, and postpartum care can be performed under more ideal circumstances, hopefully altering the outcome. Also, one cannot underestimate the effect that preparation can have for the individuals involved.

Diagnostic tests

Chorionic villus sampling and amniocentesis

Both CVS and amniocentesis have been performed for many years and can fairly safely diagnose a karyotypic or genetic abnormality. Both procedures have been studied extensively. Differences in technique, as well as timing of the procedure, affect loss rates. To fairly compare procedure-induced loss rates between the two procedures, adjustments must be made for the higher background frequency of pregnancy loss earlier in gestation.

Second trimester amniocentesis

Compared with no amniocentesis, second trimester amniocentesis is associated with a 0.8% increase in spontaneous miscarriage (2.1% vs 1.3%) but a similar incidence of perinatal deaths (0.4 vs 0.7%).[14,15]

There are insufficient data to assess the effect of polymerase chain reaction (PCR) testing (fluorescent in-situ hybridization [FISH]). In a small trial, reporting karyotype in 3 days with PCR did not affect maternal anxiety level compared with about 3 weeks later in Chinese women with an abnormal screening test for Down's syndrome.[16]

Early amniocentesis

Early amniocentesis (< 15 weeks) is not a safe alternative, because it is associated with increased (7.6 vs 5.9%) pregnancy loss rates compared with second trimester amniocentesis, and higher incidence of talipes (1.8% vs 0.2%) compared with CVS.[14,17]

Chorionic villus sampling

CVS before 10 weeks is associated with an unacceptably high incidence of limb deficiencies, and should not be performed. The optimal time for CVS is 10–12 weeks, with trials of safety performed only at this gestational age. CVS can also be performed after 12 weeks (called usually placental biopsy) in cases in which placental karyotype is needed, but there are no trials on 'late' CVS.

Compared with second trimester amniocentesis, CVS in general – transabdominal (TA) and transcervical (TC) combined – is associated with a slight increased incidence of pregnancy losses and a slight increased incidence of spontaneous miscarriages.[14]

Compared with second trimester amniocentesis, TC CVS is associated with a higher risk of pregnancy loss (14.5 vs 11%) and higher (12.9 vs 9.4%) risk of spontaneous miscarriage.[14]

Compared with second trimester amniocentesis, TA CVS is associated with a similar risk of pregnancy loss (6.3% vs 7.0%) and spontaneous miscarriage (3.0% vs 3.9%) in one study.[14,18]

Transcervical vs transabdominal chorionic villus sampling: Compared with TA CVS, TC CVS is associated with similar pregnancy loss rates (9.0 vs 7.4%) and with similar spontaneous miscarriages (7.9 vs 4.5).[14]

Transcervical chorionic villus sampling technical instrument: There is some evidence to support the use of **small forceps** compared with cannulas for TC CVS. When different types of cannulas are compared, the Portex cannula is more likely to result in an inadequate sample and a difficult or painful procedure than either the silver or aluminum cannula. The evidence is not strong enough to support change in practice for clinicians who have become familiar with aspiration cannulas.[19]

The learning curve for transabdominal and transcervical CVS has been estimated to exceed 400 cases, with post-procedure loss rates for operators having performed less than 100 cases being two to three times higher when compared to more experienced operators. **The importance of operator experience cannot be overemphasized,** particularly for route of CVS, with TC CVS requiring more experience.

While the total miscarriage rate is higher following first trimester CVS because of the higher background rate in early pregnancy, for experienced centers, the rates of procedure-induced losses secondary to CVS are similar to those of second trimester amniocentesis. The demand for CVS is projected to increase secondary to increased use of first trimester screening. The availability of experienced practitioners, as well as qualified training programs, will need to increase to meet this demand.

The future

Advances in technology have demonstrated new avenues for non-invasive diagnostic testing in utero (i.e. fetal cells from maternal circulation or cervical sampling, free fetal DNA in the maternal circulation). While different groups have demonstrated capability with these techniques, practicality for population testing is still not yet available. It is likely that routine feasibility will require the development of newer technologies.

With advancements in laboratory techniques paired with the expanding knowledge of the human genome, prenatal diagnosis will be a vibrant field of study for the future. New screening and diagnostic tests are a real possibility as we are able to obtain more information from our patient in utero.

References

1. Hook EB. Rates of chromosome abnormalities at different maternal ages. Obstet Gynecol 1981; 58(3): 282–5. [II–1]
2. Salvedt A, Almstrom H, Kublickas M et al. Screening for Down's syndrome based on maternal age or fetal nuchal translucency: a randomized controlled trial in 39,572 pregnancies. Ultrasound Obstet Gynecol 2005; 25: 537–45. [RCT, n = 39 572]
3. Wald NJ, Rodeck C, Hackshaw AK et al; SURUSS Research Group. First and second trimester antenatal screening for Down's syndrome: the results of the serum, urine and ultrasound screening study. Health Technol Assess 2003; 7: 1–77. [II–3]
4. Nicolaides KH, Spencer K, Avgidou K, Faiola S, Falcon. Multicenter study of first-trimester screening for trisomy 21 in 75,821 pregnancies: results and estimation of the potential impact of individual risk-orientated two-stage first-trimester screening. Ultrasound Obstet Gynecol 2005; 25: 221–6. [II–3]
5. Malone FD, Canick JA, Ball RH et al; First- and Second Trimester Evaluation of Risk (FASTER) Research Consortium. First-trimester or second-trimester screening, or both, for Down syndrome. N Engl J Med 2005; 353: 2001–11. [II–3]
6. Wapner R, Thom E, Simpson JL et al; First Trimester Maternal Serum Biochemistry and Fetal Nuchal Translucency Screening (BUN) Study Group. First-trimester screening for trisomies 21 and 18. N Engl J Med 2003; 349: 1405–13. [II–3]
7. Bennett KA, Crane JMC, O'Shea P et al; First trimester ultrasound screening is effective in reducing postterm labor induction rates: a randomized controlled trial. Am J Obstet Gynecol 2004; 190: 1077–81. [RCT, n = 218]
8. Haddow JE, Pabmaki GE, Knight GJ et al. Reducing the need for amniocentesis in women 35 years of age or older with serum markers for screening. N Engl J Med 1994; 330(16): 1114–18. [II–2]
9. Nyberg DA, Souter VL, EL-Bastawissi A et al. Isolated sonographic markers for detection of fetal Down syndrome in the second trimester of pregnancy. J Ultrasound Med 2001; 20(10): 1053–63. [II–2]
10. Smith-Bindman R, Hosmer W, Feldstein VA, Deeks JJ, Goldberg JD. Second-trimester ultrasound to detect fetuses with Down syndrome: a meta-analysis. JAMA 2001; 285(8): 1044–55. [II–2]
11. Nicolaides KH, Snijders RJM, Sebire N (eds). The 11–14 Week Scan: The Diagnosis of Fetal Anomalies. Taylor and Francis, London [review].
12. Snijders R, Nicolaides K. Ultrasound Markers for Fetal Markers for Chromosomal Defects. Parthenon Publishing Group; New York: 1996. [II–2]
13. Souka AP, von Kaisenberg CS, Hyett JA, Sonek JD, Nicolaides KH. Increased nuchal translucency with normal karyotype. Am J Obstet Gynecol 2005; 192: 1005–21. [review]
14. Alfirevic Z, Sundberg K, Brigham S. Amniocentesis and chorionic villus sampling for prenatal diagnosis. Cochrane Database Syst Rev 2007; 1. [meta-analysis: 14 RCTs, n = 5000]
15. Tabor A, Madsen M, Obel EB et al. Randomised controlled trial of genetic amniocentesis in 4606 low-risk women. Lancet 1986; 1: 1287–93. [RCT, n = 4606]
16. Leung WC, Lam YH, Wong Y, Lau ET, Tang MH. The effect of fast reporting by amnio-PCR on anxiety levels in women with positive biochemical screening for Down's syndrome – a randomized controlled trial. Prenat Diagn 2002; 22: 256–9. [RCT, n = 60]
17. Collaborative. Randomised trial to assess safety and fetal outcome of early and midtrimester amniocentesis. The Canadian Early and Mid-trimester Amniocentesis Trial (CEMAT) Group. Lancet 1998; 351(9098): 242–7. [RCT, n = 4334]
18. Smidt-Jensen S, Permin M, Philip J et al. Randomized comparison of amniocentesis and transabdominal and transcervical chorionic villus sampling. Lancet 1992; 340: 1237–44. [RCT, n = 2234]
19. Alfirevic Z, von Dadelszen P. Instruments for chorionic villus sampling for prenatal diagnosis. Cochrane Database Syst Rev 2007; 1. [meta-analysis: 5 RCTs, n = 472]

5

Genetic screening

Adele Schneider

KEY POINTS

- There are no trials to assess any intervention for genetic screening and testing in pregnancy.
- **Cystic fibrosis** (CF) testing should be offered to women with a family history of CF, reproductive partners of individuals with CF, and couples in whom one or both partners are Caucasian and are planning a pregnancy or are seeking prenatal care.
- **Trisomy 21** is the most common trisomy at birth, and its incidence increases with increasing maternal age.
- Appropriate counseling regarding prognosis, possible complications, long-term issues, and follow-up should be provided to every couple with a pre- or postnatal diagnosis of aneuploidy or other genetic defect.

Preconception and/or prenatal genetic counseling

Screening for aneuploidy, prenatal diagnosis, and ultrasound screening have been previously reviewed. There are no trials to assess any intervention for genetic screening and testing in pregnancy. Basic genetic counseling should be available to every pregnant woman. All couples should have a basic screen for family history of genetic disorders, with a pedigree to at least the second prior generation. Questions should also involve history of recurrent spontaneous pregnancy loss, and history of a previous fetus or child who was affected by a genetic disorder. Those patients belonging to an ethnic group at increased risk for a recessive condition (e.g. sickle cell anemia – African-American; Tay–Sachs disease and others – Jewish; α-thalassemia – southeast Asian; β-thalassemia – Mediterranean; etc.) should be offered specific screening. Women with a specific indication for genetic testing should be referred for genetic counseling and a discussion of options available for prenatal diagnosis (see Chapter 4).

Table 5.1 *Recommended core mutation panel for general population cystic fibrosis carrier screening*

107delT	711+1G>T	R117H
1717-1G>A	A455E	xR334W
1898+G>A	ΔF508	R347P
2184delA	ΔI507	R553X
2789+5G>A	G542X	R560T
3120+1G>A	G551D	W1282X
3659delC	G85E	
3849+10kbC>T	I148T	
621+G>T	N1303K	

Cystic fibrosis

Cystic fibrosis (CF) is an autosomal recessive disorder. The most common mutation is ΔF508, but >1000 other mutations have been described (Table 5.1).[1] The mutation leads to faulty chloride transport, increased sweat chloride levels, and increased thick mucus in lungs, pancreas, biliary tree, intestines. This is the most common life-limiting genetic disorder in Caucasians (Tables 5.2 and 5.3).[1]

Screening

Screening should be offered to target groups described in Table 5.4.[1] Screening can be concurrent or sequential, and both strategies are acceptable alternatives.

Concurrent.
- Both partners tested simultaneously
- Both partners' results revealed

Table 5.2 *Cystic fibrosis (CF) carrier rate by racial and ethnic group*

Racial or ethnic group	Incidence of CF	Carrier frequency	%ΔF508
Caucasians	1/3 300	1/29	70
Hispanics	1/8 000–9000	1/46	46
African-Americans	1/15 300	1/62	48
Asian Americans	1/32 000	1/90	30

Table 5.3 *Incidence and carrier risk for cystic fibrosis (CF), based on race or ethnicity*

Racial or ethnic group	Detection rate (%)	Estimated carrier risk before test	Estimated carrier risk after a (−) test
Ashkenazi Jewish	97	1/29	~1/930
European Caucasian	80	1/29	~1/140
Hispanic American	57	1/46	~1/105
African-American	69	1/65	~1/207
Asian American	–	1/90	–

Table 5.4 *Carrier screening target groups (offer screening)*

- Family history of cystic fibrosis (CF)
- Reproductive partners of individuals with CF
- Couples in whom *one or both partners are Caucasian* and are planning a pregnancy or are seeking prenatal care

- Assesses couple's risk
- Identifies couples at risk more rapidly
- More precise.

Sequential screening.
- Initial screening of one partner
- Other partner tested if first partner is positive
- Low-risk racial/ethnic groups
- Other partner not available.

Interpretation of results

- Both partners negative (−/−) – prenatal diagnostic testing not indicated

- One partner carrier (−), one not screened
  - Intermediate risk – prenatal diagnostic testing not indicated
- One partner carrier (+), one carrier (−)
  - Prenatal diagnostic testing not recommended
- One partner carrier (+), one untested
  - Partner should be tested if possible
  - Genetic counseling
  - Availability/limitations of prenatal testing
- Both partners carriers (+)
  - 25% chance of having an affected offspring
  - Genetic counseling
  - Prenatal diagnosis offered (chorionic villus sampling [CVS], amniocentesis)
  - Counseling regarding continuation vs termination of pregnancy for affected pregnancies.

Risk of affected offspring also depends on prevalence of carrier status in the specific ethnic group (Table 5.5).

Trisomy 21 (Down's syndrome)

Historic notes: First complete description in 1846 by Seguin. Report by Down in 1866 established the name of the syndrome. In 1959 LeJeune and Jacobs independently described that Down's syndrome was caused by trisomy 21.

Definition: Down's syndrome is **trisomy 21**, or the presence of an extra chromosome number 21, either as three number 21s, or as a translocation between 21 and another chromosomes, usually an acrocentric one in a Robertsonian translocation.

Epidemiology/incidence: About **1 in 800 live births**. This is the most common trisomy at birth. Incidence increases with increasing maternal age (see also Chapter 4).

Embryology: The Down's syndrome critical region on chromosome 21 is being studied extensively to identify the genes involved in the Down's syndrome phenotype. However, this region is not one small isolated spot, but most likely several areas on chromosome 21 that are not necessarily side by side.

Genetics/inheritance: Error in cell division at the time of conception (**non-disjunction**) is responsible for 92% of Down's syndrome by resulting in **full trisomy 21**. Approximately 90% of non-disjunction occurs in the eggs. The cause of the nondisjunction error isn't known, but there is definitely a connection with maternal age. The recurrence risk is empirically 1% or the age-related risk as a woman gets older, whichever is higher. Three to four percent of all cases of trisomy 21 are due to a **Robertsonian translocation,** usually between chromosomes 14 and 21. In

Table 5.5 *Risk of offspring having cystic fibrosis*

Racial or ethnic group	No test	One partner –, one untested	One partner +, one –	One partner +, one untested	Both partners –
Ashkenazi Jewish	1/3300	1/107	1/3720	1/116	1/3 459 600
European Caucasian	1/3300	1/16	1/560	1/116	1/3 459 600
Hispanic American	1/8464	1/19	1/420	1/184	1/78 400
African-American	1/16 900	1/53	1/828	1/260	1/44 100
Asian American	1/32 000	1/53	–	1/360	1/171 396

the balanced state the individual is healthy and has 45 chromosomes with a #21 attached on #14, or another acrocentric chromosome (15, 21, or 22). An individual with Down's syndrome due to a translocation has 46 chromosomes but one is actually a combination of #21 and another acrocentric like #14. Translocations resulting in trisomy 21 may be inherited, so parental chromosomes must be checked. A female carrier of a balanced Robertsonian translocation has about a 12% risk of recurrence of Down's syndrome in future pregnancies, while a male carrier has approximately a 3% risk of recurrence. **Mosaic trisomy 21** occurs when there is a mixture of cell lines, one with normal chromosomes and another with trisomy 21. It is impossible to know how the normal and trisomy 21 cells are distributed in the different organs; therefore, the percentage of mosaic to normal cells in the peripheral blood cannot be used to predict outcome. Another tissue can be examined to help determine the level of mosaicism, usually skin.

Teratology: None.

Classification: Full trisomy 21, translocation trisomy 21, and mosaic trisomy 21.

Risk factors/associations: Advanced maternal age. Individuals who are carriers of balanced Robertsonian translocations involving chromosome #21 have an increased risk.

Pregnancy management

Screening

Screening for aneuploidy and prenatal diagnosis is described in Chapter 4.

Ultrasound findings in fetus:
- Thickened nuchal translucency at 11–14 weeks (80%) (at times cystic hygroma – 10%)
- Thickened nuchal fold (≥6 mm) at 16–23 weeks
- Congenital heart disease (CHD) (40–50%)
- Duodenal atresia (2%)
- Omphalocele (2%)
- Ventriculomegaly
- Hydrops or some hydropic changes (pleural effusion, ascites, etc.)
- Several 'soft markers', such as short humerus and femur, echogenic bowel, renal pyelectasis, cardiac (usually left ventricular) echogenic focus, short middle phalanx fifth digit, 'sandal foot', iliac crest >90° angle, short ear length
- Biometry may reveal symmetric fetal growth restriction (FGR) by the third trimester
  - **Amniotic fluid:** polyhydramnios (if gastrointestinal [GI] obstruction or macroglossia present)
  - **Placenta:** normal
  - **When detectable:** at 11–14 weeks if increased nuchal translucency (NT) is detected.

Ultrasound after 14 weeks only detects ~50% of fetuses with Down's syndrome. Choroid plexus cysts do not increase the risk. Screening provides the mother and family with a risk assessment for Down's syndrome, but true diagnosis can only be achieved with CVS or amniocentesis.

Diagnosis: **CVS or amniocentesis** achieve the diagnosis by a study of the fetal chromosomes, which reveals trisomy 21. In the neonate, peripheral blood is usually cultured and karyotyped.

Counseling: The major abnormalities are increased risk of FGR, congenital heart defects, fetal and postnatal death, and developmental delay, with average IQ of 50–75. Congenital heart defects are major contributors to mortality.

Work-up/investigations and consultations: A **fetal echocardiogram** is recommended. Depending on the lesions detected, specific pediatric subspecialty consultation can be offered. Genetic counseling can be offered as well. Care in a tertiary care center is indicated if there are significant associated anomalies, or if they cannot be ruled out adequately.

Fetal intervention: None available.

Termination issues: Termination can be offered as sole intervention as regulated by local law (usually legal < 24 weeks).

Fetal monitoring/testing: No specific trials. Non-stress tests (NSTs) weekly at ≥ 32 weeks can be offered. Non-reassuring fetal heart testing (NRFHT) is common.

Delivery/anesthesia: Mode and management of delivery should not be affected by the diagnosis of Down's syndrome. NRFHT is common.

Neonatology management

Resuscitation: Providing life support as needed, as in any other infants, is generally appropriate.

Transport: Indicated if major anomalies cannot be assessed and treated adequately.

Testing and confirmation: Karyotype is usually confirmed by blood lymphocyte culture.

Nursery management

Neonatal echocardiogram, and physical examination to assess any anomaly. **Surgery** may need to be scheduled for GI or cardiac anomalies. Down's syndrome presents with a wide variety of features and characteristics. There is a wide range of mental retardation and developmental delay noted among children with Down's syndrome. There is a great deal of variability in the presence of other anomalies such as congenital heart disease, GI, and hematological problems in these children. Hypothyroidism occurs in a high percentage of children with Down's syndrome and should be monitored closely. **Early intervention** and specialized help with education and home rearing has improved the outcome in children with Down's syndrome. Many young adults with Down's syndrome move into community living arrangements and work regular jobs or in sheltered workshops.

Future pregnancy preconception counseling

With full trisomy 21, the recurrence risk is empirically 1% or the age-related risk as a woman gets older (whichever is higher). With Robertsonian translocation, parental chromosomes should be checked, with genetic counseling regarding specific future risks. There are other rare translocations leading to Down's syndrome. One is a Robertsonian translocation between two chromosomes 21s, t(21; 21); this has a 100% risk for Down's syndrome when transmitted by a carrier parent. Also rare is a non-Robertsonian translocation formed by the union of two chromosome 21s such that the translocation forms a mirror image of the normal chromosome 21. There is some literature that suggests in some families where there have been recurrent trisomies, a relationship exists with their methylene tetrahydrofolate reductase (MTHFR) status. This has not been proven in large studies.

Helpful websites

General:
http://www.ds-health.com/
Healthcare guidelines for care of individual with Down's syndrome:
http://www.denison.edu/collaborations/dsq/health96.html
Risk and recurrence risk of Down's syndrome:
http://www.nas.com/downsyn/benke.html

Trisomy 18 (Edwards' syndrome)

Historic notes: Trisomy 18 was independently described by Edwards et al and Smith et al in 1960.

Definition: Edwards' syndrome is **trisomy 18**, or the presence of an extra chromosome number 18.

Epidemiology/incidence: Incidence of 1 in 6600 live births in the USA and UK. This is the second most common trisomy at birth. Incidence increases with increasing maternal age.

Embryology: Extra chromosome 18 affects development of all organs.

Genetics/inheritance/recurrence: Extra chromosome 18 is usually (95%) secondary to de-novo meiotic nondisjunction associated with advanced maternal age. In approximately

90% of cases, the extra chromosome is maternal in origin, with meiosis II errors occurring twice as frequently as meiosis I errors. Other human trisomies have a higher frequency of nondisjunction in maternal meiosis I. Approximately 80% of nondisjunctions occur in females. **Mosaicism** occurs in approximately 10% of cases and is due to post zygotic non-disjunction or anaphase lag. The causes of meiotic and mitotic nondisjunction are unknown. **Translocations** may also result in trisomy or partial trisomy 18 with varying phenotype due to monosomy of another chromosome and variable size of piece of chromosome 18 involved. The smallest extra region necessary for expression of serious anomalies of trisomy 18 appears to be 18q11–q12.

Teratology: None.

Classification: Trisomy 18 (95%), mosaic trisomy 18, and variable partial trisomy 18 related to translocations.

Risk factors/associations: Advanced maternal age and translocation carriers have increased risk. Recurrence risk approximately 1% for full trisomy 18.

Pregnancy management

Screening

NT has a sensitivity of >80%. First trimester screening has a sensitivity of >90%. Second trimester multiple marker screening (typically low α-fetoprotein (AFP), low human chorionic gonadotropin (HCG), and low estriol) has a sensitivity of about >80%. Accurate ultrasound is usually >90% sensitive for trisomy 18 (see Chapter 4).

Ultrasound findings in fetus:
- Thickened NT at 11–14 weeks (80%) (at times cystic hygroma – 15%)
- Thickened nuchal fold (≥6 mm) at 16–23 weeks
- Congenital heart disease (CHD) (90%)
- Omphalocele (25%)
- Neural tube defects (20%)
- Clenched hands with overlapping fingers
- Clubbed or rocker-bottom feet
- Choroid plexus cysts (25%) (most commonly isolated and seen in normal fetuses; karyotyping probably not indicated if isolated)
- Enlarged (>1 cm) cisterna magna
- Single umbilical artery
- Micrognatia
- Cleft lip or palate
- Hydrops or some hydropic changes (pleural effusion, ascites, etc.)
- Biometry may reveal FGR by the third trimester

- **Amniotic fluid:** polyhydramnios (25%)
- **Placenta:** normal
- **Biometry/measurement data:** symmetric FGR (>50%); microcephaly in third trimester
- **When detectable:** at 11–14 weeks if increased NT is detected.

Diagnosis: CVS or amniocentesis.

Counseling:[2,3] **Approximately 95% of conceptuses with trisomy 18 die in embryonic or fetal life; 5–10% of affected children born alive survive beyond the first year of life.** In utero, there are decreased fetal movements. Clinical findings the parents should be informed about include severe psychomotor and growth restriction, microcephaly, microphthalmia, malformed ears, micrognathia or retrognathia, microstomia, distinctively clenched fingers, rocker-bottom feet, and other congenital malformations. **Congenital heart disease occurs in 90%,** with ventricular septal defect (VSD) and polyvalvular heart disease (pulmonary and aortic valve defects) common. Renal anomalies, GI, and brain malformations are common. Classical dermatoglyphics are seen with digital arch patterns on finger and toe tips and distal palmar triradius with hypoplastic finger tips and small nails. Central apnea is a frequent cause of death, along with cardiac, central nervous system (CNS), and renal malformations.

If diagnosed prenatally, recommend discussion with parents about how to proceed in labor and delivery, either allowing 'nature to take its course' without monitoring or specifying level of intervention desired by parents including the extent of resuscitation after delivery. Indication for cesarean section for fetal indications may be futile. **Parents need to be counseled that some children with trisomy 18 do survive and require lifelong care,** but never achieve any independence. Few milestones are reached. There is an increased incidence of Wilms' tumor in trisomy 18 children who survive. Cardiac surgery is controversial. In the first weeks it may be considered a heroic measure, but if the child is surviving it may make life more comfortable (comfort care). Apnea is a common cause of death, and can happen at home; there is the need to understand 'nobody's fault' if this happens.

Work-up/investigations and consultations required: A fetal echocardiogram is recommended. Genetic counseling can be offered. **Neonatal consultation** is extremely important, to help the couple decide regarding neonatal management; usually just comfort care for the baby and psychological support for the parents is most appropriate.

Fetal intervention: None available.

Termination issues: Termination can be offered as sole intervention, as regulated by local law (usually legal <24 weeks).

Antepartum testing: As NRFHT is very common, and prognosis poor, fetal testing is not recommended. Many pregnancies continue without spontaneous labor until post-term (>42 weeks).

Delivery/anesthesia: Fetal heart monitoring is usually declined, and not indicated. Every attempt should be made to maximize the chances of vaginal delivery to minimize maternal morbidity given frequently fatal neonatal prognosis. Cesarean delivery for fetal indications is not recommended and should be discussed.

Neonatology management

Resuscitation: Comfort care only. Allow parents to grieve appropriately. Providing life support is usually not appropriate.

Transport: Not indicated.

Testing and confirmation: Karyotype is usually confirmed by blood lymphocyte culture.

Future pregnancy preconception counseling

Test parents if due to translocation.

Helpful websites

http://www.emedicine.com/ped/topic652.htm

Trisomy 13 (Patau syndrome)

Historic notes: Patau first identified it in the laboratory in 1960, noting three of the group 13–15 chromosomes.

Definition: Patau syndrome is **trisomy 13**, or the presence of an extra chromosome number 13.

Epidemiology/incidence: **1/10 000** live births. Incidence increases with increasing maternal age. Approximately 1% of all first trimester spontaneous losses are due to trisomy 13.

Embryology: Extra chromosome 13 affects development of all organs.

Genetics/inheritance: Extra chromosome 13 results in **full trisomy 13** (80% of cases). This is due to maternal nondisjunction, usually in meiosis I. About 15% of cases are due to **translocation**, mostly Robertsonian translocation

t(13q14). In 5%, translocation is familial, with recurrence risk of 5% and risk of spontaneous abortion of 20%. The other cases are due to **mosaicism** (5%) with both trisomy 13 and normal cell lines. Mosaicism cases may have milder phenotype.

Teratology: None.

Classification: Trisomy 13, mosaic trisomy 13, and translocation trisomy or partial trisomy 13.

Risk factors/associations: Advanced maternal age. Individuals who are carriers of balanced Robertsonian translocations involving chromosome 13 have an increased risk.

Pregnancy management
Screening

First or second trimester multiple marker screening are not sensitive and clinically useful for detecting trisomy 13. Accurate ultrasound is usually 90% sensitive for trisomy 13.

Ultrasound findings in fetus:

- Thickened NT at 11–14 weeks (>70%) (at times cystic hygroma – 20%)
- Thickened nuchal fold (≥6 mm) at 16–23 weeks
- CHD (80%) (atrial septal defect [ASD] and VSD most common, but also often complex CHD)
- Holoprosencephaly (40%)
- Cleft lip and palate (45%)
- Hypotelorism/microphthalmia
- Polydactyly
- Rocker-bottom feet
- Omphalocele (10%)
- Polycystic kidneys (30%)
- Enlarged (>1 cm) cisterna magna (15%)
- Neural tube defects
- Hydrops or some hydropic changes (pleural effusion, ascites, etc.)
- Biometry may reveal symmetric FGR by the third trimester
  - **Amniotic fluid:** polyhydramnios or oligohydramnios
  - **Placenta:** normal
  - **Biometry/measurement data:** symmetric FGR (50%)
  - **When detectable:** at 11–14 weeks if increased NT is detected.

Diagnosis: **CVS or amniocentesis** achieve the diagnosis by a study of the fetal chromosomes, which reveals trisomy 13. In the neonate, peripheral blood is usually cultured and karyotyped.

Counseling:[2,3]   Most trisomy 13 conceptions result in spontaneous early pregnancy losses. Mean life expectancy is 130 days, with many infants dying in first month of life, and 95% dying within 6 months. Apnea is a cause of death, and can happen at home; there is the need to understand 'nobody's fault' if this happens. Family needs to be prepared for intense care needs and possible sudden death. Most common causes of death are cardiopulmonary arrest, 69%; congenital heart disease, 13%; and pneumonia, 4%.

Infants who survive need complete care and achieve few milestones. Survival depends on associated medical problems. Survivors with trisomy 13 have severe mental retardation and developmental delays. For survivors there are specific growth charts available for monitoring growth. Children with trisomy 13 are irritable, do not achieve milestones beyond smiling, and most need to be fed by tube.

If diagnosed prenatally, recommend discussion with parents about how to proceed, usually allowing 'nature to take its course' given the grim prognosis. Parents need to be counseled that some children with trisomy 13 do survive and require lifelong complete care, and never achieve any independence.

Work-up/investigations and consultations: A fetal echocardiogram is recommended. Genetic counseling can be offered. **Neonatal consultation** is extremely important, to help the couple decide regarding neonatal management; usually just comfort care for the baby and psychological support for the parents is most appropriate.

Fetal intervention: None available.

Termination issues: Termination can be offered as sole intervention, as regulated by local law (usually legal < 24 weeks).

Antepartum testing: As NRFHT is very common, and prognosis poor, fetal testing is not recommended. Many pregnancies continue without spontaneous labor until post-term (> 42 weeks).

Delivery/anesthesia: Fetal heart monitoring is usually declined, and not indicated. Every attempt should be made to maximize the chances of vaginal delivery to minimize maternal morbidity given almost universally fatal neonatal prognosis. Cesarean delivery for fetal indications is not recommended and should be discussed.

Neonatology management

Resuscitation: Comfort care only. Allow parents to grieve appropriately. Providing life support is usually not appropriate.

Transport: Not indicated.

Testing and confirmation: Karyotype is usually confirmed by blood lymphocyte culture.

Long-term care: Feeding issues, gastrostomy; irritability; chronic infections, aspiration pneumonia; heart failure; frequent hospitalizations; seizures; blindness and hearing loss; few milestones achieved (smile, laugh); parental stress.

Future pregnancy preconception counseling

With full trisomy 13, the recurrence risk is empirically 1% or the age-related risk as a woman gets older (whichever is higher). With Robertsonian translocation, parental chromosomes should be checked, with genetic counseling regarding specific future risks. There are other rare translocations leading to trisomy 13. Rare translocation of t(13q13q) has a risk of recurrence or SAB of 100%.

Helpful website

http://www.emedicine.com/ped/topic1745.htm

Turner syndrome

Historic notes: In 1938 Turner described the combination of sexual infantilism, webbed neck, and cubitus valgus. Ford showed in 1959 that this combination of findings was associated with a missing X chromosome.

Definition: Turner syndrome is the **presence of single X chromosome,** or **any karyotype with Xp missing** such as isochromosome Xq, ring X, or deletion Xp. Also called 45X0 or 45X syndrome.

Epidemiology/incidence: 1/2500 female births (**1/5000** total births). 98–99% of Turner fetuses are spontaneously aborted; about 20% of all spontaneous early pregnancy losses are due to Turner syndrome.

Embryology: Missing Xp leads to lymphedema usually due to congenital hypoplasia of lymphatic channels.

Genetics/inheritance: The **presence of single X chromosome,** or **any karyotype with Xp missing,** such as isochromosome Xq, ring X, or deletion Xp. The presence of a single X chromosome results from chromosomal nondisjunction. **Mosaicism** is common (40%) and may include a 46,XY cell lines, associated with ambiguous genitalia. Since features of Turner syndrome are seen in other syndromes, karyotype is essential to make the diagnosis. Chromosome studies on more than one tissue may be needed to detect mosaicism. Not associated with advanced maternal age.

Teratology: None.

Classification: 45,X in 50%. Mosaicism in >30%, 46,X,i(Xq) in 17%.

Risk factors/associations: Not associated with advanced maternal age. Differentiate from Noonan syndrome by karyotype, which is normal in Noonan syndrome.

Pregnancy management

Screening

First trimester screen with NT measurement. Biochemical screening is usually not sensitive enough for clinical use.

Ultrasound findings in fetus:

- Cystic hygroma
- Thickened nuchal fold (≥6 mm) at 16–23 weeks
- CHD (20%) (usually left side: coarctation, aortic stenosis, bicuspid aortic valve, left hypoplastic heart)
- Renal anomalies (60%)
- Hydrops or some hydropic changes (pleural effusion, ascites, etc.)
  - **Amniotic fluid:** occasionally oligohydramnios
  - **Placenta:** normal
  - **Biometry/measurement data:** usually normal
  - **When detectable:** at 10+ weeks if cystic hygroma detected.

Diagnosis: **CVS or amniocentesis** achieve the diagnosis with a study of the fetal chromosomes, which reveals 45,X or missing Xp. In the neonate, usually peripheral blood is cultured and karyotyped.

Counseling: 45,X conceptions frequently (>95%) end in spontaneous early pregnancy losses. **The presence of a cystic hygroma with the diagnosis of Turner syndrome is >99% fatal.** If cystic hygroma is not present or resolves, and fetus is still alive >20 weeks, many survive until birth. Female infants with Turner syndrome have excess nuchal skin and edema of the hands and feet (80%) due to lymphedema. Congenital heart disease, if present, most affects prognosis, usually requiring surgery and long-term care. In childhood, short stature is apparent. Teenagers have delayed puberty and primary amenorrhea (>90%), with infertility (>99%). Other clinical findings include shield-shaped chest with widely spaced nipples, low posterior hair line with webbing or shortness of neck, renal anomalies (60%), cubitus valgus, short fourth metacarpal, narrow, hyperconvex and deep-set nails, hearing loss, and thyroid dysfunction. Some girls with Turner syndrome have learning difficulties, including difficulty with math and reading maps related to a deficit in spatial ability. Intelligence and verbal skills are usually within the normal range. Mosaicism with a normal female cell line may result in a milder phenotype and spontaneous puberty with fertility but often early menopause. If there is a deleted X but the XIST locus is intact, normal random X-inactivation may occur and the phenotype may be milder. If XIST is not present in a small X chromosome marker, the phenotype may be more severe. In mosaic 45X/46,XY individuals, clitoral enlargement may be present and virilization may occur. In these cases there is an increased risk of gonadoblastoma and the gonad should be removed. Psychological impact of short stature, infertility, and learning difficulties needs to be discussed.

Work-up/investigations and consultations: A **fetal echocardiogram** is recommended. Depending on the lesions detected, specific pediatric subspecialty (in particular for cardiac anomalies) consultation can be offered. Genetic counseling can be offered as well. Care in a tertiary care center is indicated if there are significant associated anomalies, or if they cannot be ruled out adequately.

Fetal intervention: None available.

Termination issues: Termination can be offered as sole intervention, as regulated by local law (usually legal <24 weeks).

Fetal monitoring/testing: No specific trials. NSTs weekly at ≥32 weeks can be offered.

Delivery/anesthesia: Mode and management of delivery should not be affected by the diagnosis of Turner syndrome.

Neonatology management

Resuscitation: Providing life support as needed, as in any other infant, is generally appropriate.

Transport: Indicated if counseling and general care cannot be provided and/or if major anomalies cannot be assessed and treated adequately at the birth institution.

Testing and confirmation: Karyotype is usually confirmed by blood lymphocyte culture.

Nursery management

Neonatal echocardiogram, **renal ultrasound**, and physical examination are indicated to assess any anomaly. **Surgery may need to be scheduled for cardiac anomalies. Early intervention** and specialized help with education has improved the outcome in children with Turner syndrome.

Long-term care

Thyroid studies annually; hearing test if otitis and not done before; speech evaluation, if needed; blood pressure checks routinely (hypertension a complication); annual echocardiogram to measure aortic root; annual urinalysis and culture if renal anomaly; use Turner growth curve after 2 years old; monitor diet (calories and calcium); ophthalmology follow-up as indicated; psychological support; individualized education plan (IEP) at school if indicated; refer to endocrinologist in infancy, discuss growth hormone (GH) and hormone replacement therapy (HRT): GH treatment can improve growth and influence a girl's final adult height. HRT helps the girl with Turner syndrome develop the physical changes of puberty. In-vitro fertilization can make it possible for some women with Turner syndrome to become pregnant using a donor egg. It is important to discuss at what age to inform the child of her diagnosis and its implications.

Future pregnancy preconception counseling

Recurrence risk in 45,X is not increased over population risk. There is an increased risk if associated with a translocation.

Klinefelter syndrome

Historic notes: In 1942, Dr Harry Klinefelter described males who had enlarged breasts, sparse facial and body hair, small testes, and azoospermia. By the late 1950s these findings were associated initially with an extra Barr body and later the extra X chromosome was identified with the karyotype 47,XXY.

Diagnosis/definition: Chromosome study 47,XXY. There are no specific phenotypic features to identify Klinefelter syndrome in an infant.

Epidemiology/incidence: 1 in 500 to 1 in 1000 male births.

Genetics/inheritance/recurrence/future prevention: Advanced maternal age slightly increases the risk for the XXY. Recent studies have shown that half the time, the extra chromosome comes from the father.

Risk factors/associations: Advanced maternal age.

Screening: No phenotypic features noted prenatally.

Clinical features: Occasional breast enlargement, lack of facial and body hair, and a female-type body configuration. Small testes. Taller than others in their family. Delayed speech occurs in >50%. Poor gross motor coordination is present in ~27%. School difficulties are relatively common and many boys with 47,XXY need assistance at school. Many are shy and somewhat passive and easy babies to care for. The average IQ is 90; verbal IQ is higher than performance IQ. XXY boys enter puberty normally, without any delay of physical maturity. But as puberty progresses, they fail to keep pace with other males. Most XXY boys benefit from receiving an injection of testosterone every 2 weeks, beginning at puberty.

Counseling: Regular injections of the male hormone testosterone, beginning at puberty, can promote strength and facial hair growth; as well as bring about a more muscular body type.

Psychological support and therapy can help with self-esteem issues and interaction with peers. Depression also may be a problem in adults.

Boys with 47,XXY have a slightly increased risk of autoimmune disorders such as type I (insulin-dependent) diabetes, autoimmune thyroiditis, and lupus erythematosus. XXY males with enlarged breasts have the same risk of breast cancer as do women – roughly 50 times the risk of XY males. XXY males who do not receive testosterone injections may have an increased risk of developing osteoporosis in later life.

Rare/related: Variations include the XY/XXY mosaic male, who may have enough normally functioning cells in the testes to allow him to father children.

Males with two or even three additional X chromosomes have also been reported in the medical literature. In these individuals, the classic features of Klinefelter syndrome may be exaggerated, with low IQ or moderate to severe mental retardation also occurring. Testosterone injections may not be appropriate for all of them.

Helpful website

http://www.nichd.nih.gov/publications/pubs/klinefelter.htm#xwhat

47,XXX

Diagnosis/definition: Karyotype shows 47,XXX.

Epidemiology/incidence: 1: 1000 newborn females.

Genetics/inheritance/recurrence: Sporadic, increased by advanced maternal age.

Risk factors/associations: Advanced maternal age.

Screening: No identifying physical features. Must have karyotype to make diagnosis.

Clinical features: Girls with 47,XXX are usually tall. Pubertal development is usually normal and fertility is probably normal but there may be an increased incidence of offspring with chromosome abnormalities.

Counseling: Girls with 47,XXX are shy and may demonstrate immaturity. The support of a loving and understanding family can improve the outcome for these girls. Many have learning difficulties (math and reading), but they are not mentally retarded. The IQ of a girl with 47,XXX may be a few points lower than that of her siblings. Those diagnosed on amniocentesis or CVS with normal ultrasound, where indication is advanced maternal age (AMA), have better prognosis than those diagnosed postnatally because a problem has been noted.

DiGeorge syndrome (22q11.2 deletion syndrome)

Historic notes: DiGeorge syndrome, described in 1965, and velocardiofacial syndrome, described in 1978, are different manifestations of the same deletion of chromosome 22q11.2.

Diagnosis/definition: Fluorescent in-site hybridization reveals an interstitial deletion of chromosome 22q11.2.

Epidemiology/incidence: 1 in 2000–4000 births.

Embryology: Defects occur in the third and fourth pharyngeal pouches, which later develop into the thymus and parathyroid glands. Developmental abnormalities may also occur in the fourth branchial arch.

Genetics/inheritance/recurrence/future prevention: Autosomal dominant inheritance. In 6% of affected individuals, one of the parents is affected. Expression is very variable, so both parents of an affected child should be tested for the deletion.

Risk factors/associations: Other conditions have been noted to be associated with deletion 22q11.2, including conotruncal anomaly face syndrome (CAFS) (Japan) and sometimes Opitz G/BBB syndrome, CHARGE association, and Cayler cardiofacial syndrome.

Screening: All women with a fetus or neonate with a diagnosis of congenital heart defect, especially if conotruncal, can be offered testing (usually FISH) for this deletion. Testing is available from amniocytes or chorionic villi.

Clinical features: Characteristic facies; cardiovascular defects (in 85%) are mostly VSD. Cleft of secondary palate

may be submucous cleft or velopharyngeal incompetence. Nasal reflux in infants. Transient neonatal hypocalcemia. Hypotonia. Immune system dysfunction. Postnatal growth delay. Developmental delay, learning disability and psychological problems. Hypernasal speech.

Counseling (prognosis, complications, pregnancy considerations): Clinical features should be reviewed. Early death due to congenital heart defects before 6 months of age in 8%. Early intervention for speech and motor delays. Special education for older children. Chance of psychiatric disorders in 10%. Very variable phenotype, not predictable from laboratory result.

5p– syndrome (cri du chat syndrome)

Historic notes: In 1963, Lejeune et al described a syndrome of multiple congenital anomalies, developmental delay, microcephaly, dysmorphic features, and a high-pitched, cat-like cry in infants with deletion of a B group chromosome (Bp–), later identified as 5p–.

Diagnosis/definition: The 5p– syndrome is characterized at birth by a high-pitched cat-like cry, low birth weight, poor muscle tone, and microcephaly. The cry is caused by abnormal laryngeal development. The cry disappears by age 2 years in about one-third of children with 5p–.

A karyotype is needed for the diagnosis. The size of the deletion of the short arm of chromosome 5 is variable, and a very small deletion may be missed using conventional G-banding. High-resolution studies may be needed or a FISH study using a specific probe for the small deleted area of 5p that is essential for this diagnosis.

Epidemiology/incidence: Estimated prevalence is about 1 in 50 000 live births. Up to 1% of profoundly retarded individuals have 5p–.

Genetics/inheritance/recurrence/future prevention: The condition may be sporadic (80–85%) if both parents have normal chromosomes, with a recurrence risk of less that 1%. In rare cases, gonadal mosaicism in one parent may result in a recurrence. If one parent carries a balanced translocation (10–15%) involving 5p, the recurrence risk is substantially higher.

Most cases have a terminal deletion of 5p. The cat-like cry maps to 5p15.3 and the cri du chat critical region is 5p15.2, which is associated with all the clinical features of the syndrome. The deletion is paternal in origin in 80% of cases.

Affected females are fertile and have a 50% chance of passing on the deletion to their offspring, although none is documented to have reproduced.

Risk factors/associations: Increased risk if translocation carrier involving 5p.

Screening: Amniocentesis, CVS, ultrasound.

Counseling: Early feeding problems are common because of swallowing difficulties; poor suck with resultant failure to thrive. Death occurs in 6–8% of the overall population with cri du chat syndrome due to pneumonia, aspiration pneumonia, and congenital heart defects. Survival to adulthood is possible. Children who are raised at home with early intervention and schooling do better than those described in the early literature. Almost all individuals with 5p– have significant cognitive, speech, and motor delays (IQ rarely above 35). Many children can develop some language and motor skills. They may also become independent in self-care skills. Physical features include microcephaly, growth retardation, hypertelorism, epicanthal folds, down-slanting palpebral fissures, round face with full cheeks, flat nasal bridge, down-turned corners of mouth, micrognathia, low-set ears, and variable cardiac defects. Renal anomalies have been described, as have cleft lip and palate, talipes equinovarus, and gut malrotation. Treatment is symptomatic.

Helpful website

http://www.emedicine.com/ped/topic504.htm

References

1. American College of Obstetrics and Gynecology. Preconception and prenatal carrier screening for cystic fibrosis: clinical and laboratory provider guidelines American College of Obstetrics and Gynecology. 2001. [review]
2. Baty BJ, Blackburn BL, Carey JC. Natural history of trisomy 18 and trisomy 13: I. Growth, physical assessment, medical histories, survival, and recurrence risk. Am J Med Genet 1994; 49(2): 175–88. [review]
3. Baty BJ, Jorde LB, Blackburn BL. Natural history of trisomy 18 and trisomy 13: II. Psychomotor development. Am J Med Genet 1994; 49(2): 189–94. [review]

6

Before labor and first stage of labor

Vincenzo Berghella

For management of induction, meconium, oligo/polyhydramnios, intrapartum monitoring (including amnioinfusion for variables), operative vaginal delivery, shoulder dystocia, vaginal birth after cesarean (VBAC), abnormal third stage, **see appropriate distinct chapters.**

KEY POINTS

- **Before labor**
  - If **non-vertex** presentation, perform **cesarean delivery** (CD)
  - If ≥41 weeks, start **induction**
  - Antenatal education for self-diagnosis of labor is **associated with less visits to the labor suite** before the onset of labor
  - **Pelvimetry should not be performed,** as it is associated with no benefits, and it increases incidence of CDs.
- **'Home' and 'home-like' (e.g. birth center) settings for birth cannot be recommended.** They are associated with modest benefits, including reduced medical interventions and increased maternal satisfaction, at the expense of **increased perinatal mortality.**
- **Delayed hospital admission** until active labor (regular painful contractions and cervical dilatation >3 cm) **is associated with less time in the labor ward, less intrapartum oxytocics,** and **less analgesia.** There is insufficient evidence to assess effects on rate of CD and other important measures of maternal and neonatal outcome.
- Admission tests such as fetal heart rate (FHR) tracing and amniotic fluid assessment have not been associated with any benefit.
- Routine enema is not recommended.
- Perineal shaving is not recommended.
- Vaginal chlorhexidine irrigation is not recommended.
- **Universal prenatal maternal screening with anovaginal specimen at 35–37 weeks and intrapartum** (penicillin first-line) **antibiotic treatment** is the most efficacious of the current strategies for prevention of early-onset group B streptococcus (GBS) disease.
- **All women should have support throughout labor and birth,** as it is associated with less intrapartum analgesia, cesarean birth, operative birth, and dissatisfaction with the childbirth experiences, and more spontaneous vaginal birth.

- There is insufficient evidence for providing nutritional recommendations for women in labor.
- There is insufficient evidence for need or rate of intravenous fluids in labor.
- Since walking does not seem to have a beneficial or detrimental effect on labor and delivery, **women can choose freely to walk or lay in bed during labor, whichever is more comfortable for them.**
- **Water immersion** during the *first stage* of labor **reduces the use of analgesia and reported maternal pain,** without adverse maternal or neonatal outcomes. There is insufficient evidence to evaluate the safety and efficacy of immersion in water *during* the actual delivery, or in the third stage.
- **Routine early amniotomy is associated with both benefits and risks.** Amniotomy is associated with a significant reduction in labor duration, mostly due to a shorter first stage, with a decrease in the use of oxytocin. There is a **trend toward an increase in the risk of CD, especially for non-reassuring fetal heart testing (NRFHT).**
- Use of the **partogram** with aggressive early oxytocin **is associated with about one-third less incidence of CD.** As use of the partogram has not been compared to "no use" of the partogram in any trial, there is insufficient evidence to assess the effectiveness of this intervention.
- There are no trials to evaluate the frequency of cervical exams in labor per se. Most studies, including those with active management, perform cervical exams every 2 hours in active labor, but the risk of chorioamnionitis increases with increasing number of exams.
- There are no trials to evaluate the timing and dosing of oxytocin in labor per se.
- The individual interventions that are part of the **active management of labor should** be studied separately, and only those which are beneficial (e.g. support by doula) implemented. Active management of labor can consist of antenatal classes, admission not before premature rupture of membranes (PROM), or 2 cm dilatation and full effacement (active labor), early amniotomy, support by doula, use of partogram, vaginal exams every 2 hours, with oxytocin started for rate of progress off the partogram or <1 cm/h. It is associated with reduced duration of labor, possibly due to early amniotomy, less maternal fever,

no significant effect on incidence of CD, and similar perinatal morbidity and maternal satisfaction.
- **Training of traditional birth assistants** in developing countries **is associated with a trend for less maternal mortality and significantly less perinatal mortality.**
- **Before performing a CD for active-phase labor arrest, labor should be arrested for a minimum of 4 hours (if uterine activity is > 200 Montevideo units) or 6 hours (if > 200 Montevideo units could not be sustained).**

Timing of onset of labor

There is no strong association between changes in barometric pressure and onset of labor. Diurnal rhythms seem to show a higher rate of starting labor in the evening and night hours.

Before labor

Non-vertex presentation

If **non-vertex presentation** is detected, cesarean delivery (CD) is recommended (see Chapter 20).

Induction

Induction is advised at ≥ 41 weeks (see Chapter 23).

Self-diagnosis of active labor

There is not enough evidence to evaluate the use of a specific set of criteria for self-diagnosis of active labor. A **specific antenatal education program is associated with a reduction in the mean number of visits to the labor suite before the onset of labor.**[1] It is unclear whether this results in fewer women being sent home because they are not in labor.

Pelvimetry

There is not enough evidence to support the use of X-ray pelvimetry in women whose fetuses have a cephalic or non-cephalic presentation. **Women undergoing X-ray pelvimetry are more likely to be delivered by cesarean section.**[2] No significant impact is detected on perinatal outcome, but numbers are small, insufficient for meaningful evaluation (e.g. perinatal mortality 1 vs 2%). The results are similar for women with or without a prior CD.

Site of labor management

Hospital vs home

There is insufficient evidence to favor either planned hospital birth or planned home birth for low-risk pregnant women. A home birth service ought to be backed up by a modern hospital system. There are diverging opinions even in Western countries, with about 30% of Dutch births occurring at home, vs < 1% of US births. Women with risk factors for abnormal outcome should deliver in a hospital setting. All women should be aware of possible maternal and fetal risks, including severe morbidity and mortality, associated with labor and delivery even in low-risk women, and should be aware of the absence of intensive care and operative capabilities in the home setting.[3] Inference from results of 'home-like' vs conventional ward setting (see below) should warn against home birth.

Hospital: 'home-like' (birth center) vs conventional ward setting

When compared with conventional institutional settings, home-like settings for childbirth are associated with modest benefits, including reduced medical interventions and increased maternal satisfaction, at the expense of increased perinatal mortality, and therefore **'home-like' settings for birth cannot be recommended.**[4] About 50% of women allocated to home-like settings are transferred to standard care before or during labor. Home-like setting significantly increases the likelihood of: **no intrapartum analgesia/anesthesia; spontaneous vaginal birth; vaginal/perineal tears; preference for the same setting the next time; satisfaction with intrapartum care;** and **breastfeeding initiation** and **continuation** to 6–8 weeks. Allocation to a home-like setting **decreased the likelihood of episiotomy.** There was a strong trend towards an 87% **higher perinatal mortality** in the home-like setting.[4] The 1% increase in spontaneous vaginal delivery (SVD) may be secondary to less epidural anesthesia, which may in turn be secondary to lack of availability in home-like settings, and/or to less intrapartum monitoring. The increase in perinatal mortality may be secondary to lack of appropriate interventions in home-like settings and to less communication or monitoring. No firm conclusions could be drawn regarding the effects of staffing or organizational models, which can certainly influence the outcome above (e.g. midwifes vs doctors, continuity of care, etc.).

Admission

Delayed vs early hospital admission

Labor assessment programs, which aim to **delay hospital admission until active labor**, may benefit women with term pregnancies. Active labor was defined as regular painful contractions and cervical dilatation > 3 cm. Compared with direct admission to hospital, delayed admission until active labor is associated with **less time in the labor ward, less intrapartum oxytocics,** and less **analgesia.**[5] Women in the labor assessment and delayed admission group report **higher levels of control during labor.** Cesarean delivery rates are similar, with a non-significant 30% decrease. A 30–40% decrease in CD has been reported in retrospective studies with delayed vs direct admission. There is insufficient evidence (a larger trial needed) to assess the true effects on rate of CD and other important measures of maternal and neonatal outcome. Potential risks of delayed admission include unplanned out-of-hospital births and the potentially harmful effects of withholding caregiver support and attention to women in early- or latent-phase labor.

Suggested criteria for admission based on these studies are a cervix of at least 3–4 cm dilatation and regular painful contractions. Pregnant women should be informed of these evidence during prenatal care.

Fetal assessment tests upon admission
Fetal heart rate tracing for 20 minutes

Fetal heart rate (FHR) tracing for 20 minutes upon admission, followed by auscultation, is not associated with any benefits compared with intermittent auscultation, including similar neonatal morbidity and mortality.[6,7]

Amniotic fluid index

Obtaining an amniotic fluid index (AFI) in early labor is associated with a higher incidence of CD, and similar neonatal outcomes, compared with no AFI.[8]

Neither a 2×1 pocket (abnormal in 8%) nor an AFI (abnormal in 25%) upon admission for labor identifies a pregnancy at risk for adverse outcome such as non-reassuring fetal heart testing (NRFHT) or CD for NRFHT.[9]

Other tests

There is insufficient evidence to support the use of vibroacoustic stimulation or Doppler ultrasound as fetal admission tests.

First stage
Enemas

There is not enough evidence to recommend the routine use of enemas during the first stage of labor. Compared with women receiving no enemas, women receiving enemas in the first stage of labor have a trend for lower infection rates, and have significantly **less need for postpartum systemic antibiotics.**[10] Their newborn children have less lower respiratory tract infections and less need for systemic antibiotics. Length of labor and other maternal and neonatal outcomes

are not different. These benefits are very modest, as the incidence of each of these complications in the no enema group is < 3%. This intervention (enema) generates discomfort in women and increases the costs of delivery. The two randomized controlled trials (RCTs) were not blinded.[10]

Perineal shaving

The evidence to date offers **no support for routine perineal shaving** for women prior to labor. Maternal febrile morbidity is similar to women who have just selective clipping of hair.[11] The potential for complications (redness, multiple superficial scratches, burning and itching of the vulva, embarrassment and discomfort afterwards when the hair grows back) suggests that shaving should not be part of routine clinical practice. Both of the trials[11] are old (1922 and 1965), and included the clipping of long hairs in their control groups to aid in operative procedures, which is itself usually unnecessary and can lead to complications.

Chlorhexidine

Compared with placebo sterile water irrigation, vaginal chlorhexidine irrigation during labor is associated with **similar incidences of maternal and neonatal infections**, including similar chorioamnionitis, postpartum endometritis, neonatal sepsis, and perinatal mortality.[12] The effectiveness of vaginal chlorhexidine might depend on the concentration and volume of the solution used. Chlorhexidine solution is safe, not expensive, and vaginal irrigation is easy to perform but apparently not beneficial.

Group B streptococcus prophylaxis

Universal prenatal maternal screening with an anovaginal specimen at 35–37 weeks and intrapartum (penicillin first-line) antibiotic treatment is the most efficacious of the current strategies for prevention of early-onset group B streptococcus (GBS) disease.[13] It is > 50% more effective than a risk factor-based strategy. There is no prevention of late-onset GBS sepsis. **Women with GBS bacteriuria** in the current pregnancy or who had a **prior infant with GBS sepsis** are candidates for **intrapartum antibiotic prophylaxis**, and should be the only two groups **not screened. Intrapartum treatment for chorioamnionitis is recommended, regardless of GBS maternal status** (see *Maternal–Fetal Evidence-Based Guidelines*, Chapter 36 for details)

Continuous support in labor
Definition

For support, it is generally intended emotional support (continuous presence, reassurance, and praise), information about labor progress and advice regarding coping techniques, comfort measures (comforting touch, massage, warm baths/showers, promoting adequate fluid intake and output), and advocacy (helping the woman articulate her wishes to others).[14]

Mechanism of action

Anxiety during labor is associated with high levels of the stress hormone epinephrine in blood, which may in turn lead to abnormal FHR patterns in labor, decreased uterine contractility, a longer active labor phase with regular well-established contractions, and low Apgar scores. One example of possible mechanisms of action for support to reduce complications of labor and delivery is decreased anxiety.[14] This in turn can lead to a beneficial 'chain-reaction': for example, if continuous support leads to reduced use of epidural analgesia, then several complications associated with regional anesthesia (see Chapter 10) can be prevented.

Types of support

Support is provided by family members or friends (not part of hospital staff) or hospital-based people (part of hospital staff). A doula (a Greek word for 'handmaiden') is a support person with the sole job of providing support to the laboring woman. They are usually not part of the hospital staff. This member of the caregiver team may also be called a labor companion, birth companion, labor support specialist, labor assistant, or birth assistant.

Effectiveness

All women should have support throughout labor and birth. Women who have continuous intrapartum support one-to-one are less likely to have **intrapartum analgesia, cesarean birth, operative birth, or to report dissatisfaction with their childbirth experiences**, and **more likely to have a spontaneous vaginal birth**.[14]

Continuous support is not associated with significant changes in incidences of artificial oxytocin during labor; low 5-minute Apgar scores; admission of the newborn to a special care nursery; postpartum reports of severe labor pain or a significant change in labor length.[14]

In general, **continuous** intrapartum support is associated with greater benefits **when the provider is not a member of the hospital staff** (women who are not part of the staff and are there solely to provide support), **when it begins early in labor, and in settings in which epidural analgesia is not routinely available**.[14]

It may be possible to increase access to one-to-one continuous labor support worldwide by encouraging women to invite a family member or friend to commit to being present at the birth and assuming this role. The mother selects her doula during pregnancy; they establish a relationship (which is likely to involve the woman's partner, if any) and discuss the mother's and partner's preferences and concerns before labor. The doula brings her experience and training (often to the level of certification) to the labor support role during childbirth, and the mother and doula frequently have telephone and/or face-to-face contact in the early postpartum period. Other models of support, for which there are few or no data, include support by a female family member and support by the husband/partner.[14]

Nutrition in labor

There is insufficient evidence for providing nutritional recommendations for women in labor.

A carbohydrate (mean intake 44 g in 350 ml) drink in early labor is associated with an increased risk of CD compared with placebo in women allowed to drink 'at-will',[15] but a carbohydrate (25 g) drink in late (8–10 cm) labor is associated with similar rates of CD compared with placebo.[16] Umbilical cord studies revealed lactate transport to the fetal circulation with potential (but not observed) fetal acidemia.[15,16]

There are no trials evaluating solid foods.

Ice chips to moisten the mouth and sips of clear liquids are the only oral intake recommended by US authorities.[17] Some experts also allow sports drinks, yogurt, or sherbet. In the Netherlands, women in labor are allowed to eat and drink. The reason for avoiding solid food is risk of aspiration, which is rare. When there is increased gastric volume, there is increased risk of vomiting and therefore aspiration. Airway precautions in labor and delivery are paramount to avoid aspiration. Maternal glucose administration in labor is associated with increased neonatal lactic acidosis.

Intravenous fluids (or not), rate

There are **no trials comparing intravenous (IV) fluids to no IV fluids in labor**. The data on IV fluid type and infusion rate are insufficient for a strong recommendation. Compared with a rate of 125 ml/h, an infusion rate of IV fluids (lactated Ringer's or normal saline) of **250 ml/h in early labor** (2–5 cm) of term nulliparous women with vertex presentation is associated with **less labors lasting > 12 hours**.[18] Other outcomes (length of labor for vaginal deliveries, use of oxytocin, successful vaginal delivery) are not significant, but trended for benefit of 250 ml/h: e.g. a 71-min shorter labor, in particular first stage.[18] While the data in pregnancy are limited to one trial, the benefits are substantiated by the fact that several trials in non-pregnant women demonstrate that increased fluid intake improves exercise performance.

Ambulation

Compared with remaining in bed, walking in labor is associated with similar length of first stage of labor, use of oxytocin, use of analgesia, need for forceps vaginal delivery, or cesarean delivery, and also similar neonatal outcomes in women at term with cephalic presentation starting at 3–5 cm of dilatation[19] or in other groups of women.[20–23] Since walking does not seem to have a beneficial or detrimental effect on labor and delivery, women can choose freely to walk or lay in bed during labor, whichever is more comfortable for them.

Immersion in water

There is evidence that water immersion during the first stage of labor **reduces the use of analgesia** and **reported maternal pain**, without significant changes in labor duration, perineal trauma, vaginal operative delivery, cesarean delivery or neonatal outcomes such as Apgar score <7 at 5 minutes, neonatal unit admissions, or neonatal infection rates, compared with no water immersion.[24] One trial compared early vs late immersion during the first stage of labor and found significantly higher epidural analgesia rates in the early group and an increased use of augmentation of labor.[24]

Blinding is not possible. The effects of immersion in water *during* pregnancy (no trials) or in the third stage are unclear. One trial explores *birth* (second stage) in water, but is too small to determine significant differences in outcomes for women or neonates.[24]

Early artificial rupture of membranes (amniotomy)

Routine early amniotomy – artificial rupture of membranes (AROM) – is associated with both benefits and risks.[25] Amniotomy is associated with a significant **reduction in labor duration** of about 53 minutes, mostly due to a shorter first stage, and with a **decrease in the use of oxytocin**. There is a trend toward a 26% **increase in the risk of CD**.[25] Early amniotomy is not associated with an increase (or decrease) in NRFHT. An association between early amniotomy and cesarean delivery for NRFHT is noted in one large trial.[25] The likelihood of a 5 min Apgar score <7 is reduced in association with early amniotomy, but the clinical significance of this finding is questionable since other indicators of neonatal status such as arterial cord pH and neonatal intensive care unit (NICU) admissions do not differ. There is no evidence of an effect of a policy of amniotomy on the mother's satisfaction with labor. This evidence suggests that early amniotomy should not be routinely used in women in normal labor, and possibly be reserved for women with slow labor progress.[25]

Stripping membranes in labor

There are no trials to evaluate stripping the amniotic membrane during spontaneous labor.

Partogram

The general intervention with the partogram is early use of oxytocin as soon as the cervical dilatation falls to the right of the partogram on the 2 hour exams. Compared with less-aggressive (e.g. exams every 4 hours and oxytocin only about 4 hours after the cervical dilatation falls to the right of the partogram) management, **use of the partogram with aggressive early oxytocin is associated with about one-third less CD.**[26,27] As use of the partogram has not been compared to "no use" of the partogram in any trial, there is insufficient evidence to assess the effectiveness of this intervention.

Frequency of cervical examinations

There are **no trials to evaluate the frequency of cervical exams in labor per se.** Most studies, including those with active management, perform cervical exams every 2 hours in labor. The risk of chorioamnionitis, though, increases with increasing number of exams.[28]

Timing and dosing of oxytocin

There are **no trials to evaluate the timing and dosing of oxytocin in labor per se.**

Active management of labor

Active management of labor was originally devised to prevent prolonged labor. Its components have varied somewhat in the literature, but generally include antenatal classes, admission not before premature rupture of membranes (PROM) or 2 cm dilatation and full effacement (active labor), **early amniotomy**, support by doula, use of partogram, vaginal exams every 2 hours, with oxytocin started for rate of progress off the partogram or <1 cm/h. **Oxytocin** rate is started at 4–6 mu/min and increased by 4–6 mu every 15 minutes to reach contractions every 2–3 minutes (but not more than 7/15 minutes) or 40 mu/min. Early amniotomy and early use of high-dose oxytocin are the two most characteristic interventions of active management of labor.

Active management of labor is associated with: (1) a **reduced duration of labor**, of about 50–100 minutes, mostly in the first stage; (2) a **reduction in prolonged (lasting >12 hours) labor**; (3) **less maternal fever**; and (4) **no significant effect on incidence of CD, and similar perinatal** morbidity and maternal satisfaction.[29–32] The shorter labor is probably due to the early amniotomy (see early amniotomy above). The similar incidence of CD may be due to the fact that some aspects of active management, i.e. support by doula, decrease CD rate, but some others, i.e. early amniotomy, increase it. It is recommended that the individual interventions which are part of active management of labor be studied separately, and only those which are beneficial (e.g. support by doula) implemented.

Monitoring

For use of continuous vs intermittent monitoring, amnioinfusion for variables, scalp sampling, etc see Chapter 9.

Bladder catheterization

There are **no trials** to evaluate the necessity, timing, and frequency of bladder catheterization in labor per se.

Epidural or other anesthesia

See Chapter 10.

Training of birth assistants

Training of traditional birth assistants **in developing countries is associated with a trend for less maternal mortality and significantly less perinatal mortality.**[33] There are no trials in the developed world.

Abnormal progression of labor

Abnormal progression of labor, including terms such as dystocia, dysfunctional labor, failure to progress, cephalopelvic disproportion, and others, is the most common problem in labor, and the reason for the majority of CDs.[34] Risk factors for dystocia are obesity, induction, Bishop < 5 at start of labor, station higher than −2, persistent occiput posterior, macrosomia, epidural anesthesia, etc. While these variables are predictive of a higher chance for operative/cesarean delivery, **no** intervention has been tested by a **trial**.

An intrauterine pressure catheter (IUPC) can measure the intensity of uterine contractions more objectively than an external tocomonitor. It necessitates rupture of membranes (ROM). Intensity is usually calculated by Montevideo units, i.e. sum of peak pressures above baseline of all contractions in 10 minutes.

In term women in spontaneous active labor not on oxytocin and with no epidural, the fifth percentile rates of dilatation for nulliparous and parous women are 1.2 cm/h and 1.5 cm/h.[35] In term women in labor necessitating oxytocin and with epidural, the fifth percentile rate for dilatation is about 0.5 cm/h for both nulliparous and parous women.[36] Dystocia cannot be diagnosed unless ROM has occurred, and adequate oxytocin to achieve at least 3–5 adequate contractions per hour has been instituted. The majority (>60%) of women who experience 2 hours of labor arrest despite a sustained uterine contraction pattern of at least 200 Montevideo units in the first stage of labor will achieve a vaginal delivery if oxytocin is continued.[37] **Before performing a CD for active-phase labor arrest, labor should be arrested for a minimum of 4 hours (if uterine activity is > 200 Montevideo units) or 6 hours (if > 200 Montevideo units could not be sustained).**[37] These data are not from a RCT, and there was a significantly higher risk of shoulder dystocia among parturients who had arrest for 4 hours or more. VBAC and diabetics were not included in this study.

There are no trials to evaluate the use of IUPC in labor per se.

In women at term with singleton gestations and requiring oxytocin by obstetrician because of 'dystocia' at 4–6 cm, **meperidine 100 mg IV does not affect operative delivery rates and worsens neonatal outcomes compared with placebo.**[38]

References

1. Bonovich L. Recognizing the onset of labour. J Obstet Gynecol Neonatal Nurs 1990; 19(2): 141–5 [RCT, n = 245; 208 analyzed]
2. Pattinson RC, Farrell E. Pelvimetry for fetal cephalic presentations at or near term. Cochrane Database Syst Rev 2005; 4. [meta-analysis: 4 RCTs (all used X-ray pelvimetry; all not of good quality); n = 895]
3. Dowswell T, Thornton JG, Hewison J et al. Should there be a trial of home versus hospital delivery in the United Kingdom? BMJ 1996; 312: 753 [RCT, n = 11]
4. Hodnett ED, Downe S, Edwards N, Walsh D. Home-like versus conventional institutional settings for birth. Cochrane Database Syst Rev 2007; 1. [6 RCTs, n = 8677]
5. McNiven PS, Williams, JI, Hodnett E, Kaufman K, Hannah ME. An early labour assessment program: a randomised, controlled trial. Birth 1998; 25(1): 5–10. [RCT, n = 209]
6. Impey L, Reynolds M, MacQuillan K et al. Admission cardiotocography: a randomized controlled trial. Lancet 2003; 361: 466–70. [RCT, n = 8580]
7. Blix E, Reinar LM, Klovning A, Oian P. Prognostic value of the labour admission test and its effectiveness compared with auscultation only: a systematic review. Br J Obstd Gynaecol 2005; 112: 1595–604. [meta-analysis; 3 RCTs, n = 11 259]
8. Chauhan SP, Washburne JF, Magann EF et al. A randomized study to assess the efficacy of the amniotic fluid index as a fetal admission test. Obstet Gynecol 1995; 86: 9–13. [RCT, n = 883]
9. Moses J, Doherty DA, Magann EF, Chauhan SP, Morrison JC. A randomized clinical trial of the intrapartum assessment of amniotic fluid volume: amniotic fluid index versus the single deepest pocket technique. Am J Obstet Gynecol 2004; 190: 1564–70 [RCT, n = 499]
10. Cuervo LG, Rodriguez MN, Delgado MB. Enemas during labour. Cochrane Database Syst Rev 2007; 1. [meta-analysis; 2 RCTs, n = 665]

11. Basevi V, Lavender T. Routine perineal shaving on admission in labour. Cochrane Database Syst Rev 2007; 1. [meta-analysis: 2 RCTs, n = 539]

12. Lumbiganon P, Thinkhamrop J, Thinkhamrop B, Tolosa JE. Vaginal chlorhexidine during labour for preventing maternal and neonatal infections (excluding Group B Streptococcal and HIV). Cochrane Database Syst Rev 2007; 1. [meta-analysis: 3 RCTs, n = 3012]

13. Schrag S, Gorwitz R, Fultz-Butts K, Schuchat A. Prevention of perinatal group B streptococcal disease. Revised guidelines from CDC. MMWR Recomm Rep 2002; 51 (RR-11): 1–22 [review/guideline; www.cdc.gov/groupbstrep]

14. Hodnett ED, Gates S, Hofmeyr GJ, Sakala C. Continuous support for women during childbirth. Cochrane Database Syst Rev 2007; 1. [14 RCTs, n = 12 791]

15. Scheepers HCJ, Thans MCJ, de Jong PA, et al. A double-blind, placebo controlled study on the influence of carbohydrate solution intake during labor. Br J Obstet Gynaecol 2002; 109: 178–81. [RCT, n = 201]

16. Scheepers HCJ, de Jong PA, Essed GGM, Kanhai HHH. Carbohydrate solution intake during labour just before the start of the second stage: a double-blind study on metabolic effects and clinical outcome. BJOG 2004; 111: 1382–7. [RCT, n = 202]

17. Practice guidelines for obstetrical anesthesia. A report by the American Society of Anesthesiologist Task Force on Obstetrical Anesthesia. Anesthesiology 1999; 90: 600–11. [review]

18. Garite TJ, Weeks J, Peters-Phair K, Pattillo C, Brewster WR. A randomized controlled trial of the effect of increased intravenous hydration on the course of labor in nulliparous women. Am J Obstet Gynecol 2000; 183: 1544–8. [RCT, n = 195]

19. Bloom SL, McIntire DD, Kelly MA et al. Lack of effect of walking on labor and delivery. N Engl J Med 1998; 339: 76–9. [RCT, n = 1067]

20. McManus TJ, Calder AA. Upright posture and the efficiency of labour. Lancet 1978; 1: 72–4. [RCT, n = 40]

21. Flynn AM, Kelly J, Hollins G, Lynch PF. Ambulation in labour. BMJ 1978; 2: 591–3. [RCT, n = 68]

22. Read JA, Miller FC, Paul RH. Randomized trial of ambulation versus oxytocin for labor enhancement: a preliminary report. Am J Obstet Gynecol 1981; 139: 669–72. [RCT, n = 14]

23. Hemminki E, Saarikoski S. Ambulation and delayed amniotomy in the first stage of labor. Eur J Obstet Gynecol Reprod Biol 1983; 15: 129–39. [RCT, n = 630]

24. Cluett ER, Nikodem VC, McCandlish RE, Burns EE. Immersion in water in pregnancy, labour and birth. Cochrane Database Syst Rev 2007; 1. [meta-analysis: 8 RCTs, n = 2939]

25. Fraser WD, Turcot L, Krauss I, Brisson-Carrol G. Amniotomy for shortening spontaneous labour. Cochrane Database Syst Rev 2007; 1. [meta-analysis: 9 RCTs, n => 4000. All RCT specific for AROM. All RCTs included singleton, vertex, mostly at-term pregnancies]

26. Pattison RC, Howarth GR, Mdluli W et al. Aggressive or expectant management of labour: a randomized clinical trial. Br J Obstet Gynaecol 2003; 110: 457–61. [RCT, n = 694]

27. World Health Organization Maternal Health and Safe Motherhood Programme. World Heath Organization partograph in the management of labour. Lancet 1994; 343: 1399–1404. [RCT, n = 35 484]

28. Soper DE, Mayhall CG, Dalton HP. Risk factors for intraamniotic infection: a prospective epidemiologic study. Am J Obstet Gynecol 1989; 161: 562–6; discussion 566–8. [II–12]

29. Lopex-Leno JA, Peaceman AM, Adashek JA, Socol ML. A controlled trial of a program for the active management of labor. N Engl J Med 1992; 326: 450–4 [RCT, n = 705]

30. Frigoletto FD, Leiberman E, Lang JM et al. A clinical trial of active management of labor. N Engl J Med 1995; 333: 745–50. [RCT, n = 1915]

31. Rogers R, Gilson GJ, Miller AC et al. Active management of labor: does it make a difference? Am J Obstet Gynecol 1997; 599–605. [RCT, n = 405]

32. Sadler LC, Davison T, McCowan LME. A randomized controlled trial and meta-analysis of active management of labour. Br J Obstet Gynaecol 2000; 107; 909–15 [RCT, n = 651]

33. Jokhio AH, Winter HR, Cheng KK. An intervention involving traditional birth attendants and perinatal and maternal mortality in Pakistan. N Engl J Med 2005; 352: 2091–9. [1 RCT, n = 20 557]

34. Ness A, Goldberg J, Berghella V. Abnormalities of the first and second stages of labor. Obstet Gynecol Clin N Am 2005; 32: 201–20. [review]

35. Friedman EA. Primigravid labor: a graphicostatistical analysis. Obstet Gynecol 1955; 6: 567–89. 1978. [II–3]

36. Rouse DJ, Owen JO, Hauth JC. Active-phase labor arrest: oxytocin augmentation for at least 4 hours. Obstet Gynecol 1999; 93: 323–8 [II–3]

37. Rouse DJ, Owen JO, Savage KG, Hauth JC. Active-phase labor arrest: revisiting the 2-hour minimum. Obstet Gynecol 2001; 98: 550–4 [II–3]

38. Sosa CG, Balaguer E, Alonso JG et al. Meperidine for dystocia during the first stage of labor: a randomized controlled trial. Am J Obstet Gynecol 2004; 191: 1212–18. [RCT, n = 407]

7

Second stage of labor

Vincenzo Berghella

KEY POINTS

- Prophylactic intrapartum maternal oxygen in the second stage of normal labor should not be used, since it is associated with more frequent low (<7.20) cord blood pH values than the control group.
- Prophylactic intrapartum betamimetics in the second stage of normal labor should not be used, since their use is associated with an increase in forceps deliveries.
- Women should be encouraged to give birth in the position they find most comfortable, which is usually upright. Use of any upright or lateral position is associated with reductions in duration of second stage of labor, abnormal fetal heart rate patterns, assisted deliveries, episiotomies, and reporting of severe pain; and increases in; second-degree perineal tears and possibly estimated blood loss > 500 ml.
- In women at term with epidural analgesia and a singleton, cephalic fetus, delayed pushing (waiting 1–3 hours or until 'urge to push') is associated with higher incidence of spontaneous vaginal delivery compared with early (immediate upon entering second stage) pushing. The duration of the second stage is longer by about 60 minutes, so careful monitoring of both mother and fetus is necessary to allow labor to continue safely.
- Pushing using the Valsalva maneuver (closed glottis) is associated with similar duration of labor and neonatal arterial pH compared with open glottis.
- Perineal massage before labor is associated with a significantly higher chance of intact perineum compared with no massage in nulliparous women. Perineal massage and stretching of the perineum with a water-soluble lubricant in the second stage of labor is associated with similar rates of intact perineum compared with the control group, with decreased incidence of third-degree lacerations.
- There are no trials to evaluate the management of the prolonged second stage and best diagnosis of dystocia.
- 'Hands-poised' is preferred to the 'hands-on' method, since they are associated with similar incidences of perineal and vaginal tears, but the hands–on method is associated with higher incidence of episiotomies.

- The inflatable obstetric belt to place fundal pressure should not be used, as it is associated with similar incidence of spontaneous vaginal delivery, but less satisfaction with management compared with no belt.
- Routine episiotomy should not be performed, as restricting episiotomy use is associated with less posterior perineal trauma, less suturing, and fewer healing complications.

Prophylactic interventions

Prophylactic intrapartum maternal oxygen in the second stage of normal labor is associated with more frequent low (<7.20) cord blood pH values than the control group.[1] There are no other statistically significant differences between the groups. There is a tendency towards reduced cord arterial blood oxygen content and oxygen saturation in mothers treated with oxygen compared with controls. Short-term oxygenation may be beneficial and long-term oxygenation harmful.

Prophylactic tocolysis for non-reassuring fetal heart rate in labor

There is no evidence to support the prophylactic use of betamimetics during the second stage of labor. Compared with placebo, prophylactic betamimetic therapy is associated with an increase in forceps deliveries. The trial protocol required forceps to be used if the second stage of labor exceeded 30 minutes, in both groups. There are no clear effects on postpartum hemorrhage, neonatal irritability, feeding slowness, umbilical arterial pH values, or Apgar scores at 2 minutes.[2]

Maternal position

There are several benefits for upright posture (sitting – obstetric chair/stool); semi-recumbent (trunk tilted backwards 30° to the vertical); kneeling; squatting (unaided or using squatting bars); and squatting (aided with birth cushion). **Women should be encouraged to give birth in the position they find most comfortable** (which is usually upright). Use of any **upright or lateral position**, compared with supine or lithotomy positions, is associated with: small (4 minutes) **reduction in duration of second stage of labor; a reduction in assisted deliveries; a reduction in episiotomies; an increase in second-degree perineal tears; an increase in estimated blood loss > 500 ml; reduction in reporting of severe pain during second stage of labor; and fewer abnormal fetal heart rate (FHR) patterns.**[3] Use of the birth stool showed no effect and results with the birth chair were variable. Estimation of blood loss in the upright group may have been influenced by the fact that blood loss in the birth chair is collected in a receptacle. Physiological advantages for non-recumbent or upright labor may include the effects of gravity, lessened risk of aortocaval compression and improved acid–base outcomes in the neonates, stronger and more efficient uterine contractions, improved alignment of the fetus for passage through the pelvis ('drive angle'), and radiological evidence of larger anteroposterior and transverse pelvic outlet diameters, resulting in an increase in the total outlet area in the squatting and kneeling positions.[3]

Epidural or other anesthesia

See Chapter 10.

Delayed vs early pushing

In women at term with epidural analgesia and a singleton, cephalic fetus, **delayed pushing** (waiting 1–3 hours or until 'urge to push') is associated with **similar rate of operative vaginal** delivery and of cesarean delivery (CD), but **higher incidence of spontaneous vaginal delivery** compared with early (immediate upon entering second-stage) pushing.[4] The duration of the second stage is longer by about 60 minutes, the duration of pushing is similar, as are all other studied maternal outcomes. The neonatal outcomes are also similar, including incidence of admission to a neonatal intensive care unit (NICU). Women should be counseled regarding these data. The longer duration of second stage with delayed pushing has not been associated with detrimental effects on mother or fetus, but careful monitoring of both is necessary to allow labor to continue safely.

Pushing method

Most women spontaneously choose to Valsalva in the second stage of labor. Compared with encouraging a woman's own urge to push (open glottis), **pushing using the Valsalva maneuver (closed glottis:** taking a deep breath, holding it, and pushing for as long and hard as possible, i.e. 2–3 times during each contraction) is **associated with clinically similar duration of labor, neonatal arterial pH, or damage to the birth canal.**[5,6] Urodynamics 3 months after delivery are worse in the closed glottis group.[6] The duration of labor is shorter for the closed glottis group when a subanalysis according to actual method used is done[5], and in one trial by 13 minutes.[6] A labor attendant should counsel women in labor regarding these data, and probably **support the parturient in her own choice of either technique.**

Manual rotation

There is insufficient evidence (**no trials**) to evaluate the efficacy of manual rotation in labor.

Perineal massage

Perineal massage has not been associated with complications.

Before labor

Perineal massage with sweet almond oil for 5–10 minutes daily from 34 weeks until delivery is associated with a significantly **higher chance of intact perineum** compared with no massage **in nulliparous** but probably not multiparous women.[7–9]

During second stage of labor

Perineal massage and stretching of the perineum with a water-soluble lubricant in the second stage of labor is associated with **similar rates of intact perineum** compared with the control group. The incidence of **third-degree lacerations is decreased.**[10,11]

Abnormal progression of labor

There are **no trials** to evaluate the management of the prolonged second stage and best diagnosis of dystocia. Operative intervention is not warranted just because a set number of hours have elapsed in the second stage (e.g. nulliparas: 3 hours with epidural, 2 hours without an epidural; multiparas: 2 hours with epidural, 1 hour without an epidural).

The length of the second stage is not associated with poor neonatal outcome, as long as reassuring fetal testing is present. If contractions are adequate, the chance of vaginal delivery decreases progressively after 3–5 hours of pushing in the second stage.

If there are no signs of infection (maternal or fetal), no maternal exhaustion, and reassuring fetal testing, labor can be allowed to continue beyond these limits as long as some progress has been made. **Mandatory second opinion** is associated with 22 fewer intrapartum cesarean deliveries per 1000 deliveries, without affecting maternal or perinatal outcomes.[12]

Spontaneous vaginal delivery

'Hands-on' versus 'hands-poised'

The 'hands-on' method described by Ritgen in 1855 usually involves pressure on the infant's head upon crowning, and support with the other hand of the perineum, with the aim of protecting for lacerations. In the 'hands-poised' method, the fetal heads and perineum are not touched or supported by the delivering personnel. These two methods are associated with **similar incidences of perineal and vaginal tears, but the hands-on method is associated with higher incidence of episiotomies.**[13] A policy of 'hands-poised' has also been supported by a quasi-randomized study, reporting less third-degree tears compared with 'hands-on'.[14]

Fundal pressure

Manual fundal pressure to aid in vaginal delivery has **never been studied in a trial.** In the second stage of labor, fundal pressure can be provided with an obstetric belt wrapped around the woman's abdomen above the level of the uterine fundus. The belt inflates with each contraction to a maximum of 200 mHg for 30 seconds. Compared with no belt, the **inflatable obstetric belt is associated with a similar incidence of spontaneous vaginal delivery** in nulliparous women with singleton term pregnancies and an epidural at term. All other maternal and neonatal outcomes are similar, but **women with no belt have greater satisfaction.**[15]

Episiotomy

Routine episiotomy should not be performed, as restrictive episiotomy policies have a number of benefits compared with routine episiotomy policies. **Restricting episiotomy** use is associated with **less posterior perineal trauma, less suturing,** and **fewer healing complications,** with an **increased risk of anterior perineal trauma** compared with routine episiotomy.[16,17] There is no difference in severe vaginal or perineal trauma, dyspareunia, urinary incontinence, or several pain measures. Results for restrictive vs routine mediolateral vs midline episiotomy are similar to the overall comparison. There is insufficient evidence to evaluate if there are (if any) indications for the restrictive use of episiotomy, such as assisted delivery (forceps or vacuum), preterm delivery, breech delivery, predicted macrosomia, and presumed imminent tears. Episiotomy should be avoided if at all possible, but, if used, it is unknown which episiotomy technique (mediolateral or midline) provides the best (or worst) outcome.[16,17]

References

1. Fawole B, Hofmeyr GJ. Maternal oxygen administration for fetal distress. Cochrane Database Syst Rev 2007; 1. [meta–analysis: 2 RCTs, n = 245]

2. Campbell J, Anderson I, Chang A, Wood C. The use of ritodrine in the management of the fetus during the second stage of labour. Aust N Z J Obstet Gynaecolo 1978; 18: 110–13. [RCT, n = 100; normal obstetric women selected during the first stage of labor. Infusion of ritodrine 5 m/kg/min, starting when the second stage of labor is diagnosed, compared with placebo infusion (dextrose water)]

3. Gupta JK, Hofmeyr GJ. Position in the second stage of labour for women without epidural anaesthesia. Cochrane Database Syst Rev 2007; 1. [meta-analysis: 19 RCTs, n = 5764. Variable trial quality, inconsistencies within trials, and heterogeneity of subjects]

4. Roberts CL, Torvaldsen S, Cameron CA, Olive E. Delayed versus early pushing in women with epidural analgesia: a systematic review and meta-analysis. Br J Obstet Gynaecol 2004; 111: 1333–40. [meta-analysis: 9 RCTs, n = 2953]

5. Parnell C, Langhoff-Roos J, Iversen R, Damgaard P. Pushing method in the expulsive phase of labor. A randomized trial. Acta Obstet Gynecol Scand 1993; 72: 31–5. [RCT, n = 350]

6. Bloom SL, Casey BM, Schaffer JI, McIntire DD, Leveno KJ. A randomized trial of coached versus uncoached maternal pushing during the second stage of labor. Am J Obstet Gynecol 2006; 194: 10–13. [RCT, n = 320]

7. Labrecque M, Marcoux S, Pinault JJ, Laroche C, Martin S. Prevention of perineal trauma by perineal massage during pregnancy: a pilot study. Birth 1994; 21: 20–5. [RCT, n = 46]

8. Labrecque M, Eason E, Marcoux S et al. Randomized controlled trial of prevention of perineal trauma by perineal massage during pregnancy. Am J Obstet Gynecol 1999; 180: 593–600. [RCT, n = 1527]

9. Shipman MK, Boniface DR, Tefft ME, McCloghry F. Antenatal perineal massage and subsequent perineal outcomes: a randomized controlled trial. Br J Obstet Gynaecol 1997; 104: 787–91. [RCT, n = 861]

10. Beckmann MM, Garrett AJ. Antenatal perineal massage for reducing perineal trauma. Cochrane Database Syst Rev 2007; 1. [meta-analysis: 3 RCTs, n = 2434]

11. Stamp G, Kruzins G, Crowther C. Perineal massage in labour and prevention of perineal trauma: randomized controlled trial. BMJ 2001: 322: 1277–80. [RCT, n = 1340]

12. Althabe F, Belizan JM, Villar J et al. Mandatory second opinion to reduce rates of unnecessary caesarean sections in Latin America: a cluster randomised controlled trial. Lancet 2004; 363: 1934–40. [RCT, n = 149 276]

13. McCandlish R, Bower U, Van Asten, et al. A randomized controlled trial of care of the perineum during second stage of normal labor. Br J Obstet Gynaecol 1998; 105: 1262–72. [RCT, n = 5471]

14. Mayerhofer K, Bodner-Adler B, Bodner K et al. Traditional care of the perineum during birth: a prospective, randomized, multicenter study of 1,076 women. J Reprod Med 2002; 47: 477–82. [quasi-RCT, n = 1076]

15. Cox J, Cotzias CS, Siakpere O et al. Does an inflatable obstetric belt facilitate spontaneous vaginal delivery in nulliparae with epidural analgesia? Br J Obstet Gynaecol 1999; 106: 1280–6. [RCT, n = 500]

16. Carroli G, Belizan J. Episiotomy for vaginal birth. Cochrane Database Syst Rev 2007; 1. [meta-analysis: 6 RCTs, n = 4850. In the routine episiotomy group, 73% of women had episiotomies, while the rate in the restrictive episiotomy group was 28%]

17. Hartmann K, Viswanathan M, Palmieri R et al. Outcomes of routine episiotomy. A systematic review. JAMA 2005; 293: 2141–8 [meta-analysis: 7 RCTs, n = 5000]

8

Third stage of labor

Julie T Crawford and Jorge E Tolosa

For abnormal third stage, including postpartum hemorrhage, see Chapter 22.

KEY POINTS

- **Prophylactic oxytocin is the uterotonic of choice at delivery** of the anterior shoulder, as it **reduces blood loss and has less side effects** compared with other agents such as ergot alkaloids and prostaglandins.
- **Misoprostol** is helpful for treatment of primary postpartum hemorrhage but **is not recommended for routine postpartum prophylaxis.**
- **Cord traction and uterine massage shorten the third stage and reduce blood loss.**
- **Oxytocin and cord traction are the main interventions of the 'active management' of the third stage.** Compared with expectant management, active management is **associated with a shorter third stage, and reduced blood loss and postpartum hemorrhage.**
- **Vaginal/perineal lacerations should be repaired with one continuous absorbable synthetic suture, including continuous subcuticular skin repair.**
- **Rectal non-steroidal anti-inflammatory drugs (NSAIDs), topical Epifoam (hydrocortisone), and therapeutic ultrasound each decrease perineal pain and the need for additional pain therapy.**

Diagnosis/definition

Interval between delivery of neonate and expulsion of the placenta.

Epidemiology/incidence

Mean length of time of third stage is about 6 minutes, and the 97th percentile is 30 minutes.

Etiology/basic pathophysiology

- Separation of the placenta with capillary hemorrhage and shearing of placental surface when uterus contracts after delivery of infant.
- Signs of separation include gush of blood, cord lengthening, and anterior cephalic movement of the uterine fundus, which becomes more globular and firm.

Risk factors/associations

- Preterm deliveries are associated with longer third stage of labor and increased risk of retained placenta, with proportionally greater risk with decreasing gestational age.
- Longer third stage of labor is associated with greater maternal blood loss.

Complications of third stage of labor

For management of these complications, see Chapter 22.

Postpartum hemorrhage (PPH)

- Symptomatic excessive bleeding (> 500 ml for vaginal delivery)
- Three percent of all births
- Etiology: atony, lacerations, consumptive or dilutional coagulopathy, uterine inversion, uterine rupture, retained placental parts, uterine inversion.

Retained placenta

- Incidence of 1:100 to 1:200, when placenta not expelled by 30–60 minutes
- Cord avulsion occurs in up to 3% with controlled cord traction
- Risk of hemorrhage, infection, or genital tract trauma.

Uterine inversion

- Collapse of uterine fundus into the endometrial cavity
- Incidence: varies widely, approximately 1 in 2500 deliveries
- Risks: excess cord traction, fundal pressure, fundal cord insertions, abnormal placentations.

Pregnancy management

Pregnancy management covers uterotonics, cord, placenta (active management), laceration repair, and pain control (Figure 8.1).

Prophylactic uterotonics
Prophylactic oxytocics

Oxytocin (Syntocinon) **is the prophylactic uterotonic of choice in the third stage of labor. In comparison with no**

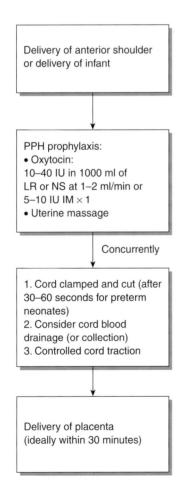

Figure 8.1
Algorithm for management of normal third stage. PPH, postpartum hemorrhage; IU, international units; LR, lactated Ringer's solution; NS, normal saline; IM, intramuscularly

uterotonics, prophylactic oxytocin **reduces blood loss > 500 ml, and the need for therapeutic oxytocics with blood loss > 1000 ml.**[1] There are similar incidences of manual removal of the placenta, and rates of blood transfusions with the use of oxytocin compared with no uterotonic.

In comparison with ergot alkaloids [ergometrine (ergonovine) or Methergine], oxytocin is associated with less manual removals of the placenta, and does not increase maternal blood pressure. There is little effect (and no benefit) from adding oxytocin to ergometrine compared with ergometrine alone.[1]

In comparison with oxytocin, ergometrine–oxytocin (Syntometrine) is associated with increased side effects with only modest benefits of minimal clinical significance. Compared with oxytocin, ergometrine–oxytocin is associated with a small reduction in PPH blood loss of at least 500 ml. This advantage is found for both 5 International Units (IU) oxytocin and 10 IU oxytocin, but is greater for the lower dose. There is no difference detected between the groups using either 5 or 10 IU for the stricter definition of PPH of blood loss of at least 1000 ml. **Adverse effects of vomiting, nausea, and hypertension are more likely to be associated with the use of ergometrine–oxytocin.** There are no significant differences in the other important maternal (e.g. blood transfusion, retained placenta, etc.) or neonatal outcomes. Most trials used intramuscular (IM) doses of oxytocics.[2]

Oxytocin:
- Oxytocin increases the strength and frequency of contractions and is specific to uterine smooth muscle.
- It may be administered before placental separation with delivery of the anterior shoulder or infant, or after placental separation; blood loss and incidence of retained placenta are similar with oxytocin administration before or after placental delivery.[3]
- Continuous infusion of intravenous (IV) 10–40 (IU) in 1,000 ml of normal saline or lactated Ringer's solution at 10 ml/min, then reduce to 1–2 ml/min or 5–10 IU IM.
- Intraumbilical injection is not superior to IV administration.[4]

Ergot alkaloids (methergine or ergometrine):
- **Little evidence in favor of ergot alkaloids alone**
- Dose: 0.2 mg IM injection
- Should not be given IV
- Contraindicated in patients with high blood pressure or pre-eclampsia.

Syntometrine:
- **Not recommended over oxytocin used alone**
- Dose: oxytocin 5 IU in combination with ergometrine 0.5 mg IM × 1
- Side-effect profile is significant for nausea, vomiting, and hypertension.

Prophylactic prostaglandins

Neither intramuscular prostaglandins ($PGF_{2\alpha}$ or PGE) nor misoprostol (prostaglandin E_1 analog) are preferable to conventional injectable uterotonics (e.g. oxytocin) as part of the active management of the third stage of labor, especially for low-risk women. Compared with no uterotonics, **oral misoprostol** does not reduce the rate of PPH or other measures of blood loss, and has more side effects.[5]

Compared with conventional injectable uterotonics, oral misoprostol 600 µg shows significantly more blood loss < 1000 ml. Shivering and elevated body temperature (> 38°C) are the main side effects of oral misoprostol and are dose-related effects. Results with rectal misoprostol are similar.[5]

Injectable prostaglandins are associated with reduced mean blood loss in the third stage of labor when compared with conventional injectable uterotonics but have more side effects. There are scarce data on severe PPH and the use of additional uterotonics.[3]

Misoprostol or injectable prostaglandins:
- **They are not recommended for routine prophylactic use in the third stage of labor.**
- Misoprostol may be given as 400–1000 µg orally or rectally for primary treatment of PPH.
- Side effects of misoprostol include fever, shivering, nausea, vomiting, diarrhea, vasospasm, and bronchospasm.
- Despite its significant side-effect profile, misoprostol may be a reasonable treatment in less-developed nations, given its ease of storage and administration.

Umbilical cord
Collection of cord blood

For fetal assessment: Cord gases are stable in a clamped segment of cord for 60 minutes, and in a heparinized syringe for 60 minutes. Umbilical artery pH, pCO_2, and base deficit may be helpful in indicating timing of insult. They should be collected in cases of non-reassuring fetal heart rate (NRFHR), thick meconium, low Apgar scores (defined as < 7 at 5 minutes), fetal growth restriction (FGR), preterm birth, or sentinel event (e.g. cord prolapse, uterine rupture, or abruptio). Umbilical vein pH may be helpful in cases of uteroplacental problems (e.g. abruption, asthma). Routine checking of umbilical cord gases is not necessary for normal labor, delivery, and Apgar score, without risk factors. Some centers mandate universal cord gases in all deliveries, with no trials available for assessing this policy. Cord blood is usually also sent for Rh status in Rh-negative women.

For stem cells: The obstetrician should support public banking of cord blood.[6] Public banks are under more stringent Food and Drug Administration (FDA) guidelines, have more legal responsibilities, allow greater access to cord blood by the general population, and are more cost-effective than private banks. Directed donation of cord blood when there is a disease in the family amenable to stem cell transplantation can be arranged through many public banks, listed in this reference.[6] The chance of a child requiring a transplant of his/her own cord blood is 1/2700, with other applications not yet proven in trials.

Timing of cord clamping

Preterm neonates: Delayed cord clamping by 30–60 (120 max) seconds is associated with **fewer transfusions** for anemia or low blood pressure, and **less intraventricular hemorrhage** than early clamping < 30 seconds.[7] There are no clear differences in other outcomes, such as respiratory diseases, death, or long-term outcomes. Positioning of the infant has not been studied in sufficient numbers for a recommendation.

Term neonates: There is insufficient evidence to assess the best timing of cord clamping for term neonates.

Placenta
Cord drainage and traction

Compared to no drainage and traction, cord drainage and traction is associated with **shorter third stage and less decline in maternal hemoglobin** when no uterotonics are used.[8]

Controlled cord traction

There is insufficient evidence to evaluate the effect of cord traction alone, as there are no specific trials. This intervention has been evaluated together with the other interventions of the active management of the third stage. Cord traction by itself has been associated with **lower mean blood loss and shorter third stage**, but insufficient data regarding PPH and retained placenta.[9]

Massage of uterus

There is insufficient evidence to evaluate the effect of massage of uterus alone, as there are no specific trials. This intervention has been evaluated only together with the other interventions of the active management of the third stage.

Injection of oxytocin in cord

There is insufficient evidence to evaluate the effect of injection of oxytocin in the umbilical cord. Umbilical injection is not superior to IV oxytocin.[4] Compared with injection of saline, injection of 20 IU of oxytocin in the umbilical vein after delivery shortens the third stage, with no effect on blood loss, in a small trial.[10]

Active management

Active management should be the routine management of choice for women expecting to deliver a baby by vaginal delivery in a maternity hospital[11] (see Figure 8.1).

Active management of the third stage usually consists of:

- **prophylactic oxytocic** at delivery of anterior shoulder or after delivery of baby
- **uterine massage/fundal manipulation**
- **controlled cord traction.**

Expectant management of the third stage usually consists of:

- Using gravity and maternal expulsive efforts.
- No cord traction, fundal pressure, or uterine massage, and no uterotonic drugs.

Compared with expectant management, **active management** (in the setting of a maternity hospital) is associated with **reduced risks** of: **maternal blood loss; PPH** of more than 500 ml; **need for blood transfusion; hemoglobin < 9 g/dl at 24–48 hours postpartum; and prolonged third stage of labor.**[11] No differences in retained placenta or need for surgical evacuation are seen. Active management with use of ergometrine is associated with an increased risk of maternal nausea, vomiting, and raised blood pressure. No advantages or disadvantages are apparent for the baby, and there are similar rates of breastfeeding at 6 weeks. Homebirths and women with bleeding disorders, anemia, prior PPH, multiparity, hypertension, and previous cesarean delivery were excluded from most studies on active management of the third stage of labor.

Repair of laceration (or episiotomy)
Closure vs non-closure

Compared with non-closure, **closure of first- and second-degree perineal lacerations after vaginal delivery is associated with similar pain scores, but better healing (at 10 days and 6 weeks).**[12, 13]

Anal ultrasound

Compared with a clinical examination only, anal endosonography with clinical examination immediately after delivery in nulliparous women with second-degree lacerations detected more sphincter tears. Anal endosonography with immediate repair of these tears is associated with less-severe fecal incontinence at 1 year compared with clinical examination only.[14]

Type of suture

Absorbable synthetic materials should be used for all layers of the repair. Compared with catgut (plain or chromic), **absorbable synthetic sutures** (polyglycolic acid [Dexon] or polyglactin [Vicryl]) for perineal repair following childbirth **decrease a woman's experience of short-term (3 days) pain.**[15] There is also **less need for analgesia, reduced rate of suture dehiscence** up to day 10, and less need for resuturing at ≤ 3 months. There is no significant difference in long-term pain. Removal of suture material is significantly more common in the polyglycolic acid and polyglactin groups, but most trials used 0 to 2-0 sutures. Although this is concerning, clinical experience has shown suture removal is necessary < 5% of the time when using 3-0 or finer sutures and performing subcuticular skin closure. There is no difference in the amount of dyspareunia experienced by women.

There is no randomized controlled trial (RCT) comparing Dexon and Vicryl. Compared with Dexon, a new monofilament suture (Bioxin) is associated with more reported problems in the suture area.[16]

Continuous vs interrupted repair

Compared with an interrupted (one stitch vagina, interrupted for perineal muscle and skin) repair, a **continuous suture** of rapidly absorbed 2-0 polyglactin 910 suture is associated with less pain at 10 days.[17]

Compared with interrupted sutures, a **continuous *subcuticular* suture technique of perineal repair is associated with less pain for up to 10 days postpartum.** No differences are seen in the need for analgesia, need for resuturing of the wound, or in dyspareunia. There are no differences in long-term pain and failure to resume pain-free intercourse within 3 months of the birth. The continuous technique is associated with **less need for the removal of sutures.**[18] Compared with a three-stage repair, including a last stage of skin closure, a two-stage repair leaving the skin unsutured is associated with less pain and dyspareunia 3 months postpartum.[19]

Third and fourth degree

Approximation (end-to-end) and overlap technique for third- or fourth-degree laceration repair are associated with similar outcomes.[20,21] Polyglactin (Vicryl) and polydioxanone (PDS) are associated with similar outcomes.[21] There are no RCTs that assess the need for prophylactic antibiotics.

Perineal pain control

Oral non-steroidal anti-inflammatory drugs

There are no RCTs to accurately assess the effectiveness of oral non-steroidal anti-inflammatory drugs (NSAIDs) for perineal pain control.

Rectal non-steroidal anti-inflammatory drugs

Compared with placebo, **NSAID rectal suppositories** (indomethacin or diclofenac) are associated with **less pain up to 24 hours after birth**, and **less requirement for additional analgesia in the first 24 hours and 48 hours** postpartum.[22] No information is available on pain experienced more than 72 hours after birth or other outcomes of importance to women such as the impact on daily activities, resumption of sexual intercourse, and the impact on the mother–baby relationship. Rectally administered NSAIDs appear to provide effective pain relief in postpartum women. Although rectal NSAIDs appear to offer adequate pain relief in the immediate postpartum period, more studies are needed to assess the acceptability of this route of administration.

Topical anesthetics

Compared with placebo, topical anesthetics applied to the perineum are associated with **similar pain relief** up to 24 hours and 24–72 hours postpartum, but women are more satisfied.[23] Compared with placebo, **Epifoam** (1% hydrocortisone acetate and 1% pramoxine hydrochloride in a mucoadhesive foam base) use is associated with **less additional analgesia**, whereas lidocaine showed no difference with regard to additional analgesia use compared with placebo.[23] Compared with indomethacin vaginal suppositories, topical anesthetics have similar mean pain scores.

Therapeutic ultrasound for perineal pain

There is not enough evidence to evaluate the use of ultrasound in treating perineal pain and/or dyspareunia following childbirth.

For acute pain: Compared with placebo, women treated with **active ultrasound for acute perineal pain** are more likely to report **improvement in pain**. Compared with pulsed electromagnetic energy (Megapulse), for acute perineal pain, women treated with ultrasound are **more likely to have bruising at 10 days, but less likely to experience perineal pain at 10 days and 3 months**.[24]

For persistent pain: Compared with placebo, women treated with ultrasound for persistent perineal pain and/or dyspareunia are **less likely to report pain with sexual intercourse**.[24]

Anesthesia

Spinal, epidural, or general anesthesia is required if complications arise such as management for retained placenta, intractable PPH, or uterine inversion.

Postpartum/breastfeeding after active management of third stage

- Hypertension and headache are associated with misoprostol and ergotamine use
- No known complications with breastfeeding after use of uterotonics.

Infant

- No advantages or disadvantages apparent for the infant with active management
- No differences in breastfeeding or onset of jaundice with active management.

Delivery note

A detailed note should address the essential and suggestive criteria for neonatal encephalopathy pertinent to immediate neonatal status, such as **assessment of fetal heart testing, Apgar scores, umbilical cord pH, and base deficit** (see Chapter 27).

References

1. Elbourne DR, Prendiville WJ, Carroli G, Wood J. McDonald S. Prophylactic use of oxytocin in the third stage of labour. Cochrane Database Syst Rev 2007; 1. [meta-analysis: vs no oxytocics: 7 RCTs, n => 3000; vs ergot alkaloids: 6 RCTs, n => 2800; 5 RCTs, n => 2800 – total 16 RCTs, different than below – see Cochrane]
2. McDonald S, Abbott JM, Higgins SP. Prophylactic ergometrine–oxytocin versus oxytocin for the third stage of labour. Cochrane Database Syst Rev 2007; 1. [meta-analysis: 6 RCTs, n = 9332 – different than RCTs in Reference 1.]
3. Jackson KW Jr, Allbert JR, Schemmer GK et al. A randomized controlled trial comparing oxytocin administration before and after placental delivery in the prevention of postpartum hemorrhage. Am J Obstet Gynecol 2001; 185: 873. [RCT, n = 1486]
4. Porter KB, O'Brien WF, Collins MK et al. A randomized comparison of umbilical vein and intravenous oxytocin during the puerperium. Obstet Gynecol 1991; 78: 254. [RCT, n = 104]

5. Gulmezoglu AM, Forna F, Villar J, Hofmeyr GJ. Prostaglandins for prevention of postpartum haemorrhage. Cochrane Database Syst Rev 2007; 1. [meta-analysis: 24 RCTs misoprostol: 5 RCTs – oral misoprostol vs no uterotonics/placebo; 8 RCTs IM prostaglandins]

6. Moise KJ. Umbilical cord stem cells. Obstet Gynecol 2005; 106: 1393–407. [review]

7. Rabe H, Reynolds G, Diaz-Rossello J. Early versus delayed umbilical cord clamping in preterm infants. Cochrane Database Syst Rev 2007; 1. [7 RCTs, n = 297. All are small trials]

8. Giacalone PL, Vignal J, Daures JP et al. A randomized evaluation of two techniques of management of the third stage of labor in women at low risk of postpartum hemorrhage. Br J Obstet Gynaecol 2000; 107: 396–400. [RCT, n = 477]

9. Kinmond S, Aitchison TC, Holland BM et al. Umbilical cord clamping and preterm infants: a randomized trial. BMJ 1993; 306: 172–5. [RCT, n = 36]

10. Kovasarach E, Rojsangruang S. Effect of umbilical vein oxytocin injection on the third stage of labor: a randomized controlled study. J Med Ass Thailand 1998; 81: 693–7. [RCT, n = 50]

11. Prendiville WJ, Elbourne D, McDonald S. Active versus expectant management in the third stage of labour. Cochrane Database Syst Rev 2007; 1. [meta-analysis: 5 RCTs, n = 6557]

12. Fleming VEM, Hagen S, Niven C. Does perineal suturing make a difference? The SUNS trial. Br J Obstet Gynaecol 2003; 110: 684–9. [RCT, n = 74]

13. Lunquist M, Olsson A, Nissen E, Norman M. Is it necessary to suture all lacerations after vaginal delivery? Birth 2000; 27: 79–85. [RCT, n = 78]

14. Flatin DL, Boulvain M, Floris LA, Irion O. Diagnosis of anal sphincter tears to prevent fecal incontinence. Obstet Gynecol 2005; 106: 6–13. [RCT, n = 752]

15. Kettle C, Johanson RB. Absorbable synthetic versus catgut suture material for perineal repair. Cochrane Database Syst Rev 2007; 1. [meta-analysis: 8 RCTs, n => 3600]

16. Dencker A, Lundgren I, Sporrong T. Suturing after childbirth – a randomised controlled study testing a new monofilament material. BJOG 2006; 113: 114–16. [RCT, n = 1139]

17. Kettle C, Hills RK, Jones P et al. Continuous versus interrupted perineal repair with standard or rapidly absorbed sutures after spontaneous vaginal birth: a randomized controlled trial. Lancet 2002; 359: 2217–23. [RCT, n = 1542]

18. Kettle C, Johanson RB. Continuous versus interrupted sutures for perineal repair. Cochrane Database Syst Rev 2007; 1. [4 RCTs, n = 1864]

19. Gordon B, Mackrodt C, Fern E et al. The Ipswich Childbirth Study: 1. A randomized evaluation of two stage postpartum perineal repair leaving the skin unsutured. Br J Obstet Gynaecol 1998; 105: 435–40. [RCT, n = 1780]

20. Fitzpatrick M, Behan M, O'Connell PR, O'Herlihy C. A randomized clinical trial comparing primary overlap with approximation repair of third-degree obstetric tears. Am J Obstet Gynecol 2000; 183: 1220–4. [RCT, n = 112]

21. Williams A, Adams EJ, Tincello DG et al. How to repair an anal sphincter injury after vaginal delivery: results of a randomised controlled trial. Br J Obstet Gynaecol 2006; 113: 201–7. [RCT, n = 112]

22. Hedayati H, Parsons J, Crowther CA. Rectal analgesia for pain from perineal trauma following childbirth. Cochrane Database Syst Rev 2007; 1. [meta-analysis: 3 RCTs, n = 249]

23. Hedayati H, Parsons J, Crowther CA. Topically applied anaesthetics for treating perineal pain after childbirth. Cochrane Database Syst Rev 2007; 1. [meta-analysis: 8 RCTs, n = 976]

24. Hay-Smith EJC. Therapeutic ultrasound for postpartum perineal pain and dyspareunia. Cochrane Database Syst Rev 2007; 1. [meta-analysis: 4 RCTs, n = 459]

9

Intrapartum fetal monitoring

Suneet P Chauhan

KEY POINTS

- Compared with intermittent auscultation, the use of continuous electronic fetal heart rate (FHR) tracing significantly increases the rate of operative interventions (vacuum, forceps, and cesarean delivery) for non-reassuring patterns, but it does decrease the likelihood of neonatal seizures and perinatal mortality secondary to hypoxia.
- With persistent non-reassuring FHR pattern, intrauterine resuscitation with tocolytics or amnioinfusion (if variable decelerations) reduces the need to proceed with emergent cesarean delivery but does not reduce the likelihood of asphyxial injury.
- The labor of women at risk for poor peripartum outcomes should be monitored with continuous electronic FHR tracing.
- Reinterpretation of the FHR tracing, especially knowing the neonatal outcome, should be done cautiously.
- There is insufficient evidence to assess computerized FHR monitoring.
- ST analysis may be beneficial in women with non-reassuring FHR on continuous monitoring. No benefit of ST analysis is observed with proper use of fetal scalp sampling.
- Fetal pulse oximetry is not associated with significant maternal or neonatal benefits compared with continuous FHR monitoring alone.

Background

In 2002, about 3.4 million (85% of approximately 4 million live births) fetuses in the USA were monitored with continuous electronic fetal heart rate (FHR) tracing, making it the most common obstetric procedure.[1]

Fetal heart definitions

Adapted from the National Institute of Child Health and Human Development Research Planning Workshop,[2] the definitions of FHR patterns are described in Table 9.1. The definitions were developed for intrapartum monitoring but can be applicable to antepartum monitoring. No distinction is made between short- and long-term variability.[2] Accelerations, decelerations, bradycardia, and tachycardia can be quantified by describing the nazir/zenith and the duration in minutes and seconds of the FHR change. A recurrent deceleration occurs with ≥ 50% of uterine contractions in any 20 minute period. The definition of reassuring FHR tracing is normal (110–160 beats/min) FHR baseline, moderate (6–25 beat/min) variability, presence of accelerations, and absence of decelerations. The definition of non-reassuring FHR testing (NRFHT) is controversial, but is usually recurrent late decelerations, bradycardia, or absent or minimal (≤ 5) variability. The pattern leading to such interpretation should be documented in the medical record.

In relation to uterine activity, hyperstimulation is defined as ≥ 6 contractions in 10 minutes (see also Chapter 17, page 159). Hypertonus is a single contraction lasting > 2 minutes.

Terms such as 'asphyxia', 'hypoxia', and 'fetal distress' should not be used in the interpretation of FHR tracing.

pH definitions

- Acidemia: increased concentration of hydrogen ions in blood.
- Acidosis: a pathologic condition marked by increased concentration of hydrogen ions in tissue.
- Hypoxemia: decreased oxygen content in blood.
- Hypoxia: a pathologic condition marked by decreased level of oxygen in tissue.
- Asphyxia: usually acidemia, hypoxia, and metabolic acidosis. All of these criteria must be present to entertain a diagnosis of possible intrauterine asphyxia: (1) pH < 7.00; (2) Apgar ≤ 3 at > 5 minutes, and (3) neonatal neurologic sequelae (e.g. seizures, coma, hypotonia, etc.).[3] This term should be used with caution, and never before birth. (see also Chapter 27)

Incidence

The prevalence of cesarean delivery (CD) for non-reassuring FHR (NRFHR) testing is 3% and it is increasing.[4]

Table 9.1 *Definitions of fetal heart rate (FHR) patterns*

Pattern	Definition
Baseline FHR	The mean FHR rounded to increments of 5 beats/min during a 10 min period The baseline must be present for a minimum of 2 min May need to compare the previous 10 min segment to determine the baseline
Baseline FHR variability	Fluctuations in the FHR over 2 cycles/min or greater Variability is quantitated as the amplitude of peak-to-trough in beats/min Absent – amplitude range undetectable Minimal – amplitude range ≤ 5 beats/min Moderate (normal) – amplitude range 6–25 beats/min Marked – amplitude range > 25 beats/min
Acceleration	An abrupt (peak within 30 s) increase in the FHR from the recently calculated baseline Acme is ≥ 15 beats/min above baseline, lasting for 15 s or more and < 2 min from the onset to return to baseline Before 32 weeks, acceleration is acme ≥ 10 beats/min over the baseline and lasting at least 10 s but < 2 min Prolonged acceleration if it lasts beyond 2 min but less than 10 min If the acceleration is for 10 min or longer, then it is a baseline change
Bradycardia	Baseline FHR < 110 beats/min
Early deceleration	In association with a uterine contraction, a visually apparent, gradual (onset to nadir ≥ 30 s) decrease in FHR with return to baseline FHR The nadir of the deceleration occurs at the same time as the peak of the contraction
Late deceleration	In association with a uterine contraction, a visually apparent, gradual (onset to nadir ≥ 30 s) decrease in FHR with return to baseline FHR The onset, nadir, and recovery of the deceleration occur after the beginning, peak, and end of the contraction, respectively
Tachycardia	Baseline FHR > 160 beats/min
Variable deceleration	An abrupt (onset to nadir < 30 s) decrease in the FHR below the baseline FHR The decrease in FHR is at least 15 beats/min, lasting for 15 s or more but less than 2 min
Prolonged deceleration	Decrease in FHR from baseline ≥ 15 beats/min, lasting ≥ 2 min but < 10 min from onset to return to baseline FHR If the deceleration is for 10 min or longer, then it is a FHR baseline change

Adapted from The National Institute of Child Health and Human Development Research Planning Workshop.[2]

Risk factors and predictors of abnormal fetal heart rate

The risk of CD for NRFHR is > 20% in women with moderate/severe asthma, severe hypothyroidism, severe pre-eclampsia, post-term or fetal growth restriction with abnormal Doppler studies.[4]

Use of likelihood ratio suggests that fetal movement count, abnormal FHR on admission, vibroacoustic stimulation, amniotic fluid index, contraction stress test, and the modified and completed biophysical profile are poor diagnostic tests to identify which patients will require emergent CD.[4] Umbilical artery systolic/diastolic ratio, however, is a reliable test to predict the need for CD for NRFHR.

Management

Continuous electronic fetal heart rate monitoring vs intermittent auscultation

The proven benefit of continuous FHR monitoring, compared with intermittent FHR monitoring, is a 39% **decrease in neonatal seizures**.[5,6] Risks with the use of continuous electronic FHR monitoring compared with intermittent auscultation are **increased rate of cesarean** and **operative vaginal** deliveries. **Perinatal mortality is similar** (0.4 vs 0.6%), with larger numbers needed to make the 34% benefit (about 0.2–0.5% decrease in perinatal mortality) significant.[6] **Perinatal mortality secondary to fetal hypoxia is decreased** (0.07 vs 0.19%).[5] The incidence of **cerebral palsy** (CP) has been evaluated only in studies which compared continuous electronic fetal monitoring *and* scalp pH vs intermittent auscultation, and is **similar** (0.4 vs 0.3%). Given the incidence of CP, and the fact that >70% of cases of CP occur before the onset of labor and only about 4–10% intrapartum, it might be difficult for intrapartum FHR monitoring to prevent CP. The benefit in reduction of seizures has been demonstrated consistently, although the long-term neurological effects of these seizures are minimal.[6] Thus, it is reasonable to discuss the options with the patients.[7] Admittedly both patients and clinicians prefer FHR monitoring as the method to evaluate the fetus during labor.[8] The explanations for the preference include the ease of use, the reassurance women derive from hearing the heart beat during labor, and the different value patients and clinicians place on the route of delivery and neonatal outcomes. Compared with pregnant patients and mothers, obstetricians overestimate the burden posed by a CD, and, contrary to obstetricians, women value a newborn with permanent neurological handicap over neonatal death.[9]

Clinicians choosing to utilize intermittent auscultation should be aware of some of the problems associated with its use. Electronic FHR monitoring has a significantly better ability to detect acidemia (umbilical arterial pH < 7.15 in this study) than intermittent auscultation: a sensitivity of 97% vs 34% and a higher positive predictive value of 37% vs 22%, respectively.[10] Continuous tracing of FHR was not only superior with detection of respiratory and mixed acidosis but also for metabolic acidosis as well. It is possible that the ominous FHR patterns are poorly assessed by intermittent auscultation. Logistically, it may not be feasible to adhere to guidelines of how frequently the heart rate should be auscultated. One prospective study noted that the protocol for intermittent auscultation was successfully completed in only 3% of the cases.[11]

Even though the use of continuous electronic monitoring of FHR does not decrease the prevalence of cerebral palsy, it assists in determining if the injury occurred during the ante- or intrapartum period. Review of the FHR tracing of neurologically injured newborns indicates that the majority of them had an abnormal pattern consistent with asphyxial injury **prior** to the onset of labor.[12] Moreover, a pregnancy with chronic fetal compromise may develop superimposed acute asphyxia, in which case the impairment may be more severe than if the sentinel event and injury occurred during labor.

Not all pregnancies should be monitored with intermittent auscultation because those at risk for adverse outcomes like cerebral palsy, neonatal encephalopathy, and perinatal death should be monitored with continuous FHR tracing during labor.[13] Thus, high-risk pregnancies that underwent antepartum surveillance should not be evaluated with intermittent auscultation, nor should those who are likely to have CD for a NRFHR pattern.[4] These include FGR, oligohydramnios, polyhydramnios, placenta previa, post-term (≥ 42 weeks), multiple gestation, isoimmunized pregnancy, prior intrauterine fetal death (IUFD), or maternal renal disease, diabetes, pre-eclampsia, collagen disorders, hemoglobinopathies, and cardiovascular disease. Additionally, parturients should be monitored with continuous tracing of FHR if they have been induced or augmented, or have dysfunctional labor, tocolytics administered more than once an hour, suspected FHR abnormalities with auscultation, abnormal fetal presentation, regional anesthesia, abruption, infection, preterm labor, prior CD (vaginal birth after cesarean [VBAC] attempt), hypertonic uterus, and meconium staining of the amniotic fluid.[7]

FHR monitoring should be continued until delivery. If CD is performed, internal scalp monitoring can be continued until delivery, while external monitoring can be discontinued when the abdominal preparation begins.

Reviewing electronic fetal heart rate monitoring

When electronic fetal monitoring is utilized during labor the nurses or physicians should review it frequently. If the patient is a low-risk pregnancy, the FHR tracing should be reviewed every

30 minutes in the first stage of labor and every 15 minutes during the second stage. The corresponding frequency for high-risk parturients is 15 and 5 minutes. The maternal pulse should be taken to make sure the FHR is indeed fetal, and not maternal. Healthcare providers should *document* that they have reviewed the tracing by a narrative note or use of comprehensive flow sheets or by placing one's initials on the monitor strip, if it is reassuring.[7] Among low-risk patients, it is more feasible to confirm that the strips are reviewed according to the guidelines, while among high-risk patients, compliance during active phase, and especially during the second stage of labor, is more demanding and difficult. The FHR tracing, as a part of medical chart, should be labeled and available for review if the need arises. Alternatives like computer storage of the FHR tracing that do not permit overwriting or revisions are reasonable, as are microfilm recordings.[7]

Due to the inter- and intraobserver variability, FHR tracing should be interpreted cautiously and preferably without knowing the neonatal outcome. When four obstetricians, for example, examined 50 cardiotocograms, they agreed on only 22% of the cases. Two months later, during the second review of the same 50 tracings, the clinicians interpreted 21% of the tracings differently than they did during the first evaluation.[14] Factors that influence the interpretation of cardiotocograms include the clinician's experience, whether the tracing is normal vs equivocal or ominous, with greater agreement if the tracing is reassuring, and the time of the day, with possibly greater error at night. With retrospective reviews, the foreknowledge of neonatal outcome alters the impressions of the tracing. Given the same intrapartum tracing but opposite neonatal outcomes, the reviewer is more likely to find evidence of fetal hypoxia and criticize the obstetrician's management if the outcome was supposedly poor vs good.[15]

The positive predictive value of NRFHR for cerebral palsy is about 0.1%.[7] The false-positive rate is extremely high (99%) for FHR tracing and abnormal neonatal outcome, especially cerebral palsy.[16]

External vs internal fetal heart rate monitoring

External FHR monitoring is accomplished via a Doppler ultrasound device applied to the maternal abdomen. An internal scalp electrode ('scalp lead') measures the R-R interval between consecutive beats. This provides an accurate representation of FHR variability. There are no randomized controlled trials (RCTs) comparing these two monitoring techniques. Internal monitoring is used in general for FHR that cannot be consistently assessed by external monitoring. Contraindications to internal monitoring include maternal infections such as human immunodeficiency virus (HIV), and active hepatitis B or C, fetal thrombocytopenia, etc. Otherwise, internal monitoring is safe.

Computerized fetal heart rate monitoring

Measured by interobserver agreement, the reliability of electronic fetal monitoring is not very good. There is insufficient evidence to assess if computerized evaluation improves perinatal outcomes, as there is no trial available.[17]

Management of abnormal fetal heart rate (Figure 9.1)

FHR should be evaluated in labor:[7]

- In low-risk women: every 30 minutes in the first stage active phase, and every 15 minutes in the second stage.
- In high-risk women (see below): every 15 minutes in the first stage active phase, and every 5 minutes in the second stage.

The best time for evaluation is after a contraction.

Gestational age, medications (Table 9.2), prior fetal assessment, and obstetric and medical conditions should be accounted for correct interpretation of FHR tracing, and clinicians should be cognizant of it.[7]

The presence of acceleration usually assures that the fetus is not acidotic (pH < 7.20). If spontaneous acceleration is not present, and/or NRFHR is present, **digital scalp or vibroacoustic stimulation** should be done to elicit an acceleration (see Figure 9.1). Even an acceleration of 10 beats over baseline is usually reassuring. Allis clamp and scalp puncture have been used to elicit acceleration, but are less safe. Digital scalp stimulation (gentle stroking of the fetal scalp for 15 seconds) is the test with the best predictive accuracy among these four.[18] There are currently no RCTs that address the safety and efficacy of digital scalp or vibroacoustic stimulation used to assess fetal well-being in labor in the presence of NRFHR. If the FHR increases, then labor should continue, since an acceleration following fetal stimulation indicates that the likelihood of low scalp pH is 2%.[18] In the absence of an acceleration, the likelihood is 38%.

With a persistent non-reassuring FHR tracing, a **scalp pH** should be attempted, if available. If the results of scalp pH is < 7.20 or lactate > 4.8 mmol/L, then delivery should be accomplished expeditiously, usually by CD[19] (see Figure 9.1). The sensitivities of abnormal scalp pH or lactate to predict moderate to severe hypoxic-ischemic encephalopathy are 50% and 66%, respectively, while the corresponding specificities are 73% and 76%.[19] If the results are scalp pH ≥ 7.20 or lactate ≤ 4.8 mmol/L, continuous careful FHR monitoring should continue, with repeat scalp stimulation and/or pH if NRFHR persists. Several RCTs of continuous vs intermittent FHR monitoring in labor used scalp pH in concomitance with continuous FHR monitoring.[6] Scalp pH

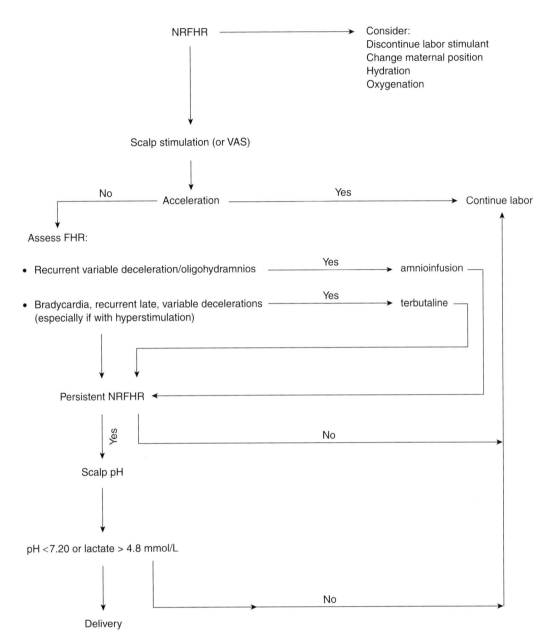

Figure 9.1
Algorithm for the management of non-reassuring fetal heart rate tracing in labor. FHR, fetal heart rate; NRFHR, non-reassuring fetal heart rate, i.e. recurrent late decelerations, bradycardia, ≤ 5 beats/min variability. VAS, vibroacoustic stimulation.

may not be feasible in cases with cervical dilatation < 3 cm. To be beneficial, the scalp pH machine needs to be reliable and readily available, with prompt results.

If neither acceleration nor a scalp pH can be obtained, then the management of NRFHR tracing depends on the abnormality.

When the FHR abnormality is **recurrent variable decelerations** (usually with preceding oligohydramnios), **amnioinfusion** to relieve cord compression should be utilized (see Figure 9.1).[20] Prophylactic (for oligohydramnios, and therefore suspicion of later variable decelerations) or therapeutic (for variable decelerations) **transcervical** amnioinfusion significantly **reduces the rate of persistent variable decelerations, cesarean delivery for suspected NRFHR, and overall CD compared with no treatment.**[20] The incidence of umbilical arterial pH < 7.20 is decreased. Postpartum endometritis is decreased, too. There is a non-significant 49% decrease in perinatal mortality.[20] Transabdominal amnioinfusion should be considered if amniotomy cannot be done and an intrauterine pressure catheter placed, since it has similar effects, relieving persistent recurrent variable decelerations and lowering the incidence of umbilical arterial pH < 7.20 in two small

Table 9.2 *Effect of medications and fetal heart rate (FHR) patterns*

Medications	Study design	Effect on FHR
Butorphanol	Case–control	Transient sinusoidal FHR pattern
Cocaine	Case–control	No characteristic changes in FHR pattern
Corticosteroid	RCT	Decrease in FHR variability with betamethasone but not dexamethasone
Magnesium sulfate	RCT and retrospective	A significant decrease in the FHR baseline and variability; inhibits the increase in accelerations with advancing gestational age
Meperidine	RCT	No characteristic changes in FHR pattern
Morphine	Case–control	Decreased number of accelerations
Nalbuphine	RCT	Decreased the number of accelerations, long- and short-term variation
Terbutaline	Retrospective	Abolishment or decrease in frequency of late and variable decelerations
Zidovudine	Case–control	No difference in the FHR baseline, variability, number of accelerations or decelerations

RCT, randomized clinical trial. Adapted from Chauhan and Macones.[7]

trials.[21,22] The limited evidence available suggests that there is no advantage to using amnioinfusion prophylactically as opposed to therapeutically (see Chapter 16). The trials reviewed are small; it is impossible to address the possibility of rare but serious maternal adverse effects of amnioinfusion.

The mechanism of effectiveness of amnioinfusion is relief of the umbilical cord compression thought to be causing the variable decelerations.

Amnioinfusion can be done by a bolus or continuous infusion technique, with similar ability to relieve recurrent variable decelerations. Neither pumps nor warmers are necessary with amnioinfusion. In fact, the use of an infusion pump during amnioinfusion significantly increases the risk of fetal compromise. Either lactated Ringer's solution or normal saline can be used to place a crystalloid solution into the uterus without altering the neonatal electrolyte imbalance.[20]

For **bradycardia, or recurrent late or variable decelerations,** tocolytics can be used to abolish uterine contractions, especially if hyperstimulation is present. During suspected NRFHR, compared with no treatment, β-mimetics (terbutaline 0.25 mg subcutaneously or hexoprenaline 10 μg intravenously) are associated with fewer failed improvements in FHR abnormalities.[23] There is insufficient evidence to evaluate the effect on important neonatal outcomes such as umbilical artery pH, given the small numbers. When terbutaline is compared with magnesium sulfate (4 g over 10 minutes), the β-mimetic is faster acting and more effective, with similar maternal cardiovascular side effects.[24] Thus, β-mimetics are a useful treatment for 'buying time'

when NRFHR is diagnosed during labor. Such time may be useful for preparing for cesarean section or operative delivery, setting up regional analgesia, transferring a woman at home or in a unit without the necessary surgical or neonatal facilities, to an appropriate hospital, or reviewing the need for urgent delivery.

In the presence of NRFHR, concomitantly with performing scalp stimulation and/or scalp pH, intrauterine resuscitation can be attempted (see Figure 9.1) with:

- **Maternal position** change to left or right lateral:
  - there is insufficient evidence (no trial) to assess by itself the effect of intrapartum maternal position change on fetal status.
- **Hydration:**
  - there is insufficient evidence (no trial) to assess by itself the effect of intrapartum maternal hydration on fetal status.
- **Oxygenation:**
  - there is insufficient evidence (no trial) to assess by itself the effect of intrapartum maternal oxygen on fetal status.
- **Labor stimulant** should be discontinued:
  - there is insufficient evidence (no trial) to assess by itself the effect of labor stimulant discontinuation on fetal status.

Intravenous fluid bolus of 1000 ml, lateral positioning, and O_2 administration at 10 L/min via non-breather facemask are (together) effective resuscitative measures to improve fetal oxygen saturation ($FSpO_2$) during labor.[25] The evidence is from patients with normal FHR, and at present it is a reasonable assumption that the findings are applicable to the non-reassuring FHR pattern.

Additional steps with the management of non-reassuring FHR tracing might include (no trials available):

- Tocomonitoring assessment for hyperstimulation.
- Cervical examination to assess rapid dilation or descent, and to ensure that the umbilical cord has not prolapsed.
- Maternal blood pressure monitoring, especially among those who have received regional anesthesia. If hypotension is present in conjunction with non-reassuring FHR pattern, ephedrine or phenylephrine may be utilized.[7]

Piracetam for non-reassuring fetal heart rate in labor

Piracetam, a derivative of γ-aminobenzoic acid, is thought to promote the metabolism of the brain cells when they are hypoxic. There is not enough evidence to evaluate the use of piracetam for NRFHT in labor. Compared with placebo, piracetam is associated with a non-significant trend to reduced need for cesarean section, and similar incidences of low Apgar scores, or neonatal respiratory problems and signs of hypoxia.[26]

Operative delivery for non-reassuring fetal heart rate in labor

There are no contemporary trials of operative vs conservative management of suspected fetal NRFHR testing. In the only old trial, there is no difference in perinatal mortality.[27]

Fetal electrocardiogram for fetal monitoring in labor

The use of the fetal electrocardiogram (ECG) has been evaluated as an adjunct to continuous electronic FHR monitoring during labor.[28] The use of internal monitoring with a scalp lead is mandatory to obtain ECG. Three studies assessed the ST segment,[29–31] whereas one the PR interval.[32]

The use of **ST** waveform analysis is associated with fewer fetal scalp samples during labor and **fewer operative** (CD and operative vaginal) deliveries. Neonatally, **fewer babies have severe metabolic acidosis at birth** (cord pH < 7.05 and base deficit > 12 mmol/L), but similar numbers have pH < 7.05 or 7.15. There is a strong trend for lower encephalopathy, and similar neonatal intensive care unit (NICU) admissions and perinatal mortality.[29,30] One recent smaller study did not observe such differences, and reported a lower incidence of fetal scalp sampling in the ST group.[31]

The use of **PR** interval analysis yields similar results to ST analysis, as it is associated with a trend towards fewer operative deliveries. There is insufficient evidence that it conveyed any benefit, which may reflect limitations of the technique or, alternatively, the smaller numbers available for analysis from the single trial.[32]

These findings (mostly in fetuses > 34 weeks old) support the use of fetal ST waveform analysis when a decision has been made to undertake continuous electronic FHR monitoring during labor. However, in most labors, technically satisfactory cardiotocographic traces can be obtained by external ultrasound monitors, which are less invasive than internal scalp electrodes (which are required for ECG analysis). The largest trial of fetal ECG analysis[29] used guidelines for clinicians that recommended no action if cardiotocography was normal, regardless of ST waveform analyses. A better approach might be to restrict fetal ST waveform analysis to those fetuses demonstrating NRFHR on FHR monitor.

Fetal pulse oximetry

A normal fetal oxygen saturation in labor is 35–65%. A fetal pulse oximetry showing $FSpO_2$ < 30% for at least > 2 minutes is associated with a higher risk for low fetal arterial pH and metabolic acidosis. The fetal oxygen sensor lies against the fetal cheek. The use of fetal pulse oximetry has been evaluated as an adjunct to continuous electronic FHR monitoring during labor.

Fetal pulse oximetry (FPO) with continuous FHR tracing is associated with a **similar overall cesarean section rate compared** to continuous FHR only.[33] There are **less cesarean and operative deliveries for non-reassuring fetal status** in the FPO plus FHR group compared with the FHR only group.[33] The only reported neonatal seizure occurred in the FHR only group. No differences are seen for endometritis, intrapartum or postpartum hemorrhage, uterine rupture, low Apgar scores, umbilical arterial pH or base excess, admission to the NICU or fetal/neonatal death.[33] No difference is seen in the overall cesarean or operative delivery rates because more CD were performed for monitoring dystocia in the FPO group. Non-reassuring fetal heart rate may predict the need for delivery by cesarean section for dystocia, despite adequate fetal oxygenation.[33] Three other trials[34–36] showed similar results, and a large trial also showed no benefit.[37] Given the above evidence, **routine use of FPO in labor is not recommended**.

References

1. Martin JA, Hamilton BE, Ventura SJ et al. Births: final data for 2002. Natl Vital Stat Rep 2003; 52(10): 1–113. [II–3].
2. National Institute of Child Health and Human Development Research Planning Workshop. Electronic fetal heart rate monitoring: research guidelines for interpretation. Am J Obstet Gynecol 1997; 177: 1385–90. [review]

3. Inappropriate use of the terms fetal distress and birth asphyxia. ACOG Committee Opinion #197, 1998. [review]

4. Chauhan SP, Magann EF, Scott JR et al. Cesarean delivery for fetal distress: rate and risk factors. Obstet Gynecol Surv 2003; 58: 337–50. [review of 392 articles published in English from 1990 to 2000]

5. Vintzileos AM, Nochimson DJ, Guzman EF et al. Intrapartum electronic fetal heart rate monitoring versus intermittent auscultation: a meta-analysis. Obstet Gynecol 1995; 85: 149–55. [meta-analysis]

6. Thacker SB, Stroup D, Chang M. Continuous electronic heart rate monitoring for fetal assessment during labor (Cochrane Review). In: Cochrane Database Syst Rev 2007, 1. [meta-analysis: 9 RCTs, n = 18 561]

7. Chauhan SP, Macones GA. ACOG Practice Bulletin Intrapartum fetal heart rate monitoring. Obstet Gynecol 2005; 105: 1161–9. [review]

8. Hundley V, Ryan M, Graham W. Assessing women's preferences for antepartum care. Birth 2001; 28: 254–63. [II–3]

9. Vandenbussche FP, De Jong-Potjer LC, Stiggelbout AM, Le Cessie S, Keirse MJ. Differences in the valuation of birth outcomes among pregnant women, mothers, and obstetricians. Birth 1999; 28: 178–83. [II–3]

10. Vintzileos AM, Nochimson DJ, Antsaklis A et al. Comparison of continuous electronic fetal heart rate monitoring versus intermittent auscultation in detecting fetal acidemia at birth. Am J Obstet Gynecol 1995; 173: 1021–4. [II–1]

11. Morrison JC, Chez BF, Davis ID et al. Intrapartum fetal heart rate assessment: monitoring by auscultation or electronic means. Am J Obstet Gynecol 1993; 168: 63–6. [II–1]

12. Phelan JP, Ahn MO. Perinatal observations in forty-eight neurologically impaired term infants. Am J Obstet Gynecol 1994; 171: 424–31. [II–3]

13. Society of Obstetricians and Gynaecologists of Canada Policy Statement. Fetal health surveillance in labour. J Soc Obstet Gynaecol Can 1995; 17: 865–901. [review]

14. Nielsen PV, Stigsby B, Nickelsen C, Nim J. Intra-and inter-observer variability in the assessment of intrapartum cardiotocograms. Acta Obstet Gynecol Scand 1987; 66: 421–4. [II–3]

15. Zain HA, Wright JW, Parrish GE, Diehl SJ. Interpreting the fetal heart rate tracing: effect of knowledge of neonatal outcome. J Reprod Med 1998; 43: 367–70. [II–3]

16. Nelson KB, Dambrosia JM, Ting TY, Grether JK. Uncertain value of electronic fetal monitoring in predicting cerebral palsy. N Engl J Med 1996; 324: 613–18. [II–2]

17. Devoe LD, McDaniel T. Visual vs. computerized analysis of FHR tracings. Cont Obstet Gynecol 2002; May: 65–80. [review]

18. Skupski DW, Rosenberg CR, Eglinton GS. Intrapartum fetal stimulation tests: a meta-analysis. Obstet Gynecol 2002; 99: 129–34 [meta-analysis: 11 studies (not RCTs)]

19. Kruger K, Hallberg B, Blennow M, Kublickas M, Westgren M. Predictive value of fetal scalp blood lactate concentration and pH markers of neurologic disability. Am J Obstet Gynecol 1999; 181: 1072–8. [II–3]

20. Hofmeyr GJ. Amnioinfusion for umbilical cord compression in labor. Cochrane Database Syst Rev 2007, 1. [meta-Analysis: 14 RCTs, most with < 200 women each]

21. Busowski J, Pendergraft JS, Parsons M, O'Brien W. Transabdominal amnioinfusion prior to induction of labor. Am J Obstet Gynecol 1995; 172: 287. [RCT, n = 31. Decreased amniotic fluid prior to induction of labor. Transabdominal amnioinfusion with 250 ml normal saline over 20 minutes under ultrasound guidance using a 22 gauge needle (n = 16), compared with no amnioinfusion (n = 15).]

22. Vergani P, Ceruti P, Strobelt N et al. Transabdominal amnioinfusion in oligohydramnios at term before induction of labor with intact membranes: a randomized clinical trial. Am J Obstet Gynecol 1996; 175: 465–70. [RCT, n = 79. Oligohydramnios (largest amniotic fluid pocket < 2 × 2 cm on perpendicular planes); no FHR abnormality. Transabdominal amnioinfusion under ultrasonographic guidance: normal saline 500 ml at 37° infused through a 20 gauge spinal needle at 30 ml per minute. Sulbactam–ampicillin 3 g given intravenously (n = 39). Compared with no amnioinfusion (n = 40).]

23. Kulier R, Hofmeyr GJ. Tocolytics for suspected intrapartum fetal distress. Cochrane Database Syst Rev 2007; 1. [meta-analysis: 3 RCTs, n = 103]

24. Magann EF, Cleveland RS, Dockery JR et al. Acute tocolysis for fetal distress: terbutaline versus magnesium sulphate. Aust N Z J Obstet Gynecol 1993; 33: 362–4. [RCT, n = 46]

25. Simpson KR, James DC. Efficacy of intrauterine resuscitation techniques in improving fetal oxygen status during labor. Obstet Gynecol 2005; 105: 1362–8. [RCT, n = 56]

26. Huaman EJ, Hassoun R, Itahashi CM, Pereda GJ, Mejia MA. Results obtained with piracetam in foetal distress during labour. J In Med Res 1983; 11: 129–36. [RCT, n = 96. Lima, Peru. Fetal distress: meconium-stained amniotic fluid and/or pathological fetal heart rate pattern. Piracetam (n = 48) vs placebo (n = 48), intravenously 6 ampoules at once and 2 ampoules hourly.]

27. Walker N. A case for conservatism in management of foetal distress. Br Med J 1959; 2: 1221–6. [RCT, n = 350. Fetal distress = meconium-stained liquor; fetal heart rate below 110/min, above 160/min, or irregular. Drawn envelop from drum for either operative delivery or expectant management.]

28. Neilson JP. Fetal electrocardiogram (ECG) for fetal monitoring during labour. Cochrane Database Syst Rev 2007; 1. [meta-analysis: 3 RCTs (good quality), n = 8357]

29. Amer-Wahlin I, Hellsten C, Noren H et al. Cardiotocography only versus cardiotocography plus ST analysis of fetal electrocardiogram for intrapartum fetal monitoring: a Swedish randomised controlled trial. Lancet 2001; 358: 534–8. [RCT, n = 4966. CTG plus ST analysis of fetal ECG (2519 women) vs CTG alone (2477). The monitoring device was the STAN S21 (Neoventa Medical, Gothenburg) which incorporates an 'expert system' to provide advice to clinical staff. In this, it constitutes a technically more advanced system than used in the Westgate 1993 trial.]

30. Westgate J, Harris M, Curnow JSH, Greene KR. Plymouth randomized trial of cardiotocogram only vs ST waveform plus cardiotocogram for intrapartum monitoring in 2400 cases. Am J Obstet and Gynecol 1993; 169: 1151–60. [RCT, n = 2434]

31. Ojala K, Vaarasmaki M, Makikallio K, Valkama M, Tekay A. A comparison of intrapartum automated fetal electrocardiography and conventional cardiography – a randomized controlled study. Br J Obstet Gynecol 2006; 113: 419–23. [RCT, n = 1483]

32. Strachan BK, van Wijngaarden WJ, Sahota D, Chang A, James DK, for the FECG Study Group. Cardiotocography only versus cardiotocography plus PR-interval analysis in intrapartum surveillance: a randomised, multicentre trial. Lancet 2000; 355: 456–9. [RCT, n = 957]

33. Garite TJ, Dildy GA, McNamara H et al. A multicenter controlled trial of fetal pulse oximetry in the intrapartum managment of nonreassuring fetal heart rate patterns. Am J Obstet and Gynecol 2000; 183(5): 1049–58. [RCT, n = 1010. Control group: fetal heart rate monitoring (CTG) (Doppler/fetal scalp electrode). Study group: CTG plus fetal pulse oximetry. Protocol for action with reassuring and non-reassuring fetal oximetry values.]

34. Kuhnert M, Schmidt S. Intrapartum management of nonreassuring fetal heart rate patterns: a randomized controlled trial of fetal pulse oximetry. Am J Obstet Gynecol 2004; 191: 1989–95. [RCT, n = 146]

35. Klauser CK, Christensen EE, Chauhan SP et al. Use of fetal pulse oximetry among high-risk women in labor: a randomized clinical trial. Am J Obstet Gynecol 2005; 192: 1810–1. [RCT, n = 360]

36. East CE, Brennecke SP, King JK et al. The effect of intrapartum fetal pulse oximetry, in the presence of nonreassuring fetal heart pattern, on operative delivery rates: a multicenter, randomized, controlled trial (the FOREMOST trial). Am J Obstet Gynecol 2006; 194: 606–16. [RCT, n = 600]

37. Bloom SL, for the NICHD MFMU Network. The MFMU Network randomized trial of fetal pulse oxymetry. Am J Obstet Gynecol 2005; 193: S2. [RCT, n = 5341 – abstract]

10

Analgesia and anesthesia in pregnancy

Rolf Alexander Schlichter and Valerie A Arkoosh

KEY POINTS

- In every hospital providing labor and delivery services, anesthesia personnel have to be available on a 24-hour basis, with the ability to perform a cesarean delivery (CD) within 30 minutes from decision, and at least one qualified anesthesiologist responsible.
- Not all laboring women desire the services of an anesthesiologist.
- Intravenous pain relief is much inferior to neuraxial analgesia, is minimally effective, and is associated with several maternal and fetal/neonatal side effects.
- Neuraxial analgesia provides the best pain relief in labor, and should be available to all laboring women upon request.
- It is not necessary to obtain a platelet count before neuroaxial analgesia. If known, women with platelet counts of $\geq 100\,000/mm^3$ can safely receive neuraxial analgesia. Women with platelet counts of $50\,000$ to $99\,000/mm^3$ are potential candidates for neuroaxial analgesia.
- As there seems to be no benefit from delaying an epidural, the decision of when to place epidural analgesia should be made individually with each woman.
- An epidural is associated with several obstetric effects, such as a 23 minute longer first and 16 minute longer second stages of labor, as well as increased use of oxytocin augmentation, a trend for increased incidence of fetal malposition, an increased risk of instrumental vaginal birth, and a strong trend for increased incidence of CD for non-reassuring fetal heart rate (NRFHR) testing.
- An epidural is also associated with increased risk of fever, hypotension, and urinary retention.
- Women should be counseled about these risks before labor.
- Neuraxial analgesia complications also include hypotension, postdural headache, hematoma, and respiratory depression from opioid use.
- Discontinuation of an epidural late in labor does not prevent obstetric effects of the epidural.
- Use of low doses of anesthetic, prophylactic prehydration, and ephedrine can decrease the incidences of hypotension and consequent NRFHR testing.
- Compared with the standard epidural approach, combined spinal epidural (CSE) has been shown to produce a quicker (by about 6 minutes) onset of analgesia, to result in a lower total dose of local anesthetic over the course of the labor, to achieve a lower median visual analog pain score earlier in labor, to increase the incidence of maternal satisfaction, to have a lower incidence of incomplete block, and possibly lower incidence of instrument-assisted deliveries, but more pruritus.
- For CD, neuraxial is the analgesia of choice. Spinal (intrathecal) anesthesia is more advantageous over epidural due to its association with quicker onset of adequate analgesia. Other advantages cited are its simplicity, lower drug doses, and superior abdominal muscle relaxation. Compared with an epidural, the spinal technique is associated with a similar failure rate, need for additional intraoperative analgesia, need for conversion to general anesthesia intraoperatively, maternal satisfaction, need for postoperative pain relief, and neonatal intervention.
- Hypotension following spinal analgesia for CD can be decreased by crystalloid or colloid administration, ephedrine or phenylephrine, and lower limb compression.
- General anesthesia for CD should be avoided if at all possible, as it is associated with a threefold risk of maternal death compared with neuraxial analgesia. The biggest risk is being unable to intubate or ventilate the patient. There are no evident advantages to general anesthesia in the absence of a contraindication to a neuraxial approach.

History

In 1847 Dr Simpson first administered ether to a woman during childbirth. The practice of obstetric anesthesia has changed markedly since. In 2004, about 60% (2.4 million) of laboring US women chose and received an epidural or combined spinal–epidural. Women in labor now receive analgesia rather than anesthesia, with the goal of enabling maternal mobility during labor. Refined anesthetic techniques for women requiring cesarean delivery (CD) have decreased substantially the number of maternal deaths directly related to anesthesia.

Definitions

Analgesia: From the Greek for 'no pain': partial or complete relief of pain sensation (absence of sensitivity to pain) without loss of consciousness.

Anesthesia: From the Greek for 'no sensation': historically defined as loss of sensation and total/partial consciousness.

Recently, the distinction between the definitions of analgesia and anesthesia has not been maintained, with these two terms used interchangeably.

General comments

Labor is associated with two sources of pain: visceral pain at T-10 through L-1 from uterine contractions and cervical dilatation, and somatic pain transmitted by the pudendal nerve at S2 through S4 from descend and consequent pressure of the fetal head on pelvic floor, vagina, and perineum.[1] This pain is amenable to safe intervention. **While not all laboring women desire the services of an anesthesiologist, maternal request is a sufficient medical indication for pain relief in labor.**

Pregnant women have a unique physiology compared with the general population. After the first trimester, they are at increased risk for aspiration of gastric contents, have decreased oxygen reserve, and are much more likely to be difficult to intubate than a non-pregnant woman. Pregnant patients should be positioned with left uterine displacement when supine after about 22–24 weeks of gestation. Left uterine displacement prevents aortocaval compression, which can result in a marked decrease in venous return to the heart and a subsequent drop in cardiac output. The ability to compensate for aortocaval compression is compromised in the presence of neuraxial analgesia or anesthesia. When considering anesthesia or analgesia, one must take into account that pregnant women are more sensitive to sedative hypnotics, local anesthetics, and the inhaled anesthetic agents than non-pregnant women. Maternal mortality associated with general anesthesia is estimated at approximately 32 per 1 000 000 live births vs 1.9 per 1 000 000 live births for neuraxial analgesia.[1] Also, the pregnant patient is, in reality, two patients and occasionally the needs of one must be prioritized over the other. An informed consent should be attempted even in case of an emergency, and the patient's wishes for an unmedicated birth always respected.

Hospitals providing labor and delivery services should have anesthesia personnel available on a 24-hour basis, with the ability to perform a CD within 30 minutes from decision.[2] Availability of licensed practitioners to administer anesthetics and support vital functions in emergencies, and of at least one qualified anesthesiologist responsible for all anesthetics administered, is recommended.[2] Breastfeeding is not affected by the choice of anesthesia.

LABOR ANALGESIA

Non-neuraxial labor analgesia

Systemic analgesia

Opioids (intravenous/intramuscular)

Numerous choices exist for systemic analgesia during the first stage of labor, including intravenous (IV) meperidine, buprenorphine (Buprenex), butorphanol (Stadol), or nalbuphine (Nubain), which are all opioid agonist–antagonists, as well as pentazocine, fentanyl (Duragesic), morphine, hydromorphone, oxycodone, their derivatives, or other opioids. Characteristics of some of these drugs are shown in Table 10.1.

Efficacy: These drugs are similarly efficacious, or better stated, similarly minimally efficacious in relief of maternal labor pain. **Compared with placebo, meperidine (Demerol) 100 mg intramuscular (IM) in early labor is associated with a very modest** (17 mm) **reduction in** visual analogue scale (VAS) **pain score at 30 minutes.**[3,4] Request for epidural is delayed to 232 compared with 75 minutes, with no further analgesia in 32 vs 4% of women in one small study.[4] Satisfaction despite more sedation, nausea, and vomiting is more common with meperidine, whereas neonatal outcomes are similar.[4]

There is not enough evidence to evaluate the comparative efficacy of the various opioids used for analgesia in labor. There are problems with methodological quality of some of the trials, and lack of consistency in the way various outcomes were reported. For instance, maternal pain relief is sometimes reported on a VAS, sometimes using a variety of categorical scoring systems, at different time points after drug administration, sometimes considered change from baseline, etc. There is no evidence of a difference between **meperidine** (Demerol) and **tramadol** (Ultram) in terms of pain relief, interval to delivery, or instrumental or operative delivery. Maternal pain relief seems almost identical between the meptazinol and meperidine groups, whether assessed as maternal satisfaction with pain relief, VAS, or use of other pain relief. Maternal satisfaction with pain relief appears similar for **pentazocine** (Talwin) and meperidine.[3] Compered with neuraxial analgesic techniques, systemic medications are much less effective at decreasing VAS pain scores, with minimal decrease in pain scores (see below).

Safety: There is not enough evidence to evaluate the comparative safety of the various opioids used for analgesia

Table 10.1 *Intravenous (IV) or intramuscular (IM) opioid agents for maternal pain relief in labor*

Agent	Usual dose	Frequency (every hour)	Onset (minutes)	Neonatal half-life (hours)*
Tramadol	50–100 mg IM or IV	4	1 (IV)	7
Pentazocine	30–60 mg IV or IM	3–4	1–5	N/A
Meperidine	25–50 mg IV	1–2	5	13–22
	50–100 mg IM	2–4	30–45	>60
Fentanyl	50–100 µg IV	1	1	5
Nalbuphine	10 mg IV or IM	3	2–3 (IV)	4
			15 (IM)	
Butorphanol	1–2 mg IV or IM	4	1–2 (IV)	4
			10–30 (IM)	
Morphine	2–5 mg IV	4	5 (IV)	7
	10 mg IM		30–40 (IM)	

Adapted from ACOG.[*] Does not include metabolites.

in labor. Common side effects include maternal sedation, nausea, hypotension, respiratory depression, and potential for neonatal respiratory depression. There appeared to be more adverse effects such as maternal nausea and vomiting and drowsiness with meptazinol compared to meperidine, and even less with **tramadol or pentazocine** compared with meperidine,[3] making these last two agents the ones with best evidence of **most efficacy and least side effects of the overall inefficacious opioid analgesic agents**.

Intravenous opioids cross the placenta and can affect the fetus/neonate. Intravenous opioids are associated with **increased incidence of non-reassuring fetal heart rate (NRFHR), lower fetal base excess, and decreased fetal respirations and tone at birth** when compared with neuraxial anesthesia. Drugs with active metabolites, such as meperidine/normeperidine, are associated with more prolonged neonatal sedation. Agonist–antagonists such as nalbuphine can result in both cardiac and respiratory depression in the baby, although there are no outcome data that show adverse outcomes. Naloxone, used preferably intravenously for fast action, is a pure opioid antagonist, and is the drug of choice in treatment of maternal or neonatal respiratory and neurobehavioral depression secondary to opioid agonist agents. Repeated doses might be necessary, but excess use can be associated with neonatal withdrawal seizures.

Regional blocks

First stage

Pain from cervical dilation (but not uterine contractions) can be blocked by a **paracervical block**. There are **no trials** to assess the effectiveness of paracervical block in labor. Risks include local anesthetic toxicity, IV injection, or fetal injection, and a strong association with fetal bradycardia.

In women with severe lower back pain, four **injections in the lumbar–sacral region of sterile water**, either 0.1 ml intracutaneously or 0.5 ml subcutaneously, are effective in reducing severe back pain.[5]

Second stage

During the second stage of labor, perineal pain (e.g. for episiotomies) can be blocked with a **pudendal block**. There are **no trials** to assess the effectiveness of pudendal block in labor. There is a small risk of local anesthetic toxicity due to accidental IV injection.

Neuraxial (regional) analgesia (epidural, spinal, or combined spinal epidural)

Overview of techniques

Neuraxial labor analgesia is also commonly called regional analgesia. It can be provided via the epidural space, the intrathecal (spinal) space, or both – combined spinal epidural (CSE).

Medications injected into the epidural space have a relatively slow analgesic onset of 8–15 minutes. Block height is determined by the volume of medication injected into the epidural space. For example, to achieve a dermatome level of T10 to L2 for early labor analgesia a volume of 8–10 ml is usually sufficient, contrasted with 20–25 ml to achieve a block height of T4 for cesarean delivery. In the epidural space, injecting low-concentration local anesthetic produces analgesia and injecting high-concentration local anesthetic produces anesthesia.

By contrast, medications injected into the intrathecal space have a quick onset of 2–5 minutes. Block height is determined

Epidural analgesia

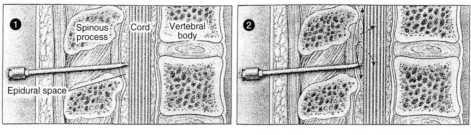

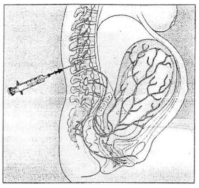

Combined spinal–epidural analgesia

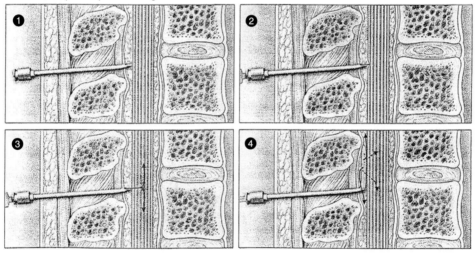

Figure 10.1

Techniques of neuraxial analgesia. Reproduced with permission, from Eltzschig HK, Lieberman ES, Camann WR. Medical Progress: Regional anesthesia and analgesia for labor and delivery. NEJM 2003; 348: 319–32. Copyright © 2003 Massachusetts Medical Society. All rights reserved.

Epidural analgesia (Panel A) is achieved by placement of a catheter into the lumbar epidural space (1). After the desired intervertebral space (e.g., between L3 and L4) has been identified and infiltrated with local anesthetic, a hollow epidural needle is placed in the intervertebral ligaments. These ligaments are characterized by a high degree of resistance to penetration. A syringe connected to the epidural needle allows the anesthesiologist to confirm the resistance of these ligaments. In contrast, the epidural space has a low degree of resistance. When the anesthesiologist slowly advances the needle while feeling for resistance, he or she recognizes the epidural space by a sudden loss of resistance as the epidural needle enters the epidural space (2). Next, an epidural catheter is advanced into the space. Solutions of a local anesthetic, opioids, or a combination of the two can now be administered through the catherer.

For combined spinal–epidural analgesia (Panel B), the lumbar epidural space is also identified with an epidural needle (1). Next, a very thin spinal needle is introduced through the epidural needle into the subarachnoid space. (2). Correct placement can be confirmed by free flow of cerebrospinal fluid. A single bolus of local anesthetic, opioid, or a combination of the two is injected through the needle into the subarachnoid space (3). Subsequently, the needle is removed, and a catheter is advanced into the epidural space through the epidural needle (4). When the single-shot spinal analgesic wears off, the epidural catheter can be used for the continuation of pain relief.

primarily by the baricity (density relative to cerebrospinal fluid [CSF]) of the injectate and, to some extent, the total volume of drug. Intrathecal analgesia is produced when small doses of local anesthetic are injected (i.e. bupivacaine 2.5 mg for labor analgesia), whereas anesthesia is produced with higher doses (i.e. bupivacaine 15 mg for CD anesthesia).

Epidural analgesia

Technique

The epidural space is located using a special needle and a loss of resistance (to air or saline) technique (Figure 10.1). A one-time injection (e.g. a caudal block) is rarely used; instead, a small catheter is placed into the epidural space through which local anesthetics and opioids can be either bolused or given as a continuous infusion.

Local anesthetics used include low-concentration bupivacaine, ropivacaine, or lidocaine. Opioids can be used alone, but are more often combined with local anesthetics. The semisynthetic opioids fentanyl and sufentanil are used most commonly. Their addition to local anesthetics produces an additive effect that results in a lower concentration of local anesthetic, producing adequate labor analgesia. A lower concentration of local anesthetic increases maternal mobility and decreases the potential for maternal toxicity. There is insufficient evidence on concentrations, type of anesthetic used, and several other technical aspects of epidural anesthesia in labor.[6]

The infusion rate can be either controlled by the anesthesiologist or the patient. **Patient-controlled epidural analgesia** (PCEA) typically employs a background infusion of local anesthetic and opioid coupled with the ability of the parturient to augment the infusion with a bolus dose every 10–15 minutes. This technique can also be used with a spinal catheter with appropriately reduced doses.

Indications

The primary indication for epidural analgesia is maternal request during labor.[1] Other indications may include prophylaxis against autonomic hyperreflexia in the woman with a high spinal cord lesion, anticipated difficulty in intubation, history of malignant hyperthermia, high risk for cesarean delivery, or the presence of a comorbidity that would benefit from the reduced catecholamine levels produced by adequate labor analgesia (e.g. selected respiratory or cardiac disease). Functioning epidural catheters can also be used to provide anesthesia for instrument delivery and extraction of a retained placenta. PCEA is very useful for patients laboring for an extended period of time. Additionally, it can be used as a manpower extender for a busy obstetric anesthesia service.

Efficacy and advantages

Compared with no analgesia or to opioids, epidural analgesia offers **much better pain relief**.[6] In >85% of cases, the pain relief is optimal. **As labor results in severe pain for many women, and epidural is the best intervention to decrease and even eliminate this pain, it should be offered when available to all women in labor. Maternal request is a sufficient justification for pain relief during labor.**[6]

Epidural analgesia is associated with **similar incidences** of **short- or long-term backache**, and **maternal satisfaction with pain relief.** Compared with systemic opioids, epidural analgesia is associated with **less incidence of neonatal pH < 7.20**, and **similar incidence of low neonatal Apgar scores at 5 minutes**.[6] Neuraxial analgesia is the least depressant method of analgesia for the fetus/neonate, except for maternal fever and subsequent increased incidence of neonatal sepsis work-ups, with no difference in the rate of neonatal infection or sepsis. In centers with structured protocols for neonatal sepsis work-ups, there are no increases in the incidence of neonatal sepsis work-ups in babies born to mothers with epidural analgesia.

There are several other advantages to epidural anesthesia. With an indwelling catheter, the block can be maintained indefinitely by intermittent injections, with a continuous infusion, or both. Modern low-dose epidural management techniques result in less impact on obstetric outcome and are least depressing for the fetus.[6]

There is insufficient evidence to assess if **delay of epidural** to more active labor and more advanced cervical dilatation reduces some of these risks. Data suggest that neuraxial analgesia can be offered as early as 2 cm without adversely affecting labor outcome or incidence of CD. Epidural at ≤2–5 cm is associated with similar maternal (instrumental delivery, CD, etc.) and neonatal outcomes compared with epidural at ≥3–5 cm or after initial narcotics in women in spontaneous labor or receiving oxytocin.[7–11] Therefore, **the decision of when to place epidural analgesia should be made individually with each woman, with relief of real pain when requested by the woman.**[1]

PCEA gives the woman control over her analgesia. Patients receive less local anesthetic overall (and therefore less motor blockade) and receive less 'top offs' (manual boluses from the anesthesiologists).[12] As patient satisfaction is high with epidural analgesia, PCEA is not associated with additional clinical or satisfaction benefits.

Safety, disadvantages, and complications

Compared with non-epidural analgesia, epidural analgesia is associated with obstetric effects, such as **a 23 minutes longer first and 16 minutes longer second stages of labor**, as well as increased use of **oxytocin** augmentation, and a trend for increased incidence of **fetal malposition**.[6] Epidural analgesia is also associated with an **increased risk of instrumental vaginal birth**. While the incidence of CD is similar, **epidural analgesia is associated with** a strong trend for 42% **increased incidence of CD for NRFHR testing.**

Epidural is associated with increased risk of **fever, hypotension,** and **urinary retention.**[6]

Although the risk of long-term backache is similar to controls, it is quite common for a woman to experience soreness or tenderness at the site of epidural insertion for 2–3 days. No studies report on rare but potentially serious adverse effects of epidural analgesia. Increased operative vaginal deliveries have been implicated in the possible increased rate of third- and fourth-degree perineal lacerations associated with epidural analgesia. The increase in maternal fever is associated with increases in maternal and neonatal antibiotic treatments, as well as neonatal sepsis evaluations. Women should be counseled about these risks before labor.

Disadvantages of epidural analgesia include a slower onset compared with intrathecal (spinal) injection, incomplete blockade of pain (in about 10–15% of patients), and inadvertent intrathecal or intravascular catheter placement. While the PCEA gives the patient more control and entails less intervention from anesthesiologists, this can lead to underdosing and therefore inadequate analgesia: for example, if the patient does not bolus herself (if she is asleep), or if there is a pump malfunction and the anesthesiologist is not immediately available.

Maternal **hypotension** following regional analgesia can occur frequently, and can affect both mothers and their babies. Maternal hypotension from neuraxial analgesia is associated with increased incidence of NRFHR testing, at times (1–2%) necessitating CD after neuraxial analgesia. Left uterine displacement might increase uterine perfusion. Prophylactic measures such as preloading with IV fluids and ephedrine have been studied in trials (see below).

Other complications include **postdural puncture headache** following accidental lumbar puncture, **hematoma, respiratory arrest** due to accidental intrathecal opioids, systemic local anesthetic toxicity due to unrecognized IV injection, or total spinal anesthesia from an unrecognized intrathecal injection of a dose of drug meant for the epidural space. See under spinal analgesia and anesthesia emergencies for further details on these effects and their prevention and treatment.

Interventions to avoid some disadvantages and complications of epidural analgesia

Obstetrical effects (discontinuation of epidural analgesia late in labor): Discontinuation of epidural analgesia late in labor (usually 8 cm or start of second stage) is not associated with a reduction in instrumental delivery rate (23 vs 28%) or other delivery outcomes, including CD (6 vs 6%).[12] The only statistically significant difference is an **increase in inadequate pain relief when the epidural is stopped** (22% vs 6%). Duration of the second stage is nonsignificantly shorter by 6 minutes. There are insufficient data to assess neonatal outcome, but rates of low pH are similar.[13]

Hypotension (preloading with IV fluids before epidural): Preloading with IV fluids (usually 500–1000 ml, or weight-based formula) prior to traditional high-dose local anesthetic blocks may have some beneficial fetal and maternal effects in healthy women.[13] Low-dose epidural and CSE analgesia techniques may reduce the need for preloading. Using **high-dose** local anesthetic, preloading with IV fluids is associated with much lower incidence of hypotension compared with traditional epidural analgesia (2 vs 28%) and a reduction in fetal heart rate abnormalities in a small trial.[14] No differences are detected in other perinatal and maternal outcomes. Using the now recommended **low-dose** anesthetic for epidural, preloading with IV fluids is associated with **no significant difference in maternal hypotension,** although only a very large effect was excluded. There is a **trend for less fetal heart rate abnormalities.**[14] There are no differences in mode of delivery, but the data are insufficient for a definite assessment.

Hypotension (prophylactic ephedrine to prevent NRFHR after epidural): Compared to with ephedrine, ephedrine 10 mg IV, followed by 20 mg continuous infusion over 60 minutes, started in the first minutes after the epidural test dose, significantly **decreases the incidence of NRFHR testing** from 15 to 3%.[15]

Spinal analgesia
Technique

Using a small-bore spinal needle (typically a pencil point-type needle that minimizes trauma to the dura and thus reduces the incidence of postdural puncture headache [PDPH]), a dural puncture is made and proper location confirmed by CSF aspiration (see Figure 10.1). A single injection of an analgesic dose (much less than for epidural analgesia) of bupivacaine, ropivacaine, or lidocaine is administered. Generally, an opioid such as fentanyl, sufentanil, or morphine is used alone or in combination with the local anesthetic.

Indications

Indications for single injection spinal analgesia for labor include labor where delivery is imminent, forceps deliveries in women without epidurals, and for patients with retained placentas.

Advantages

Advantages for single injection spinals include ease and speed of onset, completeness of block, and lower incidence of PDPH.

Disadvantages and complications

Disadvantages for single injection spinals are inability to re-dose (which can be solved with a spinal catheter or combined spinal epidural).

Postdural puncture headache can occur after 1–2% of either spinal or CSE analgesia. This low incidence of PDPH occurs when using the small-gauge pencil point needles. PDPH is believed to be caused by leak of CSF from punctured dura. The leak of CSF and subsequent decreased spinal CSF pressure lead to downward traction or stretch on the meninges, with resulting symptoms. PDPH is characterized by a frontal-occipital headache that is exacerbated by being upright (gravity worsening stretch on the meninges), improving when the patient is supine. Diploplia, tinnitus, nausea, and vomiting (from stretch on the cranial nerves) are also common. Remaining supine, hydration, caffeine, and increased abdominal pressures (e.g. from a binder) can improve symptoms. Untreated, the symptoms usually last for about 7–10 days but can persist to 4 weeks, and for some for a few months.

There are no trials for interventions to prevent or treat this complication. Usual early interventions include analgesics, supine positioning, caffeine and hydration. In about one-third of cases, the headache persists and is severe enough to require a blood patch procedure. A blood patch is performed by drawing 15–20 ml of the patient's blood and sterilely injecting it into the patient's epidural space at the level of the dural puncture. Resolution of symptoms with blood patch occurs in 70–90% of women. Side effects usually include back ache and leg pain.[16]

Respiratory depression or arrest due to intrathecal opioids occurs rarely, 1 in 5000 to 10000 patients. Naloxone reverses this complication and should be readily available, along with airway management equipment when performing labor analgesia. Patients with spinal catheters should have clearly labeled catheters so that accidental injections of epidural doses of local anesthetics aren't given intrathecally.

Hematoma after epidural or spinal analgesia is rare. A routine platelet count is not necessary before these procedures. Indications for platelet count may include severe preeclampsia, idiopathic thrombocytopenic purpura (ITP), abruption, or other risks for disseminated intravascular coagulation (DIC). A plalelet count of $\geq 100\,000/mm^3$ is safe, but several studies have also confirmed that a level of platelets of 50 000 to 99 000/mm³ is not associated with higher risk of complications.[1] Women on prophylactic unfractionated heparin or low-dose aspirin are not at increased risk for complications from regional anesthesia. Women on therapeutic unfractionated heparin can receive regional analgesia if the activated partial thromboplastin time (pTT) is normal. Women on low molecular weight heparin should not receive regional analgesia until 12–24 hours from the last dose, given a higher rate of hematomas with placement within this period. Therefore, it might be reasonable to convert women necessitating anticoagulation from low molecular weight heparin to unfractionated heparin as they approach term.

Combined spinal epidural
Technique

The anesthesiologist first identifies the epidural space. Then, a small-bore spinal needle, 1 cm longer than the epidural needle, is placed through the epidural needle into the CSF (Figure 10.1). An intrathecal dose of local anesthetic and opioids is injected through the spinal needle, which is then removed, leaving the epidural needle in place. An epidural catheter is inserted and an epidural local anesthetic and opioid infusion is started. The intrathecal dose generally lasts about 2 hours, at which point, the epidural infusion should be providing adequate analgesia.

In some cases an epidural catheter can be intentionally inserted into the intrathecal space to provide continuous spinal analgesia. However, the resulting PDPH incidence may be high. Nonetheless, this risk is acceptable in certain situations, such as the severely morbidly obese parturient with an extremely difficult or impossible airway for intubation or following an inadvertent dural puncture during a difficult epidural placement.

Indications

A CSE technique can be chosen to initiate analgesia; it provides the benefit of the immediate onset of spinal analgesia coupled with the indefinite duration of an epidural catheter technique. The CSE technique is particularly useful for women in advanced labor requesting pain relief. Indications for a CSE are the same as those for both epidural and spinal techniques.

Advantages

Both CSE and epidural techniques are shown to provide effective pain relief in labor. There is no standard CSE (or epidural) technique. The type and concentration of drugs used in the CSE or epidural technique appear more relevant with regards to mobilization and other outcomes than the technique itself.[17]

Compared with the standard epidural approach, CSE has been shown to **produce a quicker** (by about 6 minutes) **onset of analgesia, to result in a lower total dose of local anesthetic over the course of the labor, to achieve a lower median VAS pain score earlier in labor, to increase the incidence of maternal satisfaction, to have a lower incidence of incomplete block, and possibly lower the incidence of instrument-assisted deliveries.**[6,17] There are similar incidences of ambulation in labor, CD, PDPH or blood patch, hypotension, urinary retention, or neonatal outcomes such as umbilical artery pH, Apgar scores, and admission of babies to the neonatal unit compared with epidural anesthesia.[6,17]

Disadvantages

Disadvantages are similar to epidural and spinal techniques. With limited data, no differences are reported between pre-loading and no preloading groups to prevent hypotension.[14] It is not possible to draw any meaningful conclusions regarding rare complications such as nerve injury and meningitis. CSE women experience **more pruritus** than with epidural.[17] Pruritus is very common after spinal or epidural opioids. There are no trials on prevention or treatment of pruritus from neuraxial injection. Either naloxone or nalbuphine are effective interventions, as can be Benadryl (diphenhydramine) or other antipruritus drugs.

Contraindications for regional anesthesia

Coagulopathy

Parturients with *h*emolysis, *e*levated *l*iver enzymes, and *l*ow *p*latelets (HELLP) syndrome should be cautiously evaluated before starting regional anesthesia, the concern being the potential for epidural or subdural hematoma formation secondary to trauma from the needle. As stated above under hematoma, although there are no data to support absolute platelet numbers, patients with platelet counts of $100\,000/mm^3$ are acceptable candidates, whereas a platelet count of $<50\,000/mm^3$ is an absolute contraindication.[18] However, parturients with platelet counts $<50\,000/mm^3$ have safely received neuraxial analgesia and anesthesia. A risk–benefit assessment must be performed on any pregnant woman with a platelet count $<50\,000/mm^3$ and an individualized decision reached. It is important to remember that the risks of general anesthesia in pregnant women are substantial compared to those in non-pregnant women. Patients with platelets $<100\,000/mm^3$ should be examined for stigmata of coagulopathy (easy bruising, bleeding from the IV site, etc.) before instrumentation. A prothrombin time, a partial thrombin time, and a platelet count should all be reviewed before proceeding. A fibrinogen level and a D-dimer level are useful to assess the patient for the presence of DIC if any of the aforementioned tests are abnormal. A bleeding time is not indicated. Patients with known platelet dysfunction, including those on antiplatelet medication (e.g. clopidogrel), should not receive regional analgesia. Aspirin therapy is considered an acceptable risk.

Parturients on long-acting anticoagulants – e.g. for deep vein thrombosis (DVT) prophylaxis or heart valves, etc. – should be converted from their long-acting therapies (e.g. low molecular weight heparin) to subcutaneous heparin at 36 weeks gestational age. A patient on low molecular weight heparin who presents in labor must wait a minimum of 12–24 hours from the last dose before a neuraxial technique can be contemplated. Subcutaneous unfractionated prophylactic heparin is usually not a contraindication to regional anesthesia.

Infection

Systemic: Patients with suspected meningitis (bacterial or viral) or sepsis should not receive neuraxial blockade. Patients with suspected chorioamnionitis can receive regional blockade following the administration of appropriate intravenous antibiotics. HIV/AIDS is not a contraindication to spinal or epidural anesthesia.

Localized: Patients with localized skin or soft tissue infections should not be instrumented at those sites.

Anesthesia and maternal comorbidities
Hypertensive disorders
Advantages of analgesia

Patients with gestational hypertension may benefit from epidural analgesia, as it may improve uterine perfusion through several pathways (localized neuraxial vasodilatory effect, reduced catecholamine release). Epidural analgesia is the analgesia of choice in hypertensive pregnant women (see also Chapter 1 in *Maternal–Fetal Evidence Based Guidelines*).

Disadvantages

Patients with gestational hypertension, pre-eclampsia, and eclampsia are at increased risk for hemodynamic instability during both labor and surgical anesthesia. Some, but not all, studies, have found a higher incidence of hypotension in parturients receiving a spinal vs epidural. Methods to prevent hypotension as described above should be employed.

Cautions

Caution must be taken in fluid management in this population, as there is altered vascular leaking, decreased oncotic pressure, and a higher incidence of pulmonary edema. Also, there can be an exaggerated hypertensive response to ephedrine and phenylephrine. The prevention, rather than treatment, of hypotension has been associated with better outcomes for the fetus. Women with severe pre-eclampsia who must undergo general anesthesia are at risk for an extremely exaggerated hypertensive response to intubation and often benefit from pretreatment with an antihypertensive such as labetalol immediately prior to induction. Treatment with magnesium sulfate for preeclampsia/eclampsia can potentiate neuromuscular blockade in patients receiving general anesthesia, so care must be taken in women using intermediate to long-acting non-depolarizing muscle relaxants.

Maternal cardiac disease

Heart disease in the parturient is the leading cause of maternal mortality outside of obstetric complications. Understandably, the risk increases with severity of maternal disease. The normal changes in maternal cardiac physiology can either unmask subclinical or worsen clinical cardiac disease in women (see also Chapter 2 in *Maternal–Fetal Evidence Based Guidelines*).

Valvular heart disease

Women with acquired valvular disease (rheumatic fever, mitral valve prolapse, artificial valves, and endocarditis) are at increased risk for arrhythmias, pulmonary edema, and increases in maternal cardiac ischemia from the increased cardiac output, metabolic demand, and decreased oxygen reserve associated with pregnancy. Patients with arrhythmias or artificial valves may also be on heparin or low molecular weight heparin.

Advantages of neuraxial analgesia: Epidurals (and CSE) block the pain and stress of contractions, therefore reducing tachycardia and increased cardiac output. Ablation of bearing down reflex can be advantageous in patients with aortic or mitral regurgitation.

Disadvantages: Hypotension is the largest disadvantage with neuraxial analgesia; the transient hypotension can lead to coronary hypoperfusion, ischemia, arrhythmias, even arrest. This is especially dangerous in patients with moderate to severe aortic stenosis. However, parturients with aortic stenosis have safely undergone both neuraxial labor analgesia and anesthesia for cesarean delivery. Meticulous anesthetic technique and adequate time to slowly administer the medication is the key to safe provision of neuraxial anesthesia in these patients. Intravenous injection of local anesthetics is also a significant risk in patients with underlying arrhythmias due to impairment of cardiac automaticity and conduction (especially with bupivacaine).

Congenital heart disease

Women with congenital heart disease (e.g. tetralogy of Fallot and septal defects) are now surviving to childbearing years.

Depending upon the adequacy of their surgical repair, pregnancy may or may not severely complicate those patients with underlying cyanotic heart disease. The increased cardiac output, oxygen consumption, changes in systemic and pulmonary resistance, and aortocaval compression can exacerbate pre-existing right to left shunts, increasing the risk of maternal cyanosis and death.

Advantages of epidural analgesia: Although the hypotension of spinal anesthesia can be associated with risk of shunting and cyanosis, slowly administered epidural analgesia generally is advantageous to these patients by reducing catecholamine levels and preventing maternal expulsive reflexes. Additionally, if an instrumented or cesarean delivery is required, a surgical anesthetic level can be slowly produced, avoiding the risks of general anesthesia in these patients.

Disadvantages: The largest disadvantage of neuraxial analgesia is the risk of hypotension.

Previous lumbar surgery

Previous lumbar surgery (e.g. diskectomy, placement of Harrington rods) is not a contraindication for lumbar epidural or spinal analgesia or anesthesia. Successful block can be achieved, although at a lower rate (55%) than in the control population. There were no cases of spine infection, low back pain, or headaches.[19]

CESAREAN DELIVERY ANESTHESIA

Neuraxial anesthesia

Epidural

Indications

Patients with existing labor epidurals can have their level extended cephalad using a larger volume of high-concentration local anesthetic, opioids, and epinephrine (which is thought to act at α_2-receptors in the spine). For cesarean delivery, a T4 level is the goal.

Advantages

The benefit of an epidural is the ability to re-dose the epidural in the event of a delayed or prolonged surgery. Also, long-acting epidural opioids can be given to augment postoperative pain control.

Disadvantages

Disadvantages include longer onset for surgical block and the possibility of incomplete block, making epidural anesthesia a less attractive option than spinal anesthesia in the case of an emergency. The higher doses of local anesthetics used in epidural blocks (compared with spinal) increase the risk of local anesthetic toxicity.

Spinal

Indications

Spinal anesthesia can be used for elective cesarean sections and most emergencies. Intrathecal morphine can be given to augment postoperative pain control.

Advantages

Both spinal and epidural techniques are shown to provide effective anesthesia for cesarean section. Spinal anesthesia is more advantageous over epidural due to its association with **quicker onset** of adequate analgesia (by 8 minutes).[20] Other advantages cited are its simplicity, lower drug doses, and superior abdominal muscle relaxation. **Compared with epidural, the spinal technique is associated with similar failure rate, need for additional intraoperative analgesia, need for conversion to general anesthesia intraoperatively, maternal satisfaction, need for postoperative pain relief, and neonatal intervention.**[20] No conclusions can be drawn about intraoperative side effects, postoperative complications (e.g. PDPH, nausea, and vomiting, and postoperative complications needing anesthetic intervention), or breastfeeding because of their low incidence and/or the fact that they were not reported. Spinal anesthesia has developed in most L&Ds (labor and delivery floors) as the regional technique of choice for cesarean sections, owing its use in particular to rapidity of anesthetic onset, quality of anesthesia, and ease of performance of block.

Disadvantages

Hypotension, possibly profound, is increased in incidence 23% with spinal over epidural analgesia.[20] **Hypotension in labor or at CD** usually results from sympathectomy secondary to neuraxial blockade, but can also be seen from hypovolemia (from hemorrhage) or vasodilatation from general anesthesia during cesarean section.

No intervention reliably prevents hypotension during spinal anesthesia for cesarean section, but four of many tested interventions reduce the incidence of hypotension under spinal anesthesia for cesarean section: (1) **crystalloid** vs control; (2) **pre-emptive colloid administration** vs crystalloid;

(3) **ephedrine** vs control; and (4) **lower limb compression** vs control.[21] Ephedrine is associated with dose-related maternal hypertension and tachycardia, and fetal acidosis of uncertain clinical significance. Recent studies have shown that **phenylephrine** is as safe as ephedrine; in fact, fetal pH and incidence of maternal nausea are better with phenylephrine.[22]

High spinal is covered under anesthetic emergencies, 'Total spinal' section.

Limited duration is another disadvantage. CSEs and spinal catheters combine the advantages of spinal anesthesia's onset with the ability to re-dose in the case of prolonged surgical time.

General anesthesia

Indications

In the cases of failed regional anesthesia, an emergency preventing extension of an epidural or placement of a spinal, contraindication for regional, or objection by the patient to regional, general anesthesia is used. If a general anesthetic is chosen, all patients should receive acid aspiration prophylaxis, including a non-particulate oral antacid and metoclopramide. Time permitting, an H_2 blocker, which takes 45 minutes to work, can confer additional protection. Airway protection with an endotracheal tube is mandatory. Halogenated agents are potent uterine relaxants in high concentrations, and this property might be useful in the management of uterine inversion, external cephalic version (ECV), or fetal entrapment. Intravenous nitroglycerin and terbutaline are other options in these situations.

Advantages

There are no evident advantages to general anesthesia in the absence of a contraindication to a neuraxial approach.

Disadvantages

Compared with neuraxial analgesia, general anesthesia is associated with a threefold risk of maternal death. The biggest risk is being unable to intubate or ventilate the patient. Parturients have increased upper airway edema, lower pulmonary functional residual capacity, decreased lower esophageal sphincter tone, and delayed gastric emptying. These conditions increase the risk of both hypoxemia and aspiration. Airway edema can also make anesthetizing the airway more difficult for fiberoptic intubation. The use of benzodiazepines and opioids before the delivery of the fetus is controversial. Although benzodiazepines and opioids can depress the fetus, they are pharmacologically reversible. The absence of benzodiazepines increases the risk of maternal awareness under general anesthesia. Opioids effectively attenuate the hypertensive response elicited by laryngoscopy and may be necessary to safely intubate the already hypertensive patient. There are no trials on preventive measures for aspiration from general anesthesia. A fasting period of 6–8 hours and sodium citrate with citric acid are suggested before CD. General anesthesia is also associated with higher incidence of postoperative nausea and vomiting, maternal sedation, and increased time to breastfeeding.

The effect of general anesthesia on the fetus depends on the length of induction to umbilical cord clamp time, with the length of hysterotomy to clamp time also important. Fetal exposure to inhaled anesthetics of > 5–8 minutes is associated with neonatal depression. General anesthesia compared with neuraxial anesthesia has been shown to increase the incidence of acidemia and drug exposure, and lower Apgar scores. Local anesthetics, opioids, and hypnotics readily cross the placenta, whereas neuromuscular blocking agents do not. Acidemia is most closely linked to maternal hypotension. More important than which agents should be used to treat hypotension is the avoidance of hypotension in the first place.[23]

Post-cesarean delivery analgesia

First 24 hours

Preservative-free **morphine** hydrochloride 100–250 µg, placed **at the time of spinal analgesia or** after delivery when using **epidural** analgesia, provides effective pain relief in the first 12–24 hours.[1]

Another alternative is **PCEA**, which is associated though with increased motor weakness. Opioids administered via spinal or epidural routes are associated with a 35–55% incidence of maternal pruritus severe enough to require treatment.[24] The epidural catheter should be removed at 24 hours to reduce urinary retention, pruritus, and infection risks.

Intravenous patient-controlled opioids are another reasonable alternative, using morphine, hydromorphone hydrochloride, or fentanyl.

Oral analgesia with oxycodone–acetaminophen 5/325 mg two tablets every 3 hours for 12 hours and then one/two tablets every 4 hours as needed is associated with superior pain control and fewer side effects compared with morphine patient-controlled IV analgesia in one trial.[25]

After 24 hours

Non-steroidal anti-inflammatory drugs (NSAIDs) reduce maternal opioid consumption after CD, even in the first 24 hours, and should be the main intervention for pain control after the first 24 hours. Use of oral narcotics should be quickly weaned.

ANESTHETIC EMERGENCIES

Anesthetic emergencies in obstetric patients are another important time for cooperation between the anesthesia and obstetric teams. The goal should be to stabilize the mother while safely and quickly delivering the neonate, if necessary. Communication is important, as well as knowing how each team can assist one another.

Total spinal

A total spinal occurs with cephalad spread of local anesthetic to the breathing centers of the brainstem. This can occur with normal doses of spinally administered drug or be the result of an overdose of spinally administered medication. This can occur with accidental intrathecal placement of an epidural dose of medication or from subdural catheter placement with subsequent migration of the catheter. Control of the airway, often with endotracheal intubation, and blood pressure control with uterine displacement, sympathomimetic medications, and fluid should be achieved quickly. Once the airway has been secured, assessment of the fetus should be facilitated. If the fetus is stable, delivery can await maternal recovery, usually about 20–30 minutes.

Local anesthetic toxicity

Intravenous injection of local anesthetics can lead to systemic toxicity, including seizures and cardiovascular collapse. The mother's airway should be controlled as quickly as possible and delivery of the fetus is often indicated because of maternal instability. Seizures can be controlled quickly with general anesthesia as well as most sedative-hypnotic drugs. In the case of cardiovascular collapse, sympathomimetic therapy, IV fluids, and in some cases cardiopulmonary bypass should be initiated.

Failed intubation

The risk of failed intubation is increased in the parturient (about 1 in 200 for the pregnant patient vs about 1 in 800 for the general population). Increased edema in the upper airway, increased breast size, and increased friability of the mucosa increase chance of failure. In addition, parturients have decreased functional residual volume (FRV) and are at higher risk for aspiration secondary to decreased gastric emptying and increased abdominal pressure. In the case of a failed intubation, the obstetric team can assist the anesthesia team by calling for help, helping to set up emergency equipment (fiberoptic bronchoscope, laryngeal mask airway, cricothyrotomy with jet ventilation) and maintaining communication. Delivery of the fetus is indicated if the mother cannot be ventilated at all and is becoming hypoxic as evidenced by a falling pulse oximetry reading.

Cardiopulmonary resuscitation in the pregnant patient

In the rare and unfortunate case that a pregnant patient experiences cardiac arrest, cardiopulmonary resuscitation (CPR) is not as effective due to aortocaval compression by the gravid uterus. Control of the airway with subsequent immediate delivery of the fetus is the priority (with delivery of the fetus being as or more important than control of the airway). Resuscitation of a pregnant woman should never be abandoned until some period of time after the fetus is delivered.

References

1. ACOG. Obstetric analgesia and anesthesia. ACOG Practice Bulletin, No. 36, 2002. [review]

2. ACOG. Optimal goals for anesthesia care in obstetrics. ACOG Committee Opinion, 2001. [review]

3. Elbourne D, Wiseman RA. Types of intra-muscular opioids for maternal pain relief in labour. Cochrane Database Syst Rev 2007; 1. [16 RCTs, n=>5000]

4. Tsui MHY, Ngan Kee WD, Ng FF, Lau TK. A double blinded randomised placebo-controlled study of intramuscular pethidine for pain relief in the first stage of labour. Br J Obstet Gynaecol 2004; 111: 648–55. [RCT, n=112]

5. Martensson L, Wallin G. Labour pain treated with cutaneous injections of sterile water: a randomized controlled trial. Br J Obstet Gynaecol 1999; 106: 633–7. [RCT, n=99]

6. Anim-Somuah M, Smyth R, Howell C. Epidural versus non-epidural or no analgesia in labour. Cochrane Database Syst Rev 2007; 1. [meta-analysis: 21 RCTs, n=6664; 20/21 compared epidural analgesia with opiates]

7. Chestnut DH, McGrath JM, Vincent RD et al. Does early administration of epidural analgesia affect obstetric outcome in nulliparous women who are spontaneous labor? Anesthesiology 1994; 80: 1201–8. [RCT, n=344]

8. Chestnut DH, Vincent RD, McGrath JM, Choi WW, Bates JN. Does early administration of epidural analgesia affect obstetric outcome in nulliparous women who are receiving intravenous oxytocin? Anesthesiology 1994; 80: 1193–200. [RCT, n=150]

9. Luxman D, Wolman I, Groutz A et al. The effect of early epidural block administration on the progression and outcome of labor. Int J Obstet Anesth 1998; 7: 161–4. [RCT, n=60]

10. Wong CA, Scavone BM, Peaceman AM et al. The risk of cesarean delivery with neuraxial analgesia given early versus late in labor. N Engl J Med 2005; 352: 655–65. [RCT, n=750]

11. Ohel G, Gonen R, Vaida S, Barak S, Gaitini L. Early versus late initiation of epidural analgesia in labor: does it increase the risk of cesarean section? A randomized trial. Am J Obstet Gynecol 2006; 194: 600–5. [RCT, n=449]

12. Usha Kiran TS, Thakur MB, Bethel JA et al. Comparison of continuous infusion versus midwife administered top-ups of epidural bupivicaine for labour analgesia: effect on second stage of labour mode of delivery. Int J Obstet Anesth 2003: 12: 9–11. [RCT]

13. Torvaldsen S, Roberts CL, Bell JC, Raynes-Greenow CH. Meta-analysis Discontinuation of epidural analgesia late in labour for reducing the adverse delivery outcomes associated with epidural analgesia. Cochrane Database Syst Rev 2007; 1. [5 RCTs, n=462]

14. Hofmeyr GJ, Cyna AM, Middleton P, Prophylactic intravenous preloading for regional analgesia in labour. Cochrane Database Syst Rev 2007; 1. [6 RCTs, n=473]

15. Kreiser D, Katorza E, Seidmen DS, Etchin A, Schiff E. The effect of ephedrine on intrapartum fetal heart rate after epidural analgesia. Obstet Gynecol 2004; 104: 1277–81. [RCT, n=145]

16. Harrington BE. Postdural puncture headache and the development of the epidural blood patch. Reg Anesth Pain Med 2004; 29: 136–63. [review]

17. Hughes D, Simmons SW, Brown J, Cyna AM. Combined spinal–epidural versus epidural analgesia in labour. Cochrane Database Syst Rev 2007; 1. [meta-analysis: 14 RCTs, n=2047]

18. American Society of Regional Anesthesia and Pain Medicine Consensus Conference. Regional Anesthesia in the Anticoagulated Patient – Defining the Risks. American Society of Regional Anesthesia and Pain Medicine; 2002. [review]

19. Ho AM, Kee WD, Chung DC. Should laboring parturients with Harrington rods receive lumbar epidural analgesia? Int J Gynacol Obstet 1999; 67(1): 41–3. [II–3]

20. Ng K, Parsons J, Cyna AM, Middleton P. Spinal versus epidural anaesthesia for caesarean section. Cochrane Database Syst Rev 2007; 1. [meta-analysis: 10 RCTs, n=751]

21. Emmett RS, Cyna AM, Andrew M, Simmons SW. Techniques for preventing hypotension during spinal anaesthesia for caesarean section. Cochrane Database Syst Rev 2007; 1. [meta-analysis: 25 RCTs, n=1477]

22. Lee A, Ngan Kee WD, Gin T. A quantitative, systematic review of randomized controlled trials of ephedrine versus phenylephrine for the management of hypotension during spinal anesthesia for cesarean delivery. Anesth Analg 2002; 94: 920–6. [meta-analysis]

23. Littleford J. Effects on the fetus and newborn of maternal analgesia and anesthesia: a review. Can J Anesth 2004; 51: 585–609. [review]

24. Dahl JB, Jeppesen IS, Jorgensen H, Wetterslev J, Moiniche S. Intraoperative and postoperative analgesic efficacy and adverse effects of intrathecal opioids in patients undergoing cesarean section with spinal anesthesia: a qualitative and quantitative systematic review of randomized controlled trials. Anesthesiology 1999; 91: 1919–27. [meta-analysis: 11 RCTs]

25. Davis KM, Esposito MA, Meyer BA. Oral analgesia compared to intravenous patient-controlled analgesia for pain after cesarean delivery: a randomized controlled trial. Am J Obstet Gynecol 2006; 194: 967–71. [RCT, n=93]

11

Operative vaginal delivery

Ariella Baylson and Jay Goldberg

KEY POINTS

- **Vacuum and forceps assisted delivery** have the **same indications**. There are **no circumstances where operative vaginal delivery is definitely indicated.** Alternatives, including allowing the patient to labor longer, oxytocin augmentation, and cesarean delivery, should always be considered.
- When used by experienced operators, **operative vaginal delivery is safe for both mother and baby** and **effective in obtaining vaginal delivery**, with forceps having slightly higher success rates.
- There is insufficient evidence to compare different types of forceps.
- **Soft vacuum cups fail at attaining vaginal delivery more often than by rigid cups,** but have a lower rate of significant scalp trauma. Rigid cups may be better for occiput posterior and other more difficult deliveries, while soft cups may be better suited for less-complicated, routine deliveries.
- Complication rates differ between vacuum and forceps, with the predominant differences being that **neonatal injuries are more common with vacuum-assisted delivery,** and **maternal perineal/vaginal injuries are more common with forceps-assisted delivery. Failed vaginal delivery,** as well as **shoulder dystocia and postpartum hemorrhage,** are also **more common with vacuum extraction.** The choice of instrument is decided after appropriate counseling, and depends also on operator experience.
- If attempted, **vacuum application should not last more than 5 minutes,** and should be **discontinued if the vacuum cup pops off the fetal head three times.**
- **Attempting to use a different extraction instrument after failing with one should be avoided.**

Historical perspectives

Operative vaginal delivery has been practiced for centuries. Its initial function was fetal extraction during prolonged dysfunctional labor in an attempt to preserve the life of the laboring women. The invention of modern forceps can be traced back to the Chamberlain family in Europe during the 16th century. The modern evolution of vacuum delivery can be attributed to Malmström's metal cup vacuum system developed in 1954. Operative vaginal delivery has evolved significantly, and today implies a mechanism for facilitating vaginal delivery of a healthy infant while minimizing maternal risk.

Incidence

Rates of operative vaginal deliveries have been declining since 1996 in the US. The 2002 rate for birth by forceps or vacuum delivery was 5.9% compared with the 1994 rate of 9.5%.[1] Vacuum-assisted delivery accounted for 68% of all operative deliveries in 2000 (up 41% since 1990).

Indications

Both **forceps and vacuum have the same indications.** Use should depend mostly on proper evaluation of the patient's labor, risk factors, clinical pelvimetry, estimated fetal weight, and operator experience. There are no circumstances where operative vaginal delivery is definitely indicated. Alternatives, including allowing the patient to labor longer, oxytocin augmentation, and cesarean delivery, should always be considered. Operative vaginal delivery is usually considered for:

- **Maternal: inefficient maternal effort** (e.g. exhaustion or underlying medical condition precluding pushing).
- **Fetal: non-reassuring fetal heart rate tracing.**
- **Prolonged second stage:** nulliparas ≥ 2 hours without regional anesthesia or ≥ 3 hours with regional anesthesia. Multiparas ≥ 1 hour without regional anesthesia or ≥ 2 hours with regional anesthesia.[2]

'Elective' forceps delivery, i.e. without an indication, is associated with increased maternal perineal trauma, and given the other potential maternal and neonatal complications, should not be preferred to spontaneous vaginal delivery.[3]

Contraindications to operative vaginal delivery

Contraindications are non-vertex presentation, unengaged fetal head, unknown fetal head position, fetal prematurity such as < 34 weeks (especially for vacuum), known fetal coagulation disorders (e.g. hemophilia, neonatal alloimmune thrombocytopenia [NAIT]), and known fetal bone demineralization conditions (e.g. osteogenesis imperfecta). Severe scalp trauma and unexplained active bleeding may be relative contraindications in individual cases. Operative vaginal delivery should be used with extreme caution in women with maternal diabetes, prolonged labor, and fetal macrosomia, with appropriate preparations for possible shoulder dystocia.

Risks for failed operative vaginal delivery

The risks are increased maternal age, increased body mass index, diabetes, macrosomia, polyhydramnios, African-American race, induction of labor, occiput posterior (also increases rates of third- and fourth-degree perineal lacerations), dysfunctional labor, and prolonged labor.[4]

Classification of operative vaginal delivery[2]

- **Outlet:** scalp is visible at introitus without separating the labia, fetal skull has reached pelvic floor, sagittal suture is in anteroposterior diameter or right or left occiput anterior or posterior position, fetal head is at or on perineum, and rotation ≤ 45°.
- **Low:** leading point of the fetal skull is at station ≥ + 2 cm and not on the pelvis floor, rotation is ≤ 45° (left or right occiput anterior to occiput anterior, or left or right occiput posterior to occiput posterior) or rotation is > 45°.
- **Mid:** station is above + 2 cm but head is engaged.

Originally devised for forceps, this classification is valid for any operative delivery, including vacuum.[5]

Types of forceps

There are many different designs for forceps, but all consist of two separate halves that each have the same four basic components: blade, shank, lock, and handle. **There is insufficient evidence to compare different types of forceps.** In the only small trial performed, severe facial abrasion was decreased from 4.1% with the regular forceps to 1.9% with soft forceps, as were minimal markings (from 61 to 34%, respectively).[6] Unfortunately, successful delivery rates for the two different forceps were not reported, and the soft forceps were self-made. Given the paucity of data, choice of forceps type is somewhat operator-dependent.

- **Classical forceps:** have cephalic and pelvic curvatures. Usually indicated when no rotation of the fetal head is necessary before delivery. Common types include Simpson forceps (fenestrated blades, non-overlapping shanks), Tucker-McLane forceps (non-fenestrated blades, overlapping shanks), Elliot forceps (fenestrated blades, overlapping shanks, largest cephalic curvature). Many of these forceps have been modified with a Luikart pseudo-fenestration of the blade.
- **Rotational forceps:** have cephalic curvature but lack a pelvic curvature. Also have a sliding lock to allow forceps to slide to correct asynclitism of the fetal head if present. After rotation of the fetal head is accomplished, classical forceps should be used to complete the delivery. Types include Kielland, Luikart, Barton, and Salinas forceps.
- **Forceps for breech delivery:** indicated to help with the aftercoming head in a breech delivery. These forceps lack a pelvic curvature and have blades that are beneath the plane of the shank. Types include Piper and Laufe forceps.

Types of vacuum extractors

Vacuum extractors were originally designed with a rigid metal cup. Subsequently, soft cups have been developed. **Several types of rigid (metal or plastic) and soft (silicone plastic or rubber) vacuums are in clinical use. Soft vacuum cups fail at attaining vaginal delivery** more often (16 vs 9%) than rigid metal cups.[7–9] However, **soft cups have a lower rate of significant scalp trauma** (13 vs 24%) associated with their use. **Rigid cups may be better for occiput posterior** and other more difficult deliveries, whereas **soft cups are better suited for less-complicated, routine deliveries.**[7] Maternal injury, low Apgar scores at 1 or 5 minutes, umbilical artery pH < 7.20, cephalohematoma, hyperbilirubinemia/phototherapy, retinal/intracranial hemorrhage, and perinatal death do not differ between soft and rigid vacuum cups.[7] Soft vacuum cups have largely replaced the rigid cup in routine clinical practice.

Comparison of forceps- versus vacuum-assisted delivery[10]

Safety/complications

Maternal

- **Shoulder dystocia** (twofold increase) and **postpartum hemorrhage increase significantly with vacuum**-assisted deliveries compared with deliveries using forceps.

- Third- and fourth-degree perineal and vaginal wall lacerations (maternal trauma) are **significantly increased with forceps** compared with vacuum.
- **Anesthesia is needed significantly less (22 vs 31%) with vacuum-** compared with forceps-assisted deliveries.
- **Severe perineal pain at 24 hours is decreased (9 vs 15%) with vacuum-** compared with forceps-assisted deliveries.[10]
- Rates of moderate/severe pain at delivery and endoanal ultrasound abnormalities[11] are similar.

Fetal/neonatal

- **Rates of cephalohematomas** occur in 10 vs 4% in vacuum and forceps, respectively.[10] Cephalohematomas have an overall rate of 2.5% in the population.[12] However, the diagnosis of cephalohematoma can be falsely positive in up to 75% of cases.[13]
- **Retinal hemorrhages** occur in 49 vs 33% in vacuum and forceps, respectively. One study found retinal hemorrhages occurred in 18% of spontaneous vaginal deliveries.[14] The clinical significance of retinal hemorrhages remains unclear.[13]
- **Hyperbilirubinemia increases significantly with vacuum-**assisted deliveries compared to deliveries with forceps.
- An **Apgar score <7 is non-significantly increased (5 vs 3%) with vacuum**-assisted deliveries compared to deliveries with forceps.[10]
- Rates of scalp/face injury other than cephalohematoma, use of phototherapy, perinatal death, readmission to hospital, and hearing or vision disability are similar between forceps- and vacuum-assisted vaginal deliveries.[10,15]
- Other possible uncommon fetal complications associated with operative vaginal delivery include facial nerve injury, corneal abrasions, facial bruising, and lacerations. Very rare findings include facial nerve palsy, skull fractures, cervical spine injury, and intracranial hemorrhage. **With vacuum-assisted delivery,** life-threatening neonatal injuries include **subgaleal (subaponeurotic) hematoma** (0–4%) and **intracranial hemorrhage** (0–2.5%).
- Most neonatal complications, in particular intracranial hemorrhage, associated with operative vaginal delivery have been found in some studies to be similar to those of similar pregnancies who instead elect cesarean delivery.[16] Therefore, abnormal labor is the common risk factor for neonatal intracranial hemorrhage, and not the procedure itself.
- **Long-term infant outcome:** there are **no neurological or cognitive differences** in infants and children who underwent operative vaginal delivery with forceps or vacuum compared with each other or to infants delivered by spontaneous vaginal delivery.[17,18]

Efficacy

Both vacuum- and forceps-assisted delivery have high delivery success rates (vacuum, 83–94%; forceps, 85–92%).[10,13]

Failed vaginal delivery is increased significantly in vacuum- vs forceps-assisted vaginal deliveries (12 vs 7%).[10]

Management

Preoperative assessment

Counseling

Review with patient and document indication(s), absence of contraindications, type of instrument and rationale, and possible complications of operative vaginal delivery. The option of cesarean delivery should be reviewed. Obtain verbal or written informed consent prior to operative vaginal delivery.

Preparation/documentation

- **Maternal:** sufficient analgesia, clinical assessment of pelvis, lithotomy position, ± empty bladder.
- **Fetal:** vertex presentation, head engaged (lower part of bony vertex – not caput – at or lower than level of ischial spines), precise knowledge of the position of the head (consider ultrasound for confirmation), asynclitism, and estimated fetal weight.
- **Uteroplacental:** cervix completely dilated, ruptured membranes, absence of placenta previa or other contraindications.
- **Other:** alert nursing, anesthesia, and neonatology of operative vaginal delivery. Be prepared for shoulder dystocia. Be willing to discontinue the procedure if it does not proceed as planned, and ability to perform emergency cesarean delivery.[2]

Vacuum application

Vacuum application, if performed, should begin with low suction and be slowly increased to vacuum of about 0.7–0.8 kg/cc^2 (500–600 mmHg).

No torque or rocking motions should be applied to the vacuum. Traction should only be in the direct line of the vaginal canal. The risk of cephalohematoma increases as the time of vacuum application increases. Vacuum application **should not last more than 5 minutes**, and should be **discontinued if the vacuum cup pops off the fetal head three times.**[2]

Antibiotic prophylaxis

Antibiotic prophylaxis cannot be recommended solely for the indication 'operative vaginal delivery': 2 g of intravenous cefotetan at the time of vacuum or forceps delivery is associated with a non-significant decrease (0 vs 3.5%) in endometritis.[19]

It is essential to examine carefully both the fetus and the maternal perineum after operative vaginal delivery.

Attempting to use a different extraction instrument after failing with one should be avoided, as cephalopelvic disproportion may be present, and the highest incidence of neonatal intracranial hemorrhage, as well as other neonatal injuries, is among infants delivered using forceps and vacuum sequentially.[16,20,21]

References

1. Martin JA, Hamilton BE, Sutton PD et al. Births: final data for 2002. Natl Vital Stat Rep 2003; 52: 1–113. [data report]
2. American College of Obstetricians and Gynecologists. Operative vaginal delivery. The College; Washington, DC: 2000. Practice Bulletin No. 17. [review]
3. Yancey MK, Herpolsheimer A, Jordan GD, Benson WL, Brady L. Maternal and neonatal effects of outlet forceps delivery compared with spontaneous vaginal delivery in term pregnancies. Obstet Gynecol 1991; 78: 646–50. [II–2, n = 333].
4. Gopalani S, Bennett K, Critchlow. Factors predictive of failed operative vaginal delivery. Am J Obstet Gynecol 2004; 191: 896–902. [II–3]
5. Weinstein L, Calvin S, Trofatter KR. Operative vaginal delivery: risks and benefits. ACOG Update 2001; 27:5. [review]
6. Roshan DF, Petrikovski B, Sichinava L et al. Soft forceps. Int J Obstet Gynecol 2005; 88:249–52. [RCT, n = 96]
7. Johanson RB, Menon V. Soft versus rigid vacuum extractor cups for assisted vaginal delivery. Cochrane Database Syst Rev 2007; 1. [meta-analysis: 9 RCTs, n = 1375]
8. Attilakos G, Sibanda T, Winter C, Johnson N, Draycott T. A randomized controlled trial of a new handheld vacuum extraction device. Br J Obstet Gynaecol 2005; 112: 1510–15. [RCT, n = 194]
9. Groom KM, Jones BA, Miller N, Paterson-Brown S. A prospective randomized controlled trial of the Kiwi Omnicup versus conventional ventouse cups for vacuum-assisted vaginal delivery. Br J Obstet Gynaecol 2006; 113: 183–9. [RCT, n = 404]
10. Johanson RB, Menon V. Vacuum extraction versus forceps for assisted vaginal delivery. Cochrane Database Syst Rev. 1, 2007. [meta-analysis: 10 RCTs, n = 3000]
11. Fitzpatrick M, Behan M, O'Connel PR, Herlihy C. Randomized clinical trial to assess anal sphincter function following forceps or vacuum assisted vaginal delivery. Br J Obstet Gynaecol 2003; 110: 424–9. [RCT, n = 130]
12. Uhing M. Management of birth injuries. Clin Perinatol 2005; 32(1): 19–38. [II–3]
13. Williams M, Knuppel R, O'Brien W et al. A randomized comparison of assisted vaginal delivery by obstetric forceps and polyethylene vacuum cup. Obstet Gynecol 1991; 78: 789–94. [RCT, n = 99]
14. Williams M, Knuppel R, O'Brien W et al. Obstetric correlates of neonatal retinal hemorrhage. Obstet Gynecol 1993; 81: 688–94. [II-2, n = 278]
15. Bofill, JA, Rust OA, Schorr SJ et al. A randomized prospective trial of the obstetric forceps versus the M-cup vacuum extractor. Am J Obstet Gynecol 1996; 175: 1325–30. [RCT, n = 637]
16. Towner D, Castro MA, Eby-Wilkens E, Gilbert WM. Effect of mode of delivery in nulliparous women on neonatal intracranial injury. N Engl J Med 1999; 341: 1709–14. [II–2]
17. Wesley BD, van den Berg BJ, Reece EA. The effects of forceps delivery on cognitive development. Am J Obstet Gynecol 1993; 169: 1091–5. [II-2]
18. Ngan Hy, Miu P, Ko L et al. Long-term neurological sequelae following vacuum extractor delivery. Aust N Z J Obstet Gynaecol 1990; 30: 111–14. [II–2]
19. Heitmann JA, Benrubi GI. Efficacy of prophylactic antibiotics for the prevention of endomyometritis after forceps delivery. South Med J 1989; 82: 960–2. [RCT, n = 393]
20. Edozien LC, Williams JL, Chattopadhyay I, Hirsch PJ. Failed instrumental delivery: how safe is the use of a second instrument? J Obstet Gynaecol 1999; 19: 460–2. [III]
21. Demissie K, Rhoads GG, Smulian JC et al. Operative vaginal delivery and neonatal and infant adverse outcomes: population based retrospective analysis. BMJ 2004; 329: 24–9. [II–2]

12

Cesarean delivery

Vincenzo Berghella

See specific guidelines for VBAC (Chapter 13), postpartum infectious complications (Chapter 26), and anesthesia (Chapter 10).

KEY POINT

- Blunt uterine incision expansion, prophylactic antibiotics (either ampicillin or first-generation cephalosporin for just one dose), spontaneous placental removal, non-closure of both visceral and parietal peritoneum, and suture closure or drainage of the subcutaneous tissue when thickness is ≥2 cm should routinely be performed in cesarean delivery.

Historic notes

The word cesarean is probably derived either from the *Lex Regia*, later called *Cesarea*, which allowed, in ancient Rome, the postmortem abdominal delivery of the child, or from the Latin *caesare*, which means 'to cut'. Until the late 1800s, most cesarean deliveries (CDs) were done after maternal death, for attempt at fetal salvage. In 1882, the era of the modern CD began when Saenger advocated closing all uterine incisions immediately after surgery. The lower uterine segment incision was introduced by Kronig in 1912 and popularized in the USA by DeLee in 1922. The transverse uterine incision was described by Munro Kerr in 1926.[1] CD has been associated with relatively low maternal mortality for about 100 years. Safety has improved in the last 50 years, as the above techniques have become more widely used, and antibiotics have been introduced.

Diagnosis/definition

Birth via the abdominal route.

Epidemiology/incidence

Cesarean delivery is now the most common surgical procedure in the USA, with over one million performed each year. Its incidence had increased to >30% of deliveries in 2005.[2] This increase has been fueled at least in part by the increased incidence of multiple gestations, and decreased incidences of vaginal births after CD and vaginal breech deliveries. Recently, the demand of women for elective CD has increased as complications from the procedure diminish, women have fewer children, and fear and concerns about vaginal delivery do not abate.

Indications

Commonly accepted indications for CD are failure to progress (aka failure to dilate, failure to descend, cephalopelvic disproportion, dystocia, etc.), non-reassuring fetal heart testing (NRFHT), and non-vertex presentation. See relevant chapters in this book and *Maternal–Fetal Evidence Based Guidelines* for details. There is insufficient evidence (lack of any trial) to assess the benefits and risks of a policy of CD on maternal request (only indication: woman's desire) compared with trial of labor in term women with singleton gestations in cephalic presentation. As there is no such trial, there is insufficient evidence to compare the long-term maternal and neonatal morbidity and mortality of CD on maternal request vs trial of labor.

Optimal cesarean delivery rate

There is no optimal CD rate. Maternal and neonatal morbidity and mortality are the important outcomes, not CD rate per se. Increasing CD rate, if CD is performed for appropriate indications, has at times been associated with a lower mortality rate in normally formed term babies.[3] As the CD rate increases, an increasing number of CDs have to be performed to achieve smaller benefits in perinatal mortality.

Preoperative considerations

Consent

Consent should always be obtained after counseling. Counseling should include at least indication, and possible complications.

Fetal heart monitoring

1. If external monitoring has been employed, it should be continued up until the abdominal prep has begun. This includes the time when regional anesthesia is administered. If continuous fetal monitoring is not possible, reapply the external monitor for 2–3 minutes if feasible after completion of the regional anesthesia to determine the post-anesthesia fetal status.
2. If internal monitoring has been employed, the scalp electrode can be kept on until delivery of the fetal head, at which point the lead can be cut and the fetus delivered or the fetus delivered with the electrode attached. The operating room (OR) team will be responsible to document (on the count sheet) the location of the scalp electrode after delivery.
3. If the cesarean section is done for non-reassuring fetal status, all attempts should be made to perform continuous fetal monitoring until the delivery occurs. This may not apply when the cesarean section is done in an emergent manner.

Decision making

There is no trial regarding optimal time of 'decision to incision' for CD: < 30 minutes for CD for non-reassuring fetal heart rate (NRFHR), and < 60 minutes for CD for dystocia and most other indications have been proposed, but are not based on trials.[4]

Drugs

Betamethasone 12 mg × two doses 4 hours apart at 37 weeks or beyond before elective CD has been shown to reduce the incidence of respiratory distress syndrome (RDS) to 0.002% from 0.011%. The incidence of admission to special care nursery for respiratory distress is decreased to 0.024% from 0.051%.[5] Given there is only one randomized controlled trial (RCT) on this subject, and that it was not placebo-controlled, or blinded, and had very low incidence of disease in the control group, these data are insufficient for a definite recommendation. Steroids should not be given at ≥ 39 weeks, since the incidence of RDS is extremely small.

Technique of cesarean delivery[1]

See Table 12.2 for a summary of recommendations.

Lateral tilt involves tilting the woman towards her left side 10–15° to avoid vena caval compression by the gravid uterus. Compared with the supine position, lateral tilt provides a trend for less decreased Apgar scores, with similar umbilical artery pH.[7] Fetal oxygen saturation was improved with lateral tilt in a non-randomized study of women in labor.[8]

Skin cleansing techniques for CD have been studied insufficiently for an evidence-based recommendation. Compared with 7.5% povidone–iodine scrub and then povidone–iodine 10% solution, the addition of a preceding parachlorometaxylenol scrub for 5 minutes, in women who have received prophylactic antibiotics for CD, is not associated with differences in incidences of endometritis or wound infection in a small, possibly underpowered trial.[9] Skin is impossible to sterilize. In non-pregnant adults, there are no differences in wound infection with different types and times of scrubs. Therefore, the use of an iodine solution alone (better than saline) is considered reasonable. Some insist on the importance of letting the iodine dry for best infection prophylaxis.

Compared with no scrub, a **preoperative vaginal scrub with povidone–iodine** does not significantly decrease the incidence of endometritis, post-CD fever, wound, and other infections.[10,11]

Compared with matching placebo, metronidazole gel 5 g intravaginally before CD is associated with a decrease from 17% to 7% in the incidence of endometritis, but no other significant changes in important outcomes.[12]

Adhesive drapes for CD are associated with a **higher incidence of wound infection** (13.8%) compared with the control group (10.4%);[13,14] therefore, adhesive drapes should not be recommended for prevention of wound infection at CD.

Skin incision techniques for CD have not been studied separately from other aspects of CD.[15,16] In general, a **transverse skin incision** is recommended, since this is associated with less postoperative pain and improved cosmetic effect compared with a vertical incision. The Pfannenstiel (slightly curved, 2–3 cm or two fingers above the symphysis pubis, with the mid-portion of the incision lying within the shaved area of the pubic hair) and Joel-Cohen (straight, 3 cm below the line joining the anterior superior iliac spines, and therefore slightly more cephalad than the Pfannenstiel) are the preferred transverse incisions. The best trial reveals no differences in total operative time (32 vs 33 minutes), intra- and postoperative complications, and neonatal outcomes, with the extraction time 50 seconds shorter for the Joel-Cohen group.[15] Considering the absence of clinical benefits to the mother and fetus, there is no clear indication for performing a Joel-Cohen incision. A smaller, less well-designed trial[16] shows significantly shorter operating times, reduced blood loss, and postoperative discomfort associated with the Joel-Cohen incision compared with the Pfannenstiel incision.

Table 12.1 *Standard recommendation language and quality of evidence according to the method outlined by the US Preventive Services Task Force (USPSTF)*

Recommendation:

A   The USPSTF strongly recommends that clinicians provide [the service] to eligible patients. The USPSTF found good evidence that [the service] improves important health outcomes and concludes that benefits substantially outweigh harms.

B   The USPSTF recommends that clinicians provide [this service] to eligible patients. The USPSTF found at least fair evidence that [the service] improves important health outcomes and concludes that benefits outweigh harms.

C   The USPSTF makes no recommendation for or against routine provision of [the service]. The USPSTF found at least fair evidence that [the service] can improve health outcomes but concludes that the balance of benefits and harms is too close to justify a general recommendation.

D   The USPSTF recommends against routinely providing [the service] to asymptomatic patients. The USPSTF found at least fair evidence that [the service] is ineffective or that harms outweigh benefits.

I   The USPSTF concludes that the evidence is insufficient to recommend for or against routinely providing [the service]. Evidence that the [service] is effective is lacking, of poor quality, or conflicting and the balance of benefits and harms cannot be determined.

Quality of evidence:

Good: Evidence includes consistent results from well-designed, well-conducted studies in representative populations that directly assess effects on health outcomes.

Fair: Evidence is sufficient to determine effects on health outcomes, but the strength of the evidence is limited by the number, quality, or consistency of the individual studies, generalizability to routine practice, or indirect nature of the evidence on health outcomes.

Poor: Evidence is insufficient to assess the effects on health outcomes because of limited number or power of studies, important flaws in their design or conduct, gaps in the chain of evidence, or lack of information on important health outcomes.

Table 12.2 *Evidenced based recommendations for cesarean delivery*

CD technical aspect	Recommendation[b]	Quality[b]	Comment
Lateral tilt	I	Poor	15 degrees to left
Skin cleaning	I	Poor	Iodine[a]
Adhesive drapes	D	Fair	Not recommended
Skin incision:			
Type	C	Fair	Pfannenstiel or Joel–Cohen
Length	I	Poor	15 cm
Changing to a second knife	D	Fair	Not recommended
Subcutaneous incision	I	Poor	[a]
Fascial incision	I	Poor	[a]
Rectus muscle cutting	D	Fair	Not recommended
Dissection of fascia off rectus	I	Poor	[a]
Opening of peritoneum	I	Poor	[a]
Bladder flap:			
Development	D	Fair	[a]
Use of bladder blade	I	Poor	Operator preference
Uterine incision:			
Type	B	Fair	Transverse
Stapling device	D	Fair	Not recommended

(continued)

Table 12.2 *(continued)*

CD technical aspect	Recommendation[b]	Quality[b]	Comment
Expansion of uterine incision	A	Good	Bluntly
Instrumental delivery	I	Poor	[a]
Prophylactic antibiotics:			
Yes or no	A	Good	Yes (all CDs)
Antibiotic type	A	Good	Ampicillin or first-generation cephalosporin[c]
Route of administration	A	Good	Systemic/lavage (equivalent)
Multiple systemic doses	D	Good	Not recommended
Timing	I	Poor	[a]
Prevention of uterine atony:			
Oxytocin vs placebo[d]	I	Poor	Oxytocin[a]
Oxytocin infusion rate	I	Poor	Optimal rate unclear[a]
Carbetocin vs oxytocin	C	Fair	Carbetocin if available[a]
Placental removal:			
Spontaneous vs manual	A	Good	Spontaneous
Glove change	D	Fair	Not recommended
Uterine exteriorization	C	Fair	Operator preference
Cleaning of uterus	I	Poor	[a]
Closure of uterine incision:			
Two vs one layers	B	Fair	[a]
Incorporation decidua/serosa	I	Poor	[a]
Continuous vs interrupted	B	Fair	Continuous
Sharp vs blunt needles	I	Poor	[a]
Peritoneal closure	D	Good	Not recommended (for both parietal and visceral)
Intra-abdominal irrigation:			
Saline vs none	D	Fair	Not recommended
Reapproximation of rectus	I	Poor	[a]
Subcutaneous tissue:			
any thickness:			
Closure vs non-closure	D	Fair	Closure not recommended
Drain vs no drain	D	Fair	Drain not recommended
≥2 cm thickness:			
Closure vs non-closure	A	Good	Closure recommended
Drain vs no drain	A	Good	Drain recommended
Closure vs drain	C	Fair	[a]
Closure of skin:			
staples vs subcuticular	I	Poor	[a]

CD, cesarean delivery; RCTs, randomized controlled trials.
[a]See text for more details.
[b]Level of evidence was based on the US Preventive Services Task Force recommendations (Table I)[7].
[c]Ampicillin or first-generation cephalosporin for just one dose before or after cord clamping.
[d]Based on trials of women with vaginal delivery, not CD.

Skin incision length has not been studied in a trial. Abdominal surgical incision size should provide probably about 15 cm (size of a standard Allis clamp) of exposure to assure optimal outcome of both mother and term fetus.[1]

Changing to a second scalpel after the first scalpel has been used for skin incision vs no such change has never been evaluated in a trial, or in any obstetric literature. From general surgery data, one scalpel is probably adequate to use throughout the whole surgical procedure.

Subcutaneous incision/opening has not been studied separately in a trial. Most clinicians use the scalpel as little as possible, opening layers bluntly from medial to lateral to avoid injury to tissue and the inferior epigastric vessels. Blunt dissection has been associated with shorter operating times. There are no trials to evaluate the safety or efficacy of electrosurgery, electrocautery, or diathermy (Bovie) during CD.

Fascial incision has not been studied separately in a trial. A transverse incision is usually performed with the scalpel, and then extended with scissors. Digital extension can alternatively be accomplished by separating the forefingers in a cephalad–caudad direction after inserting the fingers into a small, midline transverse fascial incision.

Rectus muscle cutting with the Maylard technique is not associated with any difference in operative morbidity, difficult deliveries, postoperative complications, or pain scores compared with the Pfannenstiel (no muscle cutting) technique,[17–19] but abdominal muscle strength at 3 months tends to be better in the Pfannenstiel group.[19] Therefore, **rectus muscle cutting is probably not necessary**.

Dissection of fascia off the recti muscles has not been studied separately in a trial. There seems to be no necessity of this commonly used technical step of CD.[1]

Opening of the peritoneum has not been studied separately in a trial. The peritoneum is usually carefully opened with blunt or sharp dissection, and blunt expansion, high above the bladder, avoiding injury to organs below.

Bladder flap development (incision and opening) is associated with longer (7 minutes vs 5 minutes) incision to delivery interval, longer (40 minutes vs 35 minutes) total operating time, and greater (1 g/dl vs 0.5 g/dl) change in hemoglobin compared with just direct incision 1 cm above the bladder fold.[20] Forming a bladder flap is also associated with more (47% vs 21%) postoperative microhematuria, and greater (55% vs 26%) need for analgesia at 2 days after CD. No long-term effects (e.g. adhesions, bladder function, fertility, etc.) have been evaluated. As bladder injury at CD is an uncommon event (1–3/1000), a sample size over 40 000 women would be required to show a difference in this outcome.[20] **Developing a bladder flap at CD may be detrimental and can be avoided**.

The use of a bladder blade to protect the bladder has not been studied separately in a trial.

Uterine incision type has not been studied separately in a trial. The **transverse incision in the lower uterine segment** is usually recommended.[1] Some experts advocate the classical vertical or at least low-vertical incision if the lower uterine segment is not large enough to allow a transverse incision, e.g. for the very preterm (<28 weeks) uterus, fibroids, etc., but this has been associated with increased blood loss compared with low transverse incision.[21]

A **uterine stapling device** is associated with an ~1 minute longer total operating time, with an ~1 minute increase in the time needed to deliver the baby, 41 ml lower blood loss, and no differences in other perinatal morbidity outcomes compared with traditional opening and closure of the uterine scar.[22] There is not enough evidence to justify the routine use of stapling devices to extend the uterine incision at lower segment cesarean section, especially since there is a possibility that stapling could cause harm by prolonging the time to deliver the baby.

Expansion of uterine incision with scissors (sharp) is associated with increased estimated blood loss, change in hematocrit, incidence of postpartum hemorrhage (13% vs 9%), need for transfusion (2% vs 0.4%), and total number of extensions compared with expansion with fingers (blunt).[23,24] As it is also quicker, and associated with less risk of inadvertently cutting the neonate or cord, **blunt should be preferred to sharp expansion of the uterine incision**.

Instrumental delivery of the fetal head by either vacuum or forceps compared with manual means has been insufficiently evaluated for a firm recommendation in women with cephalic[25] or breech presentation undergoing CD. As instrumentation has been associated with maternal (especially for forceps) or fetal (especially for vacuum) harm in vaginal deliveries, the principle of 'primum non nocere' ('first do no harm') should be applied in this setting, therefore **favoring manual delivery of the fetal head whenever possible** until further data are available.

Prophylactic antibiotics for CD are associated with decrease in incidence of endometritis of >60% in both elective and non-elective CD, and a decrease in wound infection of about 25% in elective and about 65% in non-elective CD.[26] Overall, fever and urinary tract infections are also markedly decreased. These results justify **recommending prophylactic antibiotics** in women undergoing any (elective or non-elective) CD. Comparing which antibiotic to give, the **efficacy of ampicillin is equivalent to that of first-generation cephalosporins such as cefazolin** (Ancef), and later-generation, more expensive broad-spectrum agents do not improve efficacy further.[27] **Systemic vs lavage routes of antibiotic administration seem to have similar efficacy.**[27] **Multiple systemic doses do not improve efficacy over a single dose.**[27] Timing of antibiotic administration (at cord clamp vs preoperative) has not been shown to affect infectious morbidity rates.[28–31] If ampicillin or a first-generation cephalosporin has already been given in labor, there may be no need for additional prophylactic antibiotics at CD.

Prevention of uterine atony and postpartum hemorrhage has not been studied for CD, but has been studied extensively for the third stage of labor after vaginal delivery. In the setting of vaginal delivery, **both intravenous and intramuscular oxytocin effectively reduce postpartum hemorrhage** and the need for therapeutic uterotonics by at least 40% compared with placebo or no routine prophylactic agent. **Oxytocin is as effective as and has fewer side effects than ergot alkaloids**. Regarding oxytocin infusion rates, in the setting of CD, 10 units (U) of oxytocin in 500 ml (infusion rate

333 mU/minute) lactated Ringer's solution over 30 minutes after cord clamping are associated with an increased need for another uterotonic medication (39% vs 19%) and similar change in hematocrit compared with 80 U of oxytocin in 500 ml (infusion rate = 2667 mU/min).[32] Given this is the only trial on this subject, and many obstetricians use different infusion rates, **the optimal infusion rate for oxytocin at CD is still unclear.** Carbetocin as a single 100 μg dose is associated with more effective prevention of uterine atony and lower need for additional uterotonics compared with oxytocin 8 or 16 hours infusion at CD.[33,34] Carbetocin (where available) may be recommended over oxytocin for prevention of uterine atony.

Placental removal options of either spontaneous (with gentle cord traction) or manual placental removal at CD have been studied in at least 12 randomized trials, including over 3000 women.[35] Spontaneous removal is associated with a significant reduction in postoperative endometritis, a trend for reduction in wound infection (probably insufficiently studied), and less blood loss or changes in hemoglobin/hematocrit, including less feto-maternal hemorrhage. Blood loss may be increased in manual removal because dilated sinuses in the uterine wall are not closed yet. Bacterial contamination of the lower uterine segment and incision may contaminate the surgeon's dominant hand, and therefore the upper segment in manual removal or the glove itself may be contaminated. **Spontaneous placental removal should be preferred to manual removal** given the **significant decrease in blood loss and endometritis.**

Changing the operator's glove before manual removal of the placenta does not alter the incidence of endometritis.[36]

Uterine exteriorization is associated with a significant decrease in fever for more than 3 days, and similar other important outcomes, including bleeding, compared with leaving the uterus intra-abdominally for uterine incision repair.[37] For most outcomes, there are insufficient data for a definite recommendation. So the balance of the benefits and harms is too close to justify a general recommendation.

Cleaning any placental remnants or blood clots from the uterus with a sponge or other means is a technique frequently used after placental removal, but has not been studied in any trial.

Closure of uterine incision with one layer of suture is associated with a 5-minute decrease in operating time, a lower incidence of abnormal scar ('smoother healing') during hysterography at 3 months follow-up, and similar blood loss, need for transfusion and endometritis rates compared with two layers.[38] Unfortunately, the women followed up are too few to detect a significant difference in rare but extremely important long-term outcomes such as rates of rupture in the next pregnancy,[39] with contradictory results of retrospective studies. Since there is still no trial that demonstrates the benefit of two- vs one-layer uterine closure, **it might be reasonable to omit the second layer if the woman is planning no more pregnancies** (e.g. receives

tubal ligation). **For women planning future pregnancies, the uterus can be closed in two layers.** Experts usually advocate incorporating all of the muscle up to the serosa in a one-layer closure to avoid bleeding from edges, but this aspect of CD has never been studied properly. It is unclear if one needs to incorporate the decidua or not. Continuous single-layer closure may save operating time and reduce blood loss compared with interrupted single-layer closure.[40] **Blunt needles** for closure of the uterus, peritoneum, and rectus sheath are associated with similar outcome compared with sharp needles.[41]

Peritoneal non-closure is associated with a reduction in operating time (whether both or either visceral or parietal peritoneal layer was not sutured), in postoperative fever, and in postoperative stay in hospital.[42] The trend for analgesia requirement and wound infection tended to favor non-closure. Long-term follow-up[43] after 7 years showed no differences in pain, fertility, urinary symptoms, and adhesions. A review of general surgery and gynecological data concluded that 'we encourage clinicians not to close both parietal and visceral peritoneum'.[44] Observational studies have shown that the peritoneum regenerates in 5–6 days. The hypothetical benefits of closing these layers for anatomic barrier, reduction of wound dehiscence, and minimization of adhesion have not been proven, and in fact have been invalidated by trials. **There is at present no evidence to justify the time taken and cost of peritoneal closure.**

Intra-abdominal irrigation with 500–1000 ml of normal saline before abdominal wall closure **should not be routinely performed** since it provides no significant differences in blood loss, intrapartum complications, hospital stay, return of gastrointestinal function, or incidence of infectious complications vs no irrigation.[45]

Reapproximation of rectus muscles has not been studied in any trial. Most clinicians agree that they do find the right anatomic place spontaneously, and suturing them together can cause unnecessary pain when the woman starts to move postoperatively.

Techniques of fascial closure have not been studied in any trial of CD. Most experts suggest continuous non-locking closure with delayed-absorbable suture.

Irrigation of the subcutaneous tissue to minimize wound infections and other complications has not been studied vs no irrigation in a trial of CD. The type of irrigation, with saline or antibiotic solution, has also not been studied in a trial.

Subcutaneous tissue closure vs non-closure should be analyzed by the thickness of the subcutaneous tissue, which is how most trials were done.[46,47] Some studies have evaluated only drainage of subcutaneous tissue.[48] Most studies used 3-0 Vicryl for closure.

Any subcutaneous thickness: *Suture closure* of subcutaneous fat in women with *any subcutaneous thickness* is overall associated with less wound disruption vs non-closure, but the presence of women with both < 2 cm and ≥ 2 cm thickness, which can have differing outcomes, and inability to blind, represents a possible source of confounding and bias.

Drainage of subcutaneous tissue, in women with *any thickness* and who did not receive prophylactic antibiotics, with a 2 cm corrugated rubber drain, left to drain open, coming out of one end of the incision, and removed the following day, is associated with a trend towards increased wound infection.[48] Therefore, **routine subcutaneous tissue drainage in women undergoing CD cannot be recommended.**

< 2 cm subcutaneous thickness studies: Routine subcutaneous tissue closure in women with a depth < 2 cm is not associated with any effects on outcome, and therefore cannot be recommended.

≥ 2 cm subcutaneous thickness studies: *Suture closure* of subcutaneous fat in women with *≥ 2 cm thickness* is associated with a significant decrease in wound disruptions, defined as any wound complication that requires intervention, and seromas, compared with non-closure. **The evidence supports routine subcutaneous suture closure in women with a depth ≥ 2 cm.**

Drainage of subcutaneous fat versus no drainage or vs suture closure in women with *≥ 2 cm thickness,* using a 7 mm Jackson-Pratt drain with closed suction cup, is **associated with a decrease in wound complications** compared with no drainage. Drainage is therefore recommended over no drainage in these women.

Drainage is associated with an incidence of wound complications similar to suture closure. Therefore, **while suture closure or drainage in women with ≥ 2 cm thickness is associated with benefit compared with no suture or no drainage, it is not yet clear if any of these two prophylactic interventions is superior to the other.**

Closure of skin with staples in women who had received a Pfannenstiel incision is associated with decreased operative time (< 1 minute vs 10 minutes), but increased pain pills in the hospital (24.6% vs 19.7%), and increased pain scale at hospital discharge and postpartum compared with 4-0 Vicryl subcuticular suture.[49] Staples are also associated with similar appearance by the linear trend test, as rated by physician and by patient in the short-term (6 weeks) assessment. There is no blinding possible, and no long-term outcome reported. The general surgery literature seems to support the evidence that subcuticular suture is associated with less pain and better cosmesis. CD is considered a clean-contaminated procedure, with a relatively high risk of wound infection. In clean-contaminated procedures, the general surgical literature would suggest avoiding a continuous method of wound closure. In contrast with interrupted closure (with staples or sutures), continuous wound closure does not allow selective, minimal wound opening in cases of infection or collections; therefore, there is no conclusive evidence about how the skin should be closed after CD.

Complications

Disrupted (open) laparotomy wound

Compared with healing by secondary intention, **reclosure of the disrupted laparotomy wound is associated with success in >80% of women, faster healing times (16–23 days vs 61–72 days), and fewer office visits.**[50] No serious morbidity or mortality is associated with either method. There is insufficient evidence to assess optimal timing (probably 4–6 days after disruption if non-infected) and technique (superficial vertical mattress or 'en bloc' reclosure of entire wound thickness with absorbable sutures, or adhesive tape) of reclosure, as well as utility of antibiotics. **Compared with reclosure using sutures, reclosure using permeable, adhesive tape** (Cover-Roll; Biersdorf, Norwalk, CT) is associated with faster procedure, less pain scores, and similar healing times in a small RCT.[51]

Postoperative counseling

Interval until next pregnancy after a CD should be 12–24 months, as shorter intervals have been associated with increased risk of uterine rupture (see also Chapter 13).

References

1. Berghella V, Baxter JK, Chauhan SP. Evidence-based surgery for cesarean delivery. Am J Obstet Gynecol 2005; 193: 1607–17. [meta-analysis – systematic review].
2. CDC National Vital Statistics Report. Births: Preliminary data for 2005. December, 2006. (http://www.cdc.gov/nchs/data/nvsr) [data review]
3. Matthews TG, Crowley P, Chong A et al. Rising cesarean section rates: a cause for concern? Br, J Obstet Gynaecol 2003; 110: 346–9. [review]
4. Chauhan SP, Macones GA. ACOG Practice Bulletin Intrapartum fetal heart rate monitoring. Obstet Gynecol 2005; 105: 1161–9. [review]
5. Stutchfield P, Whitaker R, Russell I et al. Antenatal betamethasone and incidence of neonatal respiratory distress after elective caesarean section: pragmatic randomized trial. BMJ 2005; 331: 662. [RCT, n=942]
6. US Preventive Services Task Force. Agency for healthcare research and quality. www.ahcpr.gov/clinic/ajpmsuppl/harris3.htm. [Review]
7. Wilkinson C, Enkin MW. Lateral tilt for caesarean section. The Cochrane Database Syst Rev 2007; 1. [meta-analysis: 3 RCTs, n=293 – poor quality]
8. Carbonne B, Benachi A, Leveque ML, Cabrol D, Papiernik E. Maternal position during labor: effects on fetal oxygen saturation measured by pulse oximetry. Obstet Gynecol 1996; 88: 797–800. [II–1]
9. Magann EF, Dodson MK, Ray MA et al. Preoperative skin preparation and intraoperative pelvic irrigation: impact on post cesarean endometritis and wound infection. Obstet Gynecol 1993; 81: 922–5. [RCT, n=50]
10. Starr RV, Zurawski J, Ismail M. Preoperative vaginal preparation with povidone-iodine and the risk of postcesarean endometritis. Obstet Gynecol 2005; 105: 1024–9. [RCT, n=308]
11. Reid VC, Hartmann KE, McMahon M, Fry EP. Vaginal preparation with povidone iodine and postcesarean infectious morbidity: a randomized controlled trial. Obstet Gynecol 2001; 97: 147–52. [RCT, n=198]
12. Pitt C, Sanchez-Ramos L, Kaunitz AM. Adjunctive intravaginal metronidazole for the prevention of postcesarean endometritis: a randomized controlled trial. Obstet Gynecol 2001; 98: 745–50. [RCT, n=224]

13. Cordtz T, Schouenborg L, Lauren K et al. The effect of incision plastic drapes and redisinfection of operation site on wound infection following caesarean section. J Hospit Infect 1989; 13: 267–72. [RCT, n = 1340]

14. Ward HRG, Jennings OGN, Potgieter P, Lombard CJ. Do plastic adhesive drapes prevent post caesarean wound infection? J Hospit Infect 2001; 47: 230–4. [RCT, n = 605]

15. Franchi M, Ghezzi F, Raio L et al. Joel-Cohen or Pfannenstiel incision at cesarean delivery: does it make a difference? Acta Obstet Gynecol Scand 2002; 81: 1040–6. [RCT, n = 366]

16. Mathai M, Ambersheth, George A. Comparison of two transverse abdominal incisions for cesarean delivery. Int J Gynecol Obstet 2002; 78: 47–9. [RCT, n = 101 (411 total)]

17. Ayers JWT, Morley GW. Surgical incision for cesarean section. Obstet Gynecol 1987; 70: 706–8. [RCT, n = 97]

18. Berthet J, Peresse JF, Rosier P, Racinet C. Comparative study of Pfannesteil's incision and transverse abdominal incision in gynecologic and obstetric surgery. Presse Med 1989; 18: 1431–3. [RCT]

19. Giacalone PL, Daures JP, Vignal J et al. Pfannesteil versus Maylard incision for cesarean delivery: a randomized controlled trial. Obstet Gynecol 2002; 99: 745–50. [RCT, n = 97]

20. Hohlagschwandtner M, Ruecklinger E, Husslein P, Joura EA. Is the formation of a bladder flap at cesarean necessary? A randomized trial. Obstet Gynecol 2001; 98: 1089–92. [RCT, n = 102]

21. Lao TT, Halpern SH, Crosby ET, Huh C. Uterine incision and maternal blood loss in preterm caesarean section. Arch Gynecol Obstet 1993; 252: 113–17. [II–2]

22. Wilkinson C, Enkin MW. Absorbable staples for uterine incision at caesarean section. Cochrane Database Syst Rev 2007; 1. [meta-analysis; 4 RCTs, n = 526]

23. Rodriguez AI, Porter KB, O'Brien WF. Blunt versus sharp expansion of the uterine incision in low-segment transverse cesarean section. Am J Obstet Gynecol 1994; 171: 1022–5. [RCT, n = 286]

24. Magann EF, Chauhan SP, Bufkin L et al. Intra-operative haemorrhage by blunt versus sharp expansion of the uterine incision at caesarean delivery: a randomised clinical trial. Br J Obstet Gynaecol 2002; 109: 448–52. [RCT, n = 945]

25. Bofill JA, Lencki SG, Barhan S, Ezenagu LC. Instrumental delivery of the fetal head at the time of elective repeat cesarean: a randomized pilot study. Am J Perinatol 2000; 17(5): 265–9. [RCT, n = 44]

26. Smaill F, Hofmeyr GJ. Antibiotic prophylaxis for cesarean section. Cochrane Database Syst Rev 2007; 1. [81 RCTs, n => 2000]

27. Hopkins, Smaill F. Antibiotic prophylaxis regimens and drugs for cesarean section. Cochrane Database Syst Rev 2007; 1. [53 RCTs, n => 2000]

28. Gordon HR, Phelps D, Blanchard K. Prophylactic cesarean section antibiotics: maternal and neonatal morbidity before or after cord clamping. Obstet Gynecol 1979; 53: 151–6. [RCT, n = 114]

29. Cunningham FG, Leveno KJ, DePalma RT, Roark M, Rosenfeld CR. Perioperative antimicrobials for cesarean delivery: before or after cord clamping? Obstet Gynecol 1983; 62: 151–4. [RCT, n = 305]

30. Wax JR, Hersey K, Philput C et al. Single dose cefazolin prophylaxis for postcesarean infections: before vs. after cord clamping. J Mater Fetal Med 1997; 6: 61–5. [RCT, n = 90]

31. Thigpen BD, Hood WA, Chauhan S et al. Timing of prophylactic antibiotic administration in the uninfected laboring gravida: a randomized clinical trial. Am J Obstet Gynecol 2005; 192: 1864–71. [RCT, n = 303]

32. Munn MB, Owen J, Vincent R et al. Comparison of two oxytocin regimens to prevent uterine atony at cesarean delivery: a randomized controlled trial. Obstet Gynecol 2001; 98: 386–90. [RCT, n = 321]

33. Boucher M, Horbay GLA, Griffin P et al. Double-blind, randomized comparison of the effect of carbetocin and oxytocin on intraoperative blood loss and uterine tone of patients undergoing cesarean section. J Perinat 1998; 18: 202–7. [RCT, n = 57]

34. Dansereau J, Joshi AK, Helewa ME et al. Double-blind comparison of carbetocin versus oxytocin in prevention of uterine atony after cesarean section. Am J Obstet Gynecol 1999; 180: 670–6. [RCT, n = 694]

35. Wilkinson C, Enkin MW. Manual removal of placenta at cesarean section. Cochrane Database Syst Rev 2007; 1. [meta-analysis: not yet updated, should include 12 RCTs, n => 3000]

36. Atkinson MW, Owen J, Wren A, Hauth JC. The effect of manual removal of the placenta on post-cesarean endometritis. Obstet Gynecol 1996; 87: 99–102. [RCT, n = 643]

37. Jacobs-Jokhan D, Hofmeyr GJ. Extra-abdominal versus intra-abdominal repair of the uterine incision at caesarean section. Cochrane Database Syst Rev 2007; 1. [meta-analysis: 6 RCTs, n = 1221]

38. Enkin MW, Wilkinson C. Single versus two layer suturing for closing the uterine incision at caesarean section. Cochrane Database Syst Rev 2007; 1. [meta-analysis: 2 RCTs, n = 1006]

39. Chapman SJ, Owen J, Hauth JC. One versus two-layer closure of a low transverse cesarean: the next pregnancy. Obstet Gynecol 1997; 89: 16–18. [follow-up of RCT]

40. Hohlagschwandtner M, Chalubinski K, Nather A, Husslein P, Joura EA. Continuous vs interrupted sutures for single-layer closure of uterine incision at cesarean section. Arch Gynecol Obstet 2003; 268: 26–8. [II–2, n = 81]

41. Stafford MK, Pitman MC, Nanthakumaran N, Smith JR. Blunt-tipped versus sharp-tipped needles: wound morbidity. J Obstet Gynecol 1998; 18: 18–19. [RCT, n = 203]

42. Bamigboye AA, Hofmeyr GJ. Closure versus non-closure of the peritoneum at caesarean section. Cochrane Database Syst Rev 2007; 1. [meta-analysis: 9 RCTs, n = 1811]

43. Roset E, Boulvain M, Irion O. Nonclosure of the peritoneum during cesarean section: long term follow-up of a randomized controlled trial. Eur J Obstet Gynecol Reprod Biol 2003; 108: 40–4. [follow-up of RCT]

44. Tulandi T, Al-Jaroudi D. Nonclosure of peritoneum: a reappraisal. Am J Obstet Gynecol 2003; 189: 609–12. [review]

45. Harrigill KM, Miller HS, Haynes DE. The effect of intraabdominal irrigation at cesarean delivery on maternal morbidity: a randomized trial. Obstet Gynecol 2003; 101: 80–5. [RCT, n = 196]

46. Chelmow D, Rodriguez EF, Sabatini MM. Suture closure of subcutaneous fat and wound disruption after cesarean delivery: a meta-analysis. Obstet Gynecol 2004; 103: 974–80. [meta-analysis; 6 RCTs, n => 1,500]

47. Anderson ER, Gates S. Techniques and materials for closure of the abdominal wall in caesarean section. Cochrane Database Syst Rev 2007; 1. [meta-analysis: 6 RCTs, n => 1500]

48. Loong RLC, Rogers MS, Chang AMZ. A controlled trial on wound drainage in caesarean section. Aust NZ J Obstet Gynecol 1988; 28: 266–9. [RCT, n = 242]

49. Frishman GN, Schwartz T, Hogan JW. Closure of Pfannenstiel skin incisions: staples vs. subcuticular suture. J Reprod Med 1997; 42: 627–30. [RCT, n = 50]

50. Wechter ME, Pearlman MD, Hartmann KE. Reclosure of the disrupted laparotomy wound. Obstet Gynecol 2005; 106: 376–83. [meta-analysis: 8 RCTs, n = 324. (includes both CDs, gyn and GI laparotomies)]

51. Harris RL, Magann EF, Sullivan DL, Meeks GR. Extrafascial wound dehiscence: secondary closure with suture versus noninvasive adhesive bandage. J Pelvic Surg 1995; 1: 88–91. [RCT, n = 27]

13

Vaginal birth after cesarean

Amen Ness

KEY POINTS

- A woman with a prior cesarean delivery (CD) has two options for mode of delivery in the subsequent pregnancy: an elective repeat cesarean delivery (ERCD) or a trial of labor (TOL) to try to achieve a vaginal birth after cesarean (VBAC). There are no trials to compare the safety, complications, and maternal and fetal/neonatal morbidity and mortality between the two options.
- **Uterine rupture** is the **main complication** associated with TOL after CD.
- The **risk of uterine rupture** with a policy of TOL after CD depends on several factors: it **is 0.7 after 1 prior low transverse CD**, and is increased with > 1 prior CD, prior vertical scar, prior rupture, induction or augmentation, fetal macrosomia, and possibly interval between delivery < 18 months, maternal age > 30 years old, and fever around prior CD.
- Rates of **all maternal complications except rupture are infrequent** and similar with both TOL and ERCD.
- The **most serious fetal risk in women with prior CD is from uterine rupture during TOL.** Risks of fetal/neonatal morbidity/mortality with term uterine rupture are about 33% risk of pH < 7.00, 40% admission to a neonatal intensive care unit (NICU), 6% risk of hypoxic-ischemic encephalopathy (HIE), and 1.8% risk of neonatal death (rupture-related risk of neonatal death: 1 in 10 000) in equipped academic centers. In other centers, these risks are higher, including risk of neonatal death from rupture up to 10–25%.
- **Compared with ERCD, TOL after CD is associated with slightly higher rates of adverse perinatal outcome:** cord pH < 7.00 (1.5/1000 TOL), hypoxic-ischemic encephalopathy (8 in 10 000), and perinatal death (excluding malformations) (4.0 in 10 000 with TOL versus 1.4 in 10 000 for ERCD). The overall risk of adverse perinatal outcome is 1/2000 with TOL, slightly higher than with ERCD.
- When compared with women without a previous cesarean delivery (instead of those having an elective CD), the perinatal mortality for TOL-VBAC after CD is higher than ERCD, but this rate is only twice as high as

that of a non-VBAC multipara in labor and the same as that of a nullipara in labor.
- **Absolute contraindications to TOL after CD are:**
  - medical or obstetric complications that preclude vaginal delivery
  - inability to perform emergency CD; vertical (classical) uterine scar
  - fundal or perifundal complete (from endometrium to serosa) uterine scar from other surgery (e.g. myomectomy);
  - prior uterine rupture.
- **Successful VBAC rates in the general population of women with previous low transverse uterine incisions vary from 60 to 80%.** Women with prior CD and without prior VBAC may have success rates of ≤ 50% if they have > 2 prior CDs, weight > 300 lbs, body mass index (BMI) > 30, or macrosomia > 4000 g. **No screening tools is sensitive enough to be clinically useful** in predicting an unsuccessful trial of labor, and none has been validated prospectively to improve outcomes.
- **Appropriate counseling, including risks as described, should be provided to the woman with a prior CD deciding on subsequent mode of delivery. The ultimate decision regarding attempting TOL after CD or ERCD is up to the patient.**
- **To minimize risks, an experienced obstetrician, anesthesia, nursing and operating room (OR) personnel, and ability to perform emergency CD must be immediately available at all times (24 hours/7 days) throughout TOL after CD.**

Historical perspective

Until the late 1970s, 'Once a cesarean always a cesarean' was the general rule among most obstetricians. This phrase did not derive from formal studies and was clearly not evidence based. A classical uterine incision was used until the 1920s, when the low transverse (LT) incision was introduced in the US. The LT incision was associated with a 10-fold decreased rate of uterine rupture in labor compared with the classical

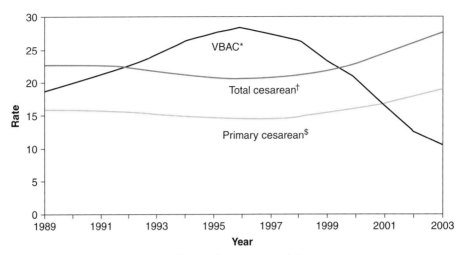

Figure 13.1
Rates of total and primary cesarean delivery and of VBAC for the period 1989–2003 in the USA. (Reproduced from Quickstats MMWR weekly,[2] with permission.)

incision. Based on studies in the 1970s when the vaginal delivery after cesarean (VBAC) rate was very low, the National Institutes of Health (NIH) in 1980 and then the American College of Obstetricians and Gynecologists (ACOG) in 1988 and in 1999 suggested that a trial of labor (TOL) after a previous LT cesarean delivery (CD) is a reasonable option.[1] In response to these recommendations, the VBAC rate in the USA increased from 3.5% in 1980 to 28.3% in 1996. As more VBACs were attempted, more ruptures were seen and litigation for complications of a TOL also increased. As a result, after declining until about 1997, cesarean rates have increased globally (21.3% in England and 29% in the USA in 2004). While VBAC rates have decreased rapidly to just 9% in the USA in 2004 (Figure 13.1), they have remained relatively high in the UK, at 33% (range 6–64%).[2,3]

Definitions

VBAC: vaginal delivery after cesarean.
TOL: trial of labor.
ERCD: elective repeat cesarean delivery (before labor).
VBAC rate: number of vaginal births after previous CD per 100 live births to all women with a previous CD (same denominator as the cesarean section rate).
TOL rate: if the average success rate of a TOL is about 70%, then the TOL rate is the VBAC rate/0.7.
Adjusted VBAC rate: number of women with prior CD and no contraindications to TOL who had a vaginal delivery per 100 live births to all women with a previous CD.
Successful VBAC rate: percentage of women with prior CD who attempted a TOL, achieving a vaginal birth (VBAC).

Successful adjusted VBAC rate: percentage of women with prior CD and no contraindications to TOL, achieving a vaginal birth (VBAC).
Failed TOL (failed VBAC): TOL after CD that results in a repeat CD.
Uterine dehiscence: disruption of the uterine muscle with intact serosa.[4] It can include asymptomatic opening of the uterine scar from prior surgery, without protrusion of fetus/fetal organs outside the uterus.
Uterine rupture: disruption or tear of the uterine muscle and visceral peritoneum, or separation of the uterine muscle with extension to the bladder or broad ligament.[4] It includes symptomatic gross rupture of the uterine scar from prior surgery, with or without protrusion of fetus/fetal organs outside the uterus.

General considerations

A woman with a prior CD has two options for mode of delivery in the subsequent pregnancy: an **ERCD or a TOL** to try to achieve a VBAC. There are **no trials** to compare the safety, complications, and maternal and fetal/neonatal morbidity and mortality between the two options. Virtually all studies on VBAC, except for a recent large prospective multicenter one,[4] are retrospective,[5–10] and often use differing criteria for patient selection and differ in their ability to correctly ascertain (make sure all cases are included) and define uterine rupture. Studies with < 1000 TOL after CD cannot adequately assess maternal and fetal/neonatal morbidity and mortality, as these complications are rare, and meta-analyses[3,11,12] might compound errors from different retrospective studies. Many studies do not differentiate between asymptomatic uterine dehiscence and true acute symptomatic uterine rupture. The main issues regarding TOL after CD (attempt at VBAC) are complications and safety (especially in regard to uterine rupture), and success rates at achieving vaginal delivery, as compared to repeat CD.

Safety/complications

Maternal–fetal

Uterine rupture is the most serious complication associated with TOL after CD. The risk of uterine rupture with a policy of TOL after CD depends on several factors, such as number of prior CD (Table 13.1), direction of scar (Table 13.1), layers of closure, induction or augmentation, maternal age, fever, prior preterm CD, and TOL at ≥ 40 weeks.

Risk factors/associations for uterine rupture

Number of prior cesareans: Women with ≥ 2 prior LT CD are at increased risk of uterine rupture compared with women with 1 prior CD.[13–15] Most of these ruptures occur in women undergoing induction or augmentation and in those without a prior vaginal delivery.[13] The overall relative risk of rupture is increased (about twofold) in women having a TOL after 2 LT CDs compared with 1. But the rupture rate in women with a prior vaginal delivery and 2 prior CDs is only 0.5%, no greater than a VBAC with only one prior CD.[13] The rate of rupture instead increases from 2% with 2 prior CDs up to 5–9% with >2 CDs, and is directly proportional to the number of prior CDs.[15]

Direction of scar: Records regarding the prior CD(s) should be obtained, with special care in documentation of direction of scar. If a woman has had a prior vertical (classical) CD, repeat CD is recommended.[1]

Layers of closure: There is insufficient evidence to assess if the numbers of layers performed at prior uterine closure affect the outcomes for future pregnancies. Randomized trials have insufficient follow-up numbers (see Chapter 12). Compared with women who had a double-layer closure, women with a single-layer closure have been reported to have either similar or up to a fourfold increased risk of uterine rupture.[3,16]

Table 13.1 *Risk of uterine rupture associated with different historic factors*		
History	Approximate risk of uterine rupture in pregnancy including TOL (%)	References
No prior uterine scars	< 0.01	
Elective repeat CD	≥ 0.1 (0.5 risk of dehiscence)	4, 7
1 prior LT CD (no prior VBAC)	0.7 (0.5–1.0)	4, 11
1 prior LT CD (prior VBAC)	< 0.5	13
2 prior LT CDs (no prior VBAC)	2 (1–3.7)	9, 13–15
2 prior LT CDs (prior VBAC)	0.5	13
> 2 prior LT CDs	5–9	15
Prior vertical (classical) CD	4–10	1
Prior low-vertical CD	1–2	3, 4
Prior 'unknown uterine scar' CD	0.5–2	4
Prior uterine rupture	6 (lower segment rupture) 32 (upper segment rupture)	1

TOL, trial of labor; LT, low transverse; CD, cesarean delivery.

Prior rupture: As prior uterine rupture is associated with **high rates (6–32%) of recurrent rupture** with TOL, these pregnancies should have an **ERCD before labor**, possibly around 38 weeks.[1]

Induction/augmentation (at or near term): There is insufficient contradicting evidence regarding the effect of **induction** on rates of complications of TOL after prior CD. Almost all studies of sufficient size report a **slight increase (up to 1–2%) in rupture with induction** of any kind.[4,8,17] One trial of women with 1 prior CD, gestational age > 37 weeks, and Bishop score < 7 did not show any rupture in either the TOL or ERCD groups, but the numbers studied were insufficient to assess the rare complications associated with VBAC.[18] The risks of uterine rupture with induction in women who had 1 prior CD may also depend on the type of induction. Risk of rupture is approximately **1.4–2.5 with induction with prostaglandin** (with or without oxytocin),[4,7] and about **1.1 with oxytocin alone.**[4] Induction with misoprostol in a woman with an unfavorable cervical examination and prior CD should be discouraged.[7] There is insufficient evidence to assess the safety of mifepristone induction in women with a prior CD.[19]

Women with prior CD should be made aware of these higher risks of rupture associated with induction.[1]

Augmentation may be associated with a very slight increased risk of rupture, e.g. up to about 1%.[4,17] In one study, compared with non-intervention, **augmentation with oxytocin** for no cervical change after 4 hours of contractions in term gravidas with 1 or 2 unknown uterine scars in early labor is associated with similar rates of CD, but an increase (5 vs 0%) in uterine scar separation; one of these occurred in a woman with 2 prior CDs, one of which vertical, requiring hysterectomy.[20]

Second trimester induction of labor: Induction of labor in the second trimester with misoprostol is associated with no or minimal risk of uterine rupture after 1 prior LT CD, but about 5% risk with ≥ 2 prior LT CDs, and about 50% risk with a prior classical CD.[21]

Macrosomia > 4000 g: Macrosomia > 4000 g is associated with a slightly increased risk of rupture.[22]

Interval between deliveries: Interval between deliveries of < 18 months is associated with an increased risk (2%) of rupture.[23]

Maternal age: Maternal age (> 30 years old) is associated with an increased risk (1.4%) of uterine rupture.[24]

Fever: The presence of both intrapartum and postpartum fever at CD, but not either alone, may increase the risk of uterine rupture in a subsequent pregnancy.[25]

Post dates: The risk of uterine rupture does not increase substantially after 40 weeks, but is increased with induction of labor regardless of gestational age.[26]

Preterm: In one study there was a trend toward a lower uterine rupture rate in preterm patients who attempted a VBAC.[27]

Twins: The risk of rupture or maternal mortality is not increased with prior CD and subsequent TOL with twins, with uncommon perinatal morbidity at ≥ 34 weeks.[28]

Maternal

- Hysterectomy: 1–2 in 1000 TOL;[4–11] similar to ERCD.[4]
- Transfusion: uncommon for TOL or ERCD, but slightly more frequent (1.7 vs 1%)[4] with TOL–VBAC (about 2 units packed red blood cells [pRBCs]/1000 TOL),[11] and related to the need for cesarean delivery following a TOL.[4]
- Thromboembolic disease: about 4 in 10 000, similar to ERCD (1 in 1000).[4]
- Endometritis: uncommon and very similar for TOL or ERCD (6 vs 7–8% – fever[12] – or 3 vs 2% in academic centers[4]), and related to the need for cesarean delivery following a TOL.
- Maternal mortality: about 2 in 100 000,[11] similar (slightly lower) to ERCD (about 4–5 in 100 000).[4–6]
- Therefore, rates of all maternal complications except rupture are infrequent and similar with both TOL and ERCD.[4,11,12] In those women who attempt a VBAC (TOL) but end up with a repeat cesarean section in labor (failed VBAC), maternal morbidity is higher than in women undergoing an elective repeat cesarean section.[10]

Fetal/neonatal

The most serious fetal risk in women with prior CD is from uterine rupture during TOL. Risks of fetal/neonatal morbidity/mortality with term uterine rupture are: 33% risk of pH < 7.00, 40% admission to a neonatal intensive care unit (NICU), 6% risk of hypoxic-ischemic encephalopathy (HIE), and 1.8% risk of neonatal death (rupture-related risk of neonatal death: 1 in 10 000) in equipped academic centers.[4] In other centers, these risks are higher, including risk of neonatal death from rupture up to 10–25%.

Compared with ERCD, **TOL after CD is associated with significantly higher rates of:**

- **Antepartum fetal death** (2–6 in 1000 vs 1–2 per 1000). This might be due to stillbirths occurring at ≥ 39 weeks with TOL, or to encouragement to TOL with diagnosis of stillbirth.[4]
- **Cord pH < 7.00** (1.5 in 1000 TOL).[11]
- **HIE:** 8 in 10 000 vs none in the ERCD.[4] The overall risk of rupture-related HIE is 1 in 2500 TOL–VBAC.

- Neonatal death rates: similar between the groups (0.08% vs 0.05%) in academic centers, with the neonatal death rate associated with a rupture at term about 1.8%.[4]
- Perinatal death (excluding malformations) rates are 4.0 in 10 000 with TOL[4,11] vs 1.4 in 10 000 for ERCD.[4]
- Overall risk of adverse perinatal outcome is 1 in 2000 with TOL, slightly higher than with ERCD.[4]

When compared with women **without a previous CD** (instead of with those having an ERCD), the overall **perinatal mortality for TOL after CD** is higher than ERCD (10 in 10 000 vs 0.4 in 10 000 births), but this rate is only twice as high as that of a non-VBAC multipara in labor and **the same as that of a nullipara in labor**.[29]

Contraindications

Absolute contraindications

- Medical or obstetric complication that precludes vaginal delivery.
- Inability to perform emergency CD.
- Vertical (classical) uterine scar.
- Fundal or perifundal complete (from endometrium to serosa) uterine scar from other surgery (e.g. myomectomy).
- Prior uterine rupture.

Relative contraindications

- Multiple uterine scars (e.g. ≥ 2 prior CDs).
- Any other factor (see above) associated with a risk of rupture of > 1%.

Successful TOL–VBAC: rates and factors affecting rates of success

Successful VBAC **rates** in the general population of women with previous LT uterine incisions vary from 60 to 80%.[4,11] In tertiary care centers, the rates may be higher, about 73–76%.[4,5] The following factors are associated with the success or failure of a TOL–VBAC.

Prior vaginal delivery after cesarean delivery

A **previously successful VBAC** is the most predictive prognostic indicator (> 90% success rate). It is more predictive of a vaginal delivery than a vaginal delivery that occurred before the prior cesarean.[30]

Prior indication

Breech presentation or other **non-recurring indication** (e.g. non-reassuring fetal monitoring) for the prior cesarean delivery significantly increases the chances for a vaginal delivery (85%). Nevertheless, about 60–70% of women undergoing a TOL after a prior CD for **dystocia** deliver vaginally.[1] There seems to be no reduction in the rates for a successful TOL–VBAC following a previous CD in the **second stage of labor** (75–80%), with no increased risk of operative vaginal delivery.[31,32]

Number of prior cesarean deliveries

About 75–80% of women attempting a VBAC with a single prior cesarean will deliver vaginally vs about **60–70% (decreased) with more than one prior cesarean**. The majority of studies have shown that the greater the number of prior cesarean deliveries, the lower are the chances for a vaginal delivery (about 10–15% lower per CD).[3]

Maternal obesity

Obese women attempting a VBAC have lower success rates, with women ≥ 300 lbs having rates of only 15%, whereas women weighing 200–300 lbs have rates of 56%.[33,34] Women ≥ 300 lbs also have a > 50% chance of infectious morbidity (vs 17.8% in women weighing 200–300 lbs). ERCD in the obese group significantly reduces the infectious morbidity by almost 50% compared with those with a TOL. In a recent study which excluded women with a prior vaginal delivery, VBAC success rates were 54.6% in women with a body mass index (BMI) ≥ 30 vs 70.5% in women with a normal BMI.[35]

Fetal macrosomia

There is conflicting evidence regarding the effect of fetal macrosomia (using actual birth weights at delivery) and the success of a VBAC.[22,36] The success rates for VBAC in women with a previous cesarean delivery and no other births is about **60% in the > 4000 g group** and **71% in the ≤ 4000 g group**.[36] There is progressive reduction in VBAC success rates as birth weight increases.[22] **With a prior VBAC or a vaginal delivery, there is no success rate below 63% for any of the birth weight strata. With no previous vaginal delivery, VBAC success rates can drop below 50% as neonatal weight exceeds 4000 g**.[22] This success rate can decrease further if the indication for the previous cesarean delivery is cephalopelvic disproportion or failure to progress. **There are no data regarding *estimated* fetal birth weight and VBAC success.**

Cervical status

The more **favorable** the **cervix**, the greater the odds for a vaginal delivery.

Induction/augmentation of labor

Women who receive oxytocin for induction or augmentation have rates of vaginal delivery about 10% lower than those that are allowed or able to labor spontaneously.[3,12]

Post dates

Few studies have addressed the issue of post-term pregnancy and the success of TOL after CD. Successful VBAC rates of 65–82% have been reported for women with gestational age >40 weeks, with the higher rates in women with prior vaginal deliveries.[1] **If VBAC is still desired after 40 weeks, awaiting the onset of spontaneous labor may be a better option than induction before 40 weeks for women planning a VBAC,** because the rate of symptomatic uterine rupture is significantly increased for women who are induced, regardless of the gestational age compared with spontaneous onset of labor after 40 weeks, and because women induced before or at 40 weeks or who enter spontaneous labor after 40 weeks have similar (30–35%) CD rates. It may be reasonable to offer an AROM (artificial rupture of membranes)/oxytocin induction around the EDC (estimated date of confinement) to women with a prior vaginal delivery and a favorable cervix (Bishop Score ≥9, or transvaginal ultrasound cervical length <20 mm).

Uterine scar type

Vaginal delivery rates appear to be **similar** for low transverse, low vertical, and for unknown incision types.[3]

Maternal age

There is an inverse association between maternal age and the likelihood of vaginal delivery, with the **odds of vaginal delivery significantly greater for younger women.**[3]

Multiple gestations

Vaginal delivery rates of both twins after prior CD range from 65 to 84%,[3–28] and do not seem to differ from success rates in singletons, without increased risk for maternal morbidity or uterine rupture.[28]

Interdelivery interval

Interdelivery interval of <19 months may be associated with similar success rates of TOL after CD compared with longer intervals, but lower rates if labor is induced.[3,37]

Preterm

Preterm patients with prior CD have a slightly higher VBAC success rate than term patients (82% vs 74%).[27]

Prediction tools for vaginal delivery

Given the associations above, several different scoring systems have been proposed to predict the likelihood of vaginal delivery or cesarean in women undergoing a VBAC.[38–41] **None of these screening tools is sensitive enough to be clinically useful in predicting an unsuccessful trial of labor, and none has been validated prospectively to improve outcomes.**[41]

Management

Patients with contraindications (see above) to VBAC should receive an ERCD at 39 weeks, or earlier if labor starts or in certain cases (e.g. prior early uterine rupture).

Patient counseling[4]

- TOL can be offered to most women with a prior CD, but several safety and success factors should be considered and discussed with the woman.
- The composite of **maternal complications** is slightly higher with TOL–VBAC compared with the ERCD group, **primarily due to the risk of rupture and the increased risks of a cesarean delivery in labor.** These estimates do not take into account the long-term increased risks of repetitive cesarean deliveries and the associated risks of placenta previa and accreta.[40] This is why **counseling should take in to account how many future pregnancies are planned.**
- The overall risks of serious perinatal complications are about 1 in 2000 TOL, which is slightly greater than that of ERCD.[4] Combining all poor perinatal outcomes, >600 ERCD would need to be performed to prevent 1 poor perinatal outcome. Although a woman with a TOL after CD is at higher risk of uterine rupture than any other group, the risk of perinatal death is similar to that of any nulliparous woman in labor.[29]
- For the approximately 60–80% of women **attempting a VBAC who will deliver vaginally,** the maternal and perinatal morbidity and mortality are lower than ERCD.
- ERCD is safer than a VBAC attempt that results in a cesarean delivery.
- Although the risks of TOL–VBAC are higher than ERCD, the absolute risks are small and comparable to other potential complications of labor.
- Efforts to reduce the frequency of the first cesarean reduce the need for a VBAC or repeat cesarean.

TOL after CD should be approached with caution in those with the lowest chance of vaginal delivery and highest risk of rupture: e.g. try to avoid induction of labor in those with an unfavorable cervix and no prior vaginal deliveries. All women with a single prior LT CD without other indications for a cesarean delivery are candidates for a TOL. Women at lowest risk for adverse outcomes and highest chance for a vaginal delivery include those with a prior vaginal delivery (especially a prior VBAC), in spontaneous labor, with a favorable cervix.

The ultimate decision regarding attempting VBAC or not is up to the patient after appropriate counseling. Most women should decide before term, and their decision should be documented in the medical record. The decision might not be made until term in women who want to assess if spontaneous labor and/or favorable cervix make their chances of complications lower and of success higher. There is no evidence that examining the adequacy of the pelvis benefits outcomes.

Prenatal education

Individualized prenatal education directed toward avoidance of a cesarean delivery does not increase the rate of vaginal birth after cesarean section.[42]

Consent

Specific consent for TOL after CD or ERCD should be signed by the woman after appropriate counseling, before term.

Non-vertex presentation

External cephalic version (ECV) can safely be performed in women with a prior CD. The success rate for ECV is similar or higher in women with a prior CD compared with controls without a prior CD (82% vs 61%).[43] Women with a successful version have successful VBAC rates of 65–76%.[43,44]

Ultrasound of lower uterine segment

Owing to the uncommon nature of rupture, several thousand women need to be studied to assess if measuring the thickness of the lower uterine segment predicts complications in women with a prior CD who elect TOL, and therefore there is insufficient evidence to assess the clinical utility of this screening test. No women with a lower uterine segment thickness of ≥ 4.5 mm seem to have dehiscence or rupture, whereas the proportion of these complications rises as this thickness decreases, with women with defects or thickness < 3.5 mm possibly benefiting from ERCD.[45]

Requirements to minimize risks[1]

To minimize risks, the following must be immediately available at all times (24 hours for 7 days) throughout TOL after CD:

- **experienced obstetrician**
- **anesthesia**
- **nursing and operating room (OR) personnel**
- **ability to perform emergency CD.**

Labor and Delivery (L&D) units with > 1000 births per year have lower risks of uterine rupture and complications compared to units with less volume.[6]

Intrapartum: detecting rupture

- Fetal heart rate (FHR) disturbances are the most common (but not universal) sign of uterine rupture (55–85%). The most commonly reported FHR disturbance is repetitive progressively severe variable decelerations and prolonged bradycardia, although in most cases they are not caused by rupture. Nevertheless, **in women with a prior cesarean delivery, in the presence of such FHR disturbances, uterine rupture must be considered.**
- Abdominal pain over the area of the prior uterine scar is a poor predictor of uterine rupture. Epidural usually does not mask rupture. Epidural should not be withheld in women attempting TOL after prior CD.
- Intrauterine pressure catheter (IUPC) monitoring has not been shown to be helpful.
- Significant loss of fetal station, especially in the second stage, may occur with rupture, but is of limited predictive value.
- There are insufficient data to assess the utility of exploring the uterus after a successful VBAC.

Cost-effectiveness

Cost savings with TOL may occur only if success rates are $\geq 70\%$.

References

1. ACOG Practice Bulletin. Vaginal birth after previous cesarean delivery. No. 54, July 2004. Clinical management guidelines for obstetrician-gynecologists. American College of Obstetricians and Gynecologists. [review]
2. Martin JA, Hamilton BE, Sutton PD et al. Births: final data for 2004. National data statistics reports; Vol 55, no. 1. National Center for Health statistics; Hyattsville, MD: 2006 [Vital statistics data]
3. Guise JM, Hashima J, Osterweil P. Evidence-based vaginal birth after caesarean section. Best Pract Res Clin Obstet Gynaecol 2005; 19(1): 117–30. [meta-analysis: 61 studies, n => 10 000]
4. Landon MB, Hauth JC, Leveno KJ et al. Maternal and perinatal outcomes associated with a trial of labor after prior cesarean delivery. N Engl J Med 2004; 351(25): 2581–9. [II–2; prospective; n = 33 699]
5. Smith GS, Pell JP, Cameron AD, Dobbie R. Risk of perinatal death associated wih labor after previous cesarean delivery in uncomplicated term pregnancies. JAMA 2002; 287: 2684–90. [II–2; n = 15515]

6. Wen SW, Rusen ID, Walker M et al. Comparison of maternal mortality and morbidity between trial of labor and elective cesarean section among women with previous cesarean delivery. Am J Obstet Gynecol 2004; 191: 1263–9. [II–2; n = 308 755]

7. Lyndon-Rochelle M, Holt VL, Easterling TR, Martin DP. Risk of uterine rupture during labor among women with a prior cesarean delivery. N Engl J Med 2001; 345(1): 3–8. [II–2; n = 20 095]

8. Rageth JC, Juzi C, Grossenbacher H; for the Swiss Working Group. Delivery after previous cesarean: a risk evaluation. Obstet Gynecol 1999; 93: 332–7. [II–2, n = 29 046]

9. Miller DA, Diaz FG, Paul RH. Vaginal birth after cesarean: a 10-year experience. Obstet Gynecol 1994; 84(2): 255–8. [II–2, n = 17 322]

10. McMahon MJ, Luther ER, Bowes WA Jr, Olshan AF. Comparison of a trial of labor with an elective second cesarean section. N Engl J Med 1996; 335(10): 689–95. [II–2, n = 6138]

11. Chauhan SP, Martin JN, Hendrichs CE, Morrison JC, Magann EF. Maternal and perinatal complications with uterine rupture in 142,075 patients who attempted vaginal birth after cesarean delivery: a review of the literature. Am J Obstet Gynecol 2003; 189: 408–17. [meta-analysis: 72 studies, n = 142 075]

12. Guise JM, Berlin M, McDonagh M et al. Safety of vaginal birth after cesarean: a systematic review. Obstet Gynecol 2004; 103(3): 420–9. [meta-analysis: n = 20 studies]

13. Macones GA, Cahill A, Pare E et al. Obstetric outcomes in women with two prior cesarean deliveries: is vaginal birth after cesarean delivery a viable option? Am J Obstet Gynecol 2005; 192: 1223–9. [II–2]

14. Caughey AB, Shipp TD, Repke JT et al. Rate of uterine rupture during a trial of labor in women with one or two prior cesarean deliveries. Am J Obstet Gynecol 1999; 181(4): 872–6. [II–2, n = 3891 TOL with 1 or 2 prior CD]

15. Asakura H, Myers SA. More than one previous cesarean delivery: a 5-year experience with 435 patients. Obstet Gynecol 1995; 85: 924–9. [II–2, n = 435 TOL with >1 prior CD]

16. Bujold E, Bujold C, Hamilton EF, Harel F, Gauthier RJ. The impact of a single-layer or double-layer closure on uterine rupture. Am J Obstet Gynecol 2002; 186(6): 1326–30. [II–2, n = 1980 with 1 or 2 layers]

17. McDonagh MS, Osterweil P, Guise J-M. The benefits and risks of inducing labour in patients with prior caesarean delivery: a systematic review. Br J Obstet Gynecol 2005; 112: 1007–15. [meta-analysis: 14 studies (only 2 RCTs)]

18. Rayburn WF, Gittens LN, Lucas MJ, Gall SA, Martin ME. Weekly administration of prostaglandin E$_2$ gel compared to expectant management in women with previous cesareans. Obstet Gynecol 1999; 94: 250–4. [RCT, n = 294]

19. Lelaidier C, Baton C, Benifla JL et al. Mifepristone for labour induction after pervious caesarean section. Br J Obstet Gynecol 1994; 101: 501–3. [RCT, n = 32]

20. Grubb DK, Kjos SL, Paul RH. Latent labor with an unknown uterine scar. Obstet Gynecol 1996; 88: 351–5. [RCT, n = 197].

21. Airoldi J, O'Neill AM, Einhorn K, Hoffman M, Berghella V. Misoprostol for second trimester labor induction in women with prior cesarean deliveries: does the type and number of incisions matter? Obstet Gynecol 2006; 107: 59–60s. [II–2 and review of the literature]

22. Elkousy MA, Sammel M, Stevens E, Peipert JF, Macones G. The effect of birth weight on vaginal birth after cesarean delivery success rates. Am J Obstet Gynecol 2003; 188(3): 824–30. [II–2]

23. Shipp TD, Zelop C, Repke JT, Cohen A, Lieberman E. Interdelivery interval and risk of symptomatic uterine rupture. Obstet Gynecol 2001; 97: 175–7. [II–2, n = 2409]

24. Shipp TD, Zelop C, Repke JT et al. The association of maternal age and symptomatic uterine rupture during a trial of labor after prior cesarean delivery. Obstet Gynecol 2002; 99(4): 585–8. [II–2, n = 3015]

25. Shipp TD, Zelop C, Cohen A, Repke JT, Lieberman E. Post-cesarean delivery fever and uterine rupture in a subsequent trial of labor. Obstet Gynecol 2003; 101(1): 136–9. [II–2]

26. Zelop CM, Shipp TD, Cohen A, Repke JT, Lieberman E. Trial of labor after 40 weeks' gestation in women with prior cesarean. Obstet Gynecol 2001; 97(3): 391–3. [II–2]

27. Quinones JN, Stamilio DM et al. The effect of prematurity on vaginal birth after cesarean delivery: success and maternal morbidity. Obstet Gynecol 2005; 105(3): 519–24. [II–2, n = 971 preterm TOL after CD]

28. Varner MW, Leindecker S, Spong CY et al. The maternal-fetal medicine unit cesarean registry: trial of labor with twin gestation. Am J Obstet Gynecol 2005; 193: 135–40. [II–2, n = 186 women with prior CD and subsequent TOL]

29. Smith GS, Pell JP, Cameron AD, Dobbie R. Risk of perinatal death associated with labor after previous cesarean delivery in uncomplicated term pregnancies. JAMA 2002; 287: 2684–90. [II–2, n = > 300 000 singleton term births]

30. Hendler I, Bujold E. Effect of prior vaginal birth after cesarean delivery on obstetric outcomes in women undergoing trial of labor. Obstet Gynecol 2004; 104(2): 273–7. [II–2]

31. Bujold E, Gauthier RJ. Should we allow a trial of labor after a previous cesarean for dystocia in the second stage of labor? Obstet Gynecol 2001; 98(4): 652–5. [II–2, n = 214]

32. Jongen VH, Halfwerk MG, Brouwer WK. Vaginal delivery after previous cesarean section for failure of second stage of labour. Br J Obstet Gynecol 1998; 105: 1079–81. [II–2]

33. Chauhan SP, Magann EF, Carroll CS et al. Mode of delivery for the morbidly obese women with prior cesarean delivery: vaginal versus repeat cesarean section. Am J Obstet Gynecol 2001; 185: 349–54. [II–2, n = 30 women > 300 lbs with TOL after CD]

34. Durnwald CP, Ehrenberg HM, Mercer BM. The impact of maternal obesity and weight gain on vaginal birth after cesarean section success. Am J Obstet Gynecol 2004; 191(3): 954–7. [II–2]

35. Edwards RK, Harnsberger DS, Johnson IM, Treloar RW, Cruz AC. Deciding on route of delivery for obese women with a prior cesarean delivery. Am J Obstet Gynecol 2003; 189(2): 385–9; discussion 389–90. [II–2]

36. Zelop CM, Shipp TD, Repke JT, Cohen A, Lieberman E. Outcomes of a trial of labor following previous cesarean delivery among women with fetuses weighing >4000 g. Am J Obstet Gynecol 2001; 185: 903–5. [II–2]

37. Huang WH, Nakashima DK, Rumney PJ, Keegan KA Jr, Chan K. Interdelivery interval and the success of vaginal birth after cesarean delivery. Obstet Gynecol 2002; 99(1): 41–4. [II–2, n = 81 with interdelivery interval < 19 months]

38. Flamm BL, Geiger AM. Vaginal birth after cesarean delivery: an admission scoring system. Obstet Gynecol 1997; 90(6): 907–10. [review: prediction]

39. Hashima JN, Eden KB, Osterweil P, Nygren P, Guise JM. Predicting vaginal birth after cesarean delivery: a review of prognostic factors and screening tools. Am J Obstet Gynecol 2004; 190(2): 547–55. [review: prediction]

40. Silver RM, Landon MB, Rouse DJ et al. Maternal morbidity associated with multiple repeat caesarean deliveries. Obstet Gynecol 2006; 107: 1226–32.

41. Dinsmoor MJ, Brock EL. Predicting failed trial of labor after primary cesarean delivery. Obstet Gynecol 2004; 103(2): 282–6. [review: prediction]

42. Fraser W, Maunsell E, Hodnett E, Moutquin JM. Randomized controlled trial of a prenatal vaginal birth after cesarean section education and support program. Childbirth Alternatives Post-Cesarean Study Group. Am J Obstet Gynecol 1997; 176(2): 419–25. [RCT, n = 1,275]

43. Flamm BL, Freid MW, Lonky NM, Giles WS, External cephalic version after previous cesarean section. Am J Obstet Gynecol 1991; 165: 370–2. [II–2]

44. de Meeus JB, Ellia F, Magnin G. External cephalic version after previous cesarean section: a series of 38 cases. Eur J Obstet Gynecol Reprod Biol 1998; 81(1): 65–8. [II–2]

45. Rozenberg P, Goffinet F, Philippe HJ, Nisand I. Ultrasonographic measurement of lower uterine segment to assess risk of defects of scarred uterus. Lancet 1996; 347: 281–4. [II–2, n = 642 women with prior CD with ultrasound of lower uterine segment]

Part II

Pregnancy complications

14

Recurrent pregnancy loss

Michele Berghella

KEY POINTS

- Diagnosis of recurrent early pregnancy loss (REPL) is ≥ 2 consecutive losses of pregnancy < 14 weeks.
- **Work-up** includes **uterine study, antiphospholipid antibodies (APA),** and **parental karyotypes,** as well as **karyotype of products of conception** (if available).
- Prognosis with negative work-up is for a 60–70% subsequent successful pregnancy in women < 35 years old, and 40–50% in women ≥ 35 years old.
- Women with **REPL and APA** should be **treated** with **low-dose aspirin (ASA) and heparin** in subsequent pregnancy.
- Women with **REPL and uterine septum, synechiae or submucous myomata** can have **hysteroscopic resection** of these abnormalities.
- Couples with abnormal parental karyotype can be offered genetic counseling, prenatal diagnosis, and/or gamete donation.
- There is insufficient evidence for universal screening for diabetes, thyroid disease, progesterone deficiency (luteal phase defect), infections, thrombophilia, etc.
- Women should **not be tested for alloimmunization or receive any of the immune therapies,** since they are ineffective and at times detrimental.
- Women should **not receive estrogen supplementation,** as this is unsafe, being detrimental to the future offspring and ineffective.
- There is very limited evidence that supportive care and progesterone are beneficial interventions.
- There is insufficient evidence to support human chorionic gonedotropin (HCG), aspirin, and vitamins as interventions.

Diagnoses/definitions

- **Pregnancy loss (PL):** spontaneous loss of pregnancy from conception to < 20 weeks. The term spontaneous abortion (SAB) is equivalent, but should be avoided since

women associate negative feeling with this term. Miscarriage is a lay term for PL.
  - anembryonic PL – no embryo identified (e.g. missed abortion, blighted ovum)
  - embryonic PL – embryo identified, but then non-viable.
- **First trimester** PL: pregnancy loss from conception to < 14 weeks. This guideline concerns mostly this type of recurrent loss (recurrent early pregnancy loss [REPL]).
  - early first trimester PL – loss of pregnancy between conception and 9 6/7 weeks
  - late first trimester PL – loss of pregnancy between 10 and 13 6/7 weeks.
- **Second trimester** (late, or fetal) PL: pregnancy loss between ≥ 14 and 19 6/7 weeks (see end of chapter).
- **Recurrent** PL (RPL): ≥ 2 consecutive losses.

Incidence

The incidence is 1% of reproductive-age women.

Etiology/basic pathophysiology

The etiology is not established in at least 50% of cases after work-up.

Classification

Primary REPL, no intervening live births.
Secondary REPL, intervening live births.

Risk factors/associations

Maternal age < 20 years old, ≥ 35 years old, maternal medical diseases, especially poorly controlled (e.g. hypertension, diabetes mellitus).

Table 14.1 *Natural history of pregnancies following prior pregnancy loss (PL)*

	Prior PL (*n*)	Probability of liveborn (%)
Women with prior liveborn	0	90
	1	80
	2	75
	3	70
	4	60–65
Women without prior liveborn	≥3	55–60

Pregnancy considerations

Human reproduction is relatively inefficient (Table 14.1). Only 30% of fertilized eggs result in a viable pregnancy. Sporadic early PL is very common in humans. At least 15–20% of clinically identified pregnancies (implanted) physiologically end with early PL, and only 50–60% of all conceptions advance to ≥20 weeks.[1] Most PLs represent failure of implantation, and are difficult to recognize clinically. The prognosis after 1 uncomplicated early PL in a healthy young woman is for >70–80% chance of a viable pregnancy in the successive pregnancy. Therefore no work-up or therapy is usually indicated after 1 PL. Oocyte quality and normal karyotype are most important for normal implantation, a lot more than uterine factors.

Pregnancy management

Appropriate diagnostic work-up is essential for choosing the proper intervention. Screening tests should not only discover diagnosis (etiology) but also lead to interventions effective in increasing incidence of subsequent live birth.

Work-up (screening)

The following women should be offered evaluation:
- women with ≥2 primary REPLs
- women with ≥3 secondary REPLs.

Initial part of work-up consists of **history** (smoking, alcohol, caffeine, illicit drug use, environmental exposures, working conditions, as well as detailed obstetric and gynecological history) and **physical examination** (pelvic). Often obstetric history is mixed, with early PL, second trimester PL, preterm birth (PTB) and/or fetal death, so that work-up may include other tests (see specific chapters).

Recommended screening tests

Mother/father

Maternal uterine study

Maternal **uterine study:** e.g. 3D sonohysterography (recommended on day 8–10 of follicular phase), hysterosalpingogram (HSG), hysteroscopy, 2D sonohysterography, or magnetic resonance imaging (MRI).

A total of 10–15% of women with REPL have uterine anomalies. Most common associated anomaly is septate uterus, followed by didelphys and bicornuate. Arcuate uterus has not been consistently associated with REPL. Uterine synechiae (Asherman's syndrome) and DES exposure are associated with REPL. Myomata have not been consistently associated with REPL. Available intervention is hysteroscopic resection of septum, synechiae, or submucous myomata. Surgical correction of these and other uterine anomalies has not been studied in trials.

Maternal antiphospholipid antibodies – anticardiolipin antibodies (ACA), lupus anticogulant (LA) and anti β2 glycoprotein-I

It is found that 3–15% of women with REPL have antiphospholipid antibodies (APAs). Tests should be positive twice, ≥12 weeks apart. See Chapter 23 on antiphospholipid syndrome (APS) in *Maternal–Fetal Evidence Based Guidelines* for tests and effective intervention, which is low-dose aspirin and prophylactic heparin.

Parental karyotype

It is found that 2–4% of couples with REPL have one parent with a balanced translocation, or less commonly a chromosome inversion. Available intervention is donor gametes.

Other Tests

- If family history or clinical suspicion of diabetes: fasting glucose.
- If clinical symptoms/suspicion of thyroid disease: thyroid-stimulating hormone (TSH), free thyroxine (T_4).

Products of conception (POC)

POC karyotype

It is found that 50–60% of early PL tested women have POC aneuploidy, especially if prior PL with aneuploidy and/or advanced maternal age (AMA) (70–80%). Aneuploidy is present in > 50% of embryos tested preimplantation in women with REPL. Over 50% of aneuploidies are trisomies; the most common single aneuploidy is 45,XO. The 46,XX karyotype is often associated with maternal cell contamination, so that caution is necessary; microsatellite analysis decreases this confusion. This test can identify probable etiology; decrease further work-up; and provide the couple with an explanation, which decreases self-blame.[2]

Tests that cannot be routinely recommended

Mother

Endometrial biopsy or progesterone levels

Hypothetically, the corpus luteum fails to make enough progesterone to sustain early decidua for placentation, leading to luteal phase defect (LPD). It is normal to have at least two consecutive out-of-phase (≥ 2 days discrepancy) biopsies (diagnosis of LPD) on endometrial histology (late luteal phase – day 25 or 26 – after presumed ovulation) in 50% of menstrual cycles. There is also high interobserver variation on interpretation of endometrial biopsies. There is insufficient evidence that intervention [such as progesterone supplementation – hydroxyprogesterone caproate (17P), micronized progesterone tablets 100 mg po bid or Crinone cream (8%) one application per vagina daily (beginning 2 days after ovulation until 10 weeks' gestation or menses)] improves outcomes specifically in women with REPL and LPD.[3,4] 17P is efficacious in improving pregnancy outcomes in women with in vitro fertilization (IVF), and in decreasing PTB in women with prior PTB (see Chapter 15).

Alloimmune tests (includes father of baby)

No consistent association, and no efficacious intervention – see below.

Thyroid antibodies

No consistent association, and no intervention studies.

ANA (antinuclear antibody)

No consistent association, and no intervention studies.

Products of conception

- POC molecular genetic abnormalities (e.g. X-chromosome inactivation, etc.). Commercially available tests are not widely available for this testing.

Both

Inherited thrombophilia

Thrombophilic mutations (factor V Leiden, prothrombin G20210, fasting hyperhomocysteinemia (methylene tetrahydrofolate reductase [MHTHFR]), antithrombin III deficiency, protein S, protein C) have not been consistently associated with REPL – see Chapter 27 in *Maternal–Fetal Evidence Based Guidelines*. Second trimester PL has been associated with thrombophilic mutations. There is insufficient evidence regarding any interventions in women with PL and inherited thrombophilias.

Infections

No infectious agent has been proven to cause REPL. *Listeria*, *Toxoplasma gondii*, and many viruses have been associated with sporadic early PL. *Chlamydia*, *Mycoplasma/Ureaplasma* (proposed diagnosis with endometrial biopsy, with treatment of woman and partner with either doxycycline 100 mg orally twice daily (po bid) or ciprofloxacin 250 mg po bid), and bacterial vaginosis are associated with sporadic PL, not REPL.

Management

Prevention

Optimize preconception medical care of all maternal diseases.

Preconception care

Informative and sympathetic counseling. Work-up is best done preconceptionally. When work-up is positive, counsel regarding specific association. If work-up is negative (> 50% of couples), counseling should include the fact that 60–70% of couples with unexplained REPL have successful pregnancies in the next gestation (see Table 14.1). This percentage decreases to 40–50% in women ≥ 35 years old. Offer all women with REPL a support group (Unite, etc).

Prenatal care

See preconception care above.

Therapy: specific for abnormal work-up

Abnormal uterine cavity

Septum, synechiae, and/or submucous myomata can be resected hysteroscopically, but there are no trials regarding this intervention. Consider referral to reproductive endocrinology specialist.

Antiphospholipid syndrome

- Heparin and aspirin (see Chapter 23 of *Maternal–Fetal Evidence Based Guidelines*).
- Therapy is usually begun once fetal viability is established.
- Low-dose aspirin dose is usually about 75–100 mg daily.
- Heparin used in trials was unfractioned heparin, but low molecular weight heparin is associated with less side effects in non-pregnant adults.
- For phophylactic unfractionated heparin: 5000–7500 U first trimester, 7500–10 000 U second trimester, 10 000 U third trimester subcutaneous (SQ) every 12 hours.
- For prophylactic low molecular weight heparin: enoxaparin (Lovenox) 30–40 mg SQ every 12 hours or dalteparin (Fragmin) 5000 U SQ every 12 hours (may adjust prophylaxis in high-risk cases to heparin [antiXa] level range 0.2–0.3).

Abnormal parental chromosomes

Offer genetic counseling, prenatal diagnosis, gamete donation.

Diabetes, thyroid disease

If a **medical condition** is identified (e.g. diabetes mellitus, thyroid disease), treat as indicated.

If the work-up is negative

Supportive care

Consider intensive supportive early prenatal care, focusing on antenatal counseling and psychological support. There are no properly controlled trials to assess the effect of this intervention. Three studies showed improved outcome vs standard or no prenatal care.[5–7]

Progesterone

In women who had ≥ 3 consecutive miscarriages, progestogen treatment shows a statistically significant 61% decrease in miscarriage rate compared with placebo or no treatment in three small trials.[8–11] No statistically significant differences were found between the route of administration of progestogen (oral, intramuscular, vaginal) vs placebo or no treatment.[8–11]

Not sufficient evidence

Human chorionic gonadotropin

There is not enough evidence to evaluate the use of human chorionic gonadotrophin (HCG) during pregnancy in order to prevent miscarriage in women with a history of unexplained recurrent spontaneous miscarriage because the trials are small and have significant (especially two studies) limitations.[12–16] HCG is associated with a 74% reduced risk of miscarriage for women with a history of recurrent miscarriage.[13–16] All studies showed at least a trend favoring benefit of HCG. This result should be interpreted cautiously because the apparent effect is greatly influenced by the two methodologically weaker studies.

Low-dose aspirin

Similar live-birth rates are observed with low-dose (50 mg/day) aspirin vs placebo in pregnant women with recurrent spontaneous abortion without detectable ACA.[17,18]

Vitamins

There is no specific adequate trial on multivitamin supplementation of any kind for women with prior REPL. In non-high-risk women, multivitamin supplementation before 20 weeks is associated with similar total fetal loss (early/late miscarriage and stillbirth), early or late miscarriage or stillbirth, and most other outcomes compared with controls.[19] Multivitamin supplementation is associated, compared with controls, with a 32% lower incidence of pre-eclampsia, possibly linked to vitamin C and D supplementation (see also Chapter 1 of *Maternal–Fetal Evidence Based Guidelines*). Multivitamin supplementation is associated with a 38% higher incidence of a multiple pregnancy, probably associated with vitamin A as well as folic acid supplementation.

Do not use (detrimental interventions)

Estrogen (mainly diethylstilbestrol)

Estrogen, mainly diethylstilbestrol (DES), should not be used in pregnancy for any indication. Data are mostly from studies of women without risk factors, women with 'threatened abortion' in the current pregnancy, or diabetics (mostly women with also recurrent PL). DES given in the first trimester leads to a 37% increased rate of miscarriage and 61% increased rate of PTB.[20–27] There is also a 48% increase in the numbers of babies weighing less than 2500 g. Fetal and neonatal deaths are not influenced by the intervention (DES) compared with the control group. Pre-eclampsia is similar in the two groups. Exposed female offspring have a non-significant trend towards more cancer of the genital tract and cancer other than of the genital tract. Primary infertility, adenosis of the vagina/cervix in female offspring, and testicular abnormality in male offspring are significantly higher in those exposed to DES before birth.

The vast use in the 1950s–1970s of a medication with no benefit proven by evidence based medicine is the best example of the importance of using data from trials and meta-analyses to guide effective practice.

Immunotherapy

The various forms of immunotherapy did not show significant differences between treatment and control groups in terms of subsequent live births:[28]

- paternal cell immunization (11 trials, 596 women), odds ratio (OR) = 1.05, 95% confidence interval (CI) 0.75–1.47[29–39]
- third-party donor cell immunization (3 trials, 156 women), OR = 1.39, 95% CI 0.68–2.82[40–41]
- trophoblast membrane infusion (1 trial, 37 women), OR = 0.40, 95% CI 0.11–1.45[42]
- intravenous immune globulin (IVIG), OR = 0.98, 95% CI 0.61–1.58 [7 trials, n = 303][43–49]

Immunization using viable mononuclear cells carries the risk of any blood transfusion such as hepatitis B virus or human immunodeficiency virus (HIV). Reactions have been uncommon, but include soreness and redness at the injection site, fever, maternal platelet alloimmunization, blood group sensitization, and cutaneous graft-versus-host-like reaction. Women who have received lymphocyte immune therapy may have a higher incidence of subsequent miscarriage than women who did not receive such cellular products.[36] The Director of the Office of Therapeutics Research and Review, US Food and Drug Administration (FDA), sent a letter on January 30, 2002, to physicians believed to be using lymphocyte immune therapy to prevent miscarriages. He informed them that the injectable products used in lymphocyte immune therapy do not have the required FDA approval and are considered investigational new drugs that pose several significant safety concerns. Administration of such cells or cellular products in humans can only be performed in the USA as part of clinical investigations, and then only if there is an investigational new drug (IND) application in effect.

IVIG therapy is expensive and in relatively short supply.

Women should be spared the pain and grief associated with false expectations that an ineffective treatment might work. These therapies should no longer be offered as treatment for unexplained recurrent pregnancy loss.

Antepartum testing

No specific testing indicated.

Delivery

No specific precaution.

Anesthesia

No specific precaution.

Postpartum/breastfeeding

No specific precaution.

Future

Effective treatment of an alleged alloimmune cause of recurrent miscarriage awaits more complete knowledge of the underlying pathophysiology. A specific assay to diagnose immune-mediated early pregnancy loss and a reliable method to determine which patients might benefit from manipulation of the maternal immune system are urgently needed. It is not presently known exactly how many recurrent early pregnancy losses are the result of anembryonic or chromosomally abnormal conceptuses, anatomic or structural abnormalities and how many are embryonic or fetal deaths. It is likely that some unexplained early losses are due to as yet undefined subchromosomal genetic abnormalities impairing early development of the conceptus. New molecular techniques should be directed at understanding the factors responsible for successful pregnancy as well as pregnancy loss.

Second trimester pregnancy loss

If loss ≥ 14 weeks and < 20 weeks, obtain any available autopsy, chromosome, work-up from that loss (see also Chapter 46 of *Maternal–Fetal Evidence Based Guidelines*). Placental pathology from previous pregnancies may be re-examined by an expert in placentas.

≥ 10 week loss

In women who have had a previous fetal loss after the 10th week and had a thrombophilic defect (heterozygous factor V Leiden, prothrombin 20210, or protein S deficiency), enoxaparin 40 mg daily treatment is associated with a 10-fold increased live-birth rate, as compared with low-dose aspirin in just one trial.[50]

References

1. ACOG Practice Bulletin. Management of recurrent early pregnancy loss. ACOG, No. 24, 2001. [review]
2. Nikcevic AV, Tunkel SA, Kuczmierczyk, Nicolaides KH. Investigation of the cause of miscarriage and its influence on women's psychological distress. Br J Obstet Gynaecol 199; 106: 808–13. [II-2]
3. Karamardian LM, Grimes DA. Luteal phase deficiency: effect of treatment on pregnancy rates. Am J Obstet Gynecol 1992; 167: 1391–8. [meta-analysis: 1 RCT, n = 44, and 3 controlled studies]
4. Balasch J, Vanrell J, Marquez M, Burzaco I, Gonzalez-Merlo J. Dehydrogesterone versus vaginal progesterone in the treatment of the endometrial luteal phase deficiency. Fertil Steril 1982; 37: 751–4. [RCT, n = 44]
5. Stray-Pedersen B, Stray-Pedersen S. Recurrent abortion: the role of psychotherapy. In: Beard RW, Sharp F, eds. Early Pregnancy Loss. Springer-Verlag; London: 1988: 433–40. [II-2]
6. Liddell HS, Pattison NS, Zanderigo A. Recurrent miscarriage – outcome after supportive care in early pregnancy. Aust NZ Obstet Gynecol 1991; 31: 320–2. [II-1]
7. Clifford K, Rai R, Regan L. Future pregnancy outcome in unexplained recurrent first trimester miscarriage. Hum Reprod 1997; 12: 387–9. [II-2]
8. Oates-Whitehead RM, Haas DM, Carrier JAK. Progestogen for preventing miscarriage. Cochrane Database Syst Rev 2007; 1. [3 RCTs for REPL, n = 93 with recurrent SAB]
9. Goldzieher JW. Double-blind trial of a progestin in habitual abortion. JAMA 1964; 188(7): 651–4. [RCT, n = 16. Women who had either never had a term pregnancy and who had had 2 or more miscarriages or who had had 1 or more term pregnancy followed by a minimum number of 2 consecutive miscarriages. All women had to have a urinary pregnanediol of less than 5 mg/day before 8 weeks gestation and/or less than 7 mg/day by 14 weeks' gestation; 10 mg/day of oral medroxyprogesterone. Placebo: yes. Duration: not stated]
10. Le Vine L. Habitual abortion. A controlled clinical study of progestational therapy. West J Surg 1964; 72: 30–6. [RCT, n = 30. Women who had had 3 consecutive miscarriages, were less than 16 weeks gestation and with no signs of threatened miscarriage in the current pregnancy. 500 mg/week IM of hydroxyprogesterone caproate. Duration: until miscarriage or the 36th week of gestation. Placebo: yes]
11. Swyer GIM, Daley D. Progesterone implantation in habitual abortion. BMJ 1953; 1: 1073–86. [RCT, n = 47 (out of 113 total). Women having had 2 or more consecutive miscarriages before 12 weeks gestation. 6 × 25 mg progesterone pellets inserted within the gluteal muscle either (a) as soon as pregnancy was confirmed or (b) not later than 10th week of gestation or (c) not later than the earliest previous miscarriage. Placebo: no, but had a no-treatment control group]
12. Scott, JR. Pattison, N. Human chorionic gonadotrophin for recurrent miscarriage. Cochrane Database Syst Rev 2007; 1. [meta-analysis: 4 RCTs, n = 180, variable quality trials]
13. Harrison RF. Treatment of habitual abortion with human chorionic gonadotrophin: results of open and placebo-controlled studies. Eur J Obstet Gynecol Reprod Biol 1985; 20: 159–68. [RCT, n= spontaneous miscarriage of 3 previous consecutive pregnancies without evidence of a cause (normal investigative profile included: chromosomal analysis of both partners, no systemic disease, normal bacteriological investigations of semen and cervical secretions, normal HSG, normal serum FSH, LH, estradiol, prolactin; normal or low progesterone). Initially 10 000 IU HCG by IM injection followed by 5000 IU twice weekly up to 12 weeks, followed by 5000 IU weekly until 20 weeks]
14. Harrison RF. Human chorionic gonadotrophine (HCG) in the management of recurrent abortion; results of a multi-centre placebo-controlled study. Eur J Obstet Gynecol Reprod Biol 1992; 47: 175–9. [RCT. 'Modus operandi' described as identical to Harrison 1985 study. HCG 10 000 IU IM starting before 8 weeks. HCG 5000 IU IM twice weekly until 12 weeks. HCG 5000 IU IM once weekly from 12 to 16 weeks. Identically packaged vs placebo vials given as same regimen]
15. Quenby S, Farquharson R. Human chorionic gonadotropin supplementation in recurring pregnancy loss: a controlled trial. Fertil Steril 1994; 62: 708–10. [RCT, n = 104. Two or more consecutive first trimester miscarriages. Profasi (Serono) 10 000 units IM initially and 5000 units twice weekly until 14 weeks gestation. Control group: placebo of normal saline IM 'in an identical fashion']
16. Svigos J. Preliminary experience with the use of human chorionic gonadotrophin therapy in women with repeated abortion. Clin Reprod Fertil 1982; 1: 131–5. [RCT. Two unexplained (normal genital tract and chromosomes) miscarriages. Treatment group managed in one of two ways according to serum progesterone. A low progesterone precipitated compliance with the intended treatment. A normal progesterone precipitated no treatment (i.e. managed as a control). Groups analysed on an intention to treat basis. 9000 IU IM. × 3 per week from 6–7 weeks until 12 weeks vs no treatment]
17. Di Nisio M, Peters LW, Middeldorp S. Anticoagulants for the treatment of recurrent pregnancy loss in women without antiphospholipid syndrome. Cochrane Database Syst Rev 2007; 1. [meta-analysis: 2 RCTs; n = 74 – subgroup analyses; only Tulppala is pertinent for this analysis]
18. Tulppala M, Marttunen M, Soderstrom-Anttila V et al. Low-dose aspirin in the prevention of miscarriage in women with unexplained or autoimmune related recurrent miscarriage: effect on prostacyclin and thromboxane A$_2$ production. Hum Reprod 1997; 12(7): 1567–72. [RCT, n = 54 with negative ACA – subcategory of 82 women with a history of at least 3 consecutive miscarriages in whom no obvious cause for their previous pregnancy losses was found. Interventions: aspirin (50 mg/daily) vs placebo, started as soon as a urinary pregnancy test became positive]
19. Rumbold A, Middleton P, Crowther CA. Vitamin supplementation for preventing miscarriage. Cochrane Database Syst Rev 2007; 1. [meta-analysis: 17 RCTs, n = 35 812]
20. Bamigboye AA, Morris J. Oestrogen supplementation, mainly diethyl-stilbestrol, for preventing miscarriages and other adverse pregnancy outcomes. Cochrane Database Syst Rev 2007; 1. [meta-analysis: 7 RCTs, n = 2897]
21. Bender S. The effect of diethylstilboestrol on recurrent miscarriage. Personal communication February 1988 [RCT, n = 58 women with prior SAB. DES in 1 clinic vs control in another clinic]
22. Crowder RE, Bills ES, Broadbent JS. The management of threatened abortion. A study of 100 cases. Am J Obstet Gynecol 1950; 60(4): 896–9. [RCT, n = 100. Women admitted for threatened abortion and diabetic. DES 25 mg every 30 minutes for 6 hours, then 100 mg daily until asymptomatic for 24 hours, then 50 mg daily until 28 weeks of pregnancy. Both DES and control group had phenobarbitone and Demerol (meperidine)]
23. Dieckmann WJ, Davis ME, Rynkiewcz SM, Pottinger RE. Does the administration of diethylstilbestrol during pregnancy have therapeutic value? Am J Obstet Gynecol 1953; 66(5): 1062–81. [RCT, n = 1646 (all women). 5 mg of DES administered from 7–8 weeks in graduated fashion up to 150 mg at 34–35 weeks vs placebo. Many long-term follow up manuscripts]
24. Ferguson JH. Effect of stilbestrol on pregnancy compared to the effect of a placebo. Am J Obstet Gynecol 1953; 65(3): 592–601. [RCT, n = 393

(all women). DES 6.3 mg to 137.5 mg, depending on gestational age vs placebo]

25. Medical Research Council. The use of hormones in the management of pregnancy in diabetics. Lancet 1955; 2: 833–6. [RCT, n = 147 (high-risk diabetic women). Incremental doses of 50 mg to 200 mg DES daily from about 16 weeks to term. Ethisterone, 25 mg/day from 16 weeks, incrementally to 250 mg/day at 32 weeks to term. Ethisterone was given incrementally. Graduated dosing with stilbestrol from 50 mg at ≤ 19 weeks to 200 mg at ≥ 32 weeks. Ethisterone from 25 mg/day at ≤ 19 weeks to 250 mg/day at ≥ 32 weeks or more vs placebo]

26. Robinson D, Shettles LB. The use of diethylstilboestrol in threatened abortion. Am J Obstet Gynecol 1952; 63(6): 1330–3. [RCT, n = 93. Women admitted for threatened abortion. DES 5 mg to 125 mg, depending on gestational age vs placebo]

27. Swyer GIM, Law RG. An evaluation of the prophylactic ante-natal use of stilboestrol. Preliminary report. Proceedings of the Society for Endocrinology. J Endocrinol 1954; 10: 36–7. [RCT, n = 460 (all primigravidas). 5 mg of DES administered from 7–8 weeks in graduated fashion up to 150 mg at 34–35 weeks vs placebo (as Dieckmann et al)]

28. Scott JR. Immunotherapy for recurrent miscarriage. Cochrane Database Syst Rev 2007; 1. [meta-analysis: 19 RCTs – see below]

29. Cauchi MN, Lim D, Young DE, Kloss M, Pepperell RJ. Treatment of recurrent aborters by immunization with paternal cells – controlled trial. Am J Reprod Immunol 1991; 25: 16–17. [RCT]

30. Christiansen OB, Mathiesen O, Husth M, Lauritsen JG, Grunnet J. Placebo-controlled trial of active immunization with third party leukocytes in recurrent miscarriage. Acta Obstet Gynecol Scand 1994; 3: 261–8. [RCT]

31. Gatenby PA, Cameron K, Simes RJ et al. Treatment of recurrent spontaneous abortion by immunization with paternal lymphocytes: results of a controlled trial. Am J Reprod Immunol 1993; 29: 88–94. [RCT]

32. Ho HN, Gill TJ, Hsieh HJ et al. Immunotherapy for recurrent spontaneous abortions in a Chinese population. Am J Reprod Immunol 1991; 25: 10–15. [RCT]

33. Illeni MT, Marelli G, Parazzini F et al. Immunotherapy and recurrent abortion: a randomized clinical trial. Hum Reprod 1994; 9: 1247–9. [RCT]

34. Kilpatrick DC, Liston W. Abstracts of contributors' individual data submitted to the Worldwide Prospective Observation Study on Immunotherapy for Treatment of Recurrent Spontaneous Abortion. Am J Reprod Immunol 1994; 32: 264. [RCT]

35. Mowbray JF, Gibbings C, Liddell H et al. Controlled trial of treatment of recurrent spontaneous abortion by immunisation with paternal cells. Lancet 1985; 1: 941–3. [RCT]

36. Ober C, Karrison T, Odem RB et al. Mononuclear-cell immunisation in prevention of recurrent miscarriages: a randomised trial. Lancet 1999; 354: 365–9. [RCT, n = 183]

37. Reznikoff-Etievant MF. Abstracts of contributors' individual data submitted to the Worldwide Prospective Observation Study on Immunotherapy for Treatment of Recurrent Spontaneous Abortion. Am J Reprod Immunol 1994; 32: 266–7. [RCT]

38. Scott JR, Branch WD, Dudley DJ, Hatasaka HH. Immunotherapy for recurrent pregnancy loss: the University of Utah perspective.

In: Dondero F, Johnson P eds Reproductive Immunology. Serono Symposium Publications, Raven Press, 1997; pp. 255–7. [RCT]

39. Stray-Pederson S. Department of Obstetrics and Gynecology, University of Oslo, Oslo, 1 Norway. Personal communication 1994 (in 2007, reference 29 above). [RCT]

40. Christiansen OB, Mathiesen O, Husth M, Lauritsen JG, Grunnet J. Placebo-controlled trial of active immunization with third party leukocytes in recurrent miscarriage. Acta Obstet Gynecol Scand 1994; 3: 261–8. [RCT]

41. Ho HN, Gill TJ, Hsieh HJ et al. Immunotherapy for recurrent spontaneous abortions in a Chinese population. Am J Reprod Immunol 1991; 25: 10–15. [RCT]

42. Johnson PM, Ramsden GH, Chia KV et al. A combined randomised double-blind and open study of trophoblast membrane infusion (TMI) in unexplained recurrent miscarriage. In: Chaouat G, Mowbray J eds. Cellular Molecular Biology of the Materno-Fetal Relationship. Vol 212, Colleque INSERM/John Libbey Eurotext LTD, 1991: 277–84. [RCT]

43. Christiansen OB, Mathieson O, Husth M, et al. Placebo-controlled trial of treatment of unexplained secondary recurrent spontaneous abortions and recurrent late spontaneous abortions with iv immunoglobulin. Hum Reprod 1995; 10: 2690–5. [RCT, n = 34]

44. Christiansen OB, Pedersen B, Rosgaard A, Husth. A randomized, double-blind, placebo-controlled trial of intravenous immunoglobulin in the prevention of recurrent miscarriage: evidence for a therapeutic effect in women with secondary recurrent miscarriage. Hum Reprod 2002; 17(3): 809–16. [RCT, n = 58]

45. Coulam CB, Krysa L, Stern JJ, Bustillo M. Intravenous immunoglobulin for treatment of recurrent pregnancy loss. Am J Reprod Immunol 1995; 34: 333–7. [RCT, n = 95]

46. German RSA/IVIG Group. Intravenous immunoglobulin for treatment of recurrent miscarriage. Br J Obstet Gynaecol 1994; 101: 1072–7. [RCT]

47. Jablonowska B, Selbing A, Palfi M et al. Prevention of recurrent spontaneous abortion by intravenous immunoglobulin: a double-blind placebo-controlled study. Hum Reprod 1999; 14: 838–41. [RCT, n = 41]

48. Perino A, Vassiliadis A, Vuceticha R et al. Short-term therapy for recurrent abortion using intravenous immunoglobulins: results of a double-blind placebo-controlled Italian study. Hum Reprod 1997; 12: 2388–92. [RCT, n = 46]

49. Stephenson MD, Dreher K, Houlihan E, Wu V. Prevention of unexplained recurrent spontaneous abortion using intravenous immunoglobulin: a prospective, randomized, double blinded, placebo controlled trial. Am J Reprod Immunol 1998; 39: 82–8. [RCT, n = 62]

50. Gris J-C, Mercier E, Quere I et al. Low-molecular-weight heparin versus low-dose aspirin in women with one fetal loss and a constitutional thrombophilic disorder. Blood 2004; 103: 3695–9. [RCT, n = 160. Open-label, quasi-random. Women with a history of one fetal loss after the 10th week of gestation and factor V Leiden, FII 20210A mutation, or protein S deficiency. Subcutaneous enoxaparin (40 mg/day from the 8th week of amenorrhea after a positive pregnancy test) vs aspirin (100 mg/day from the 8th week of amenorrhea after a positive pregnancy test)]

15

Prevention of preterm birth

Vincenzo Berghella

KEY POINTS

- Gestational age (GA) determination is of outmost importance in prevention of preterm birth (PTB) and management of presumed threatened PTB.
- PTB is defined as birth between 20 0/7 and 36 6/7 weeks. It is the number one cause of perinatal morbidity and mortality in developed countries, and these complications are inversely proportional to GA at birth.
- An accurate history should be taken regarding risk factors for PTB, especially obstetric-gynecological history, maternal lifestyle, and pre-pregnancy weight (see Table 15.1).
- Primary prevention for PTB aimed at the general population has been insufficiently studied. It includes family planning, avoidance of lifestyle risks, and proper nutrition.
- Management for prevention of PTB is therefore mostly based on identification and treatment of risk factors (secondary prevention) or treatment of symptomatic women with preterm labor (PTL) or premature preterm rupture of membranes (PPROM) (tertiary prevention).

Secondary prevention of PTB has been effective in the following groups for the following interventions:

- In women who smoke, smoking cessation counseling/support programs.
- In women with ≥ 1 prior spontaneous PTBs, now carrying a singleton gestation, for the following interventions:
  - 17α-hydroxyprogesterone caproate 250 mg IM every week starting at 16–20 weeks until 36 weeks
  - cerclage if the cervical length is < 25 mm between 14 and 23 6/7 weeks
  - omega-3 fatty acids.
- In women with ≥ 3 prior PTBs or second trimester losses, history-indicated cerclage.
- In women with asymptomatic bacteriuria of > 100 000 bacteria/ml, appropriate antibiotics.
- In women with asymptomatic group B streptococcus (GBS) bacteriuria of any colony count, appropriate antibiotics (usually penicillin).

- All other screening and treatment interventions for secondary prevention of PTB are not supported by enough evidence for recommending their clinical use.

Preterm labor

- Women with PTL but negative fetal fibronectin (fFN) and transvaginal ultrasound (TVU) cervical length (CL) ≥ 30 mm have a ≤ 2% chance of delivering within 1 week, and a > 95% chance of delivering ≥ 35 weeks without therapy, and should therefore not receive any treatment.
- Corticosteroids (betamethasone 12 mg IM every 24 hours × 2 doses between 24 and 33 6/7 weeks is preferred if available) given to the mother prior to preterm birth (either spontaneous or indicated) are effective in preventing respiratory distress syndrome, intraventricular hemorrhage (IVH), and neonatal mortality.
- Tocolytics should not be used without concomitant use of corticosteroids for fetal maturity.
- No tocolytic has been shown to improve perinatal mortality.
- There is no tocolytic agent that is most safe and efficacious. Cyclo-oxygenase (COX) inhibitors are the only class of primary tocolytics shown to decrease PTB < 37 weeks compared with placebo. COX inhibitors, beta-mimetics, and oxytocin receptor antagonists (ORA) have been shown to significantly prolong pregnancy at 48 hours and 7 days compared with placebo. COX inhibitors, calcium channel blockers (CCB), and ORAs have significantly less side effects than β-mimetics.
- There is no maintenance tocolytic that prevents PTB or perinatal morbidity/mortality. There is insufficient evidence to evaluate multiple tocolytic agents for primary tocolysis, refractory (primary agent is failing, so another is started) tocolysis, or repeated (after successful primary tocolysis) tocolysis.
- All other interventions studied to prevent PTB in women with PTL, including bedrest, hydration, and sedation, have not been shown to be beneficial in the management of PTL.

Table 15.1	*Risk factors for spontaneous preterm birth*

History:

- Obstetric-gynecological history: prior spontaneous PTB (sPTB of twins is a minor risk factor for PTB when the next pregnancy is a singleton pregnancy); prior STL; prior ≥ 2 D&Es; prior cone biopsy; uterine anomalies; DES exposure; myomata; extremes of interpregnancy interval; ART
- Maternal lifestyle (smoking, drug abuse, STIs, etc.)
- Maternal pre-pregnancy weight <120 lb (<50 kg) or low BMI; poor nutritional status
- Maternal age (<19 years old; >35 years old)
- Race (especially Afro-American)
- Education (<12 grades)
- Certain medical conditions (e.g. DM, HTN)
- Low socioeconomic status
- Limited prenatal care
- Family history of spontaneous PTB (poorly studied)
- Vaginal bleeding (especially during second trimester)
- Stress (mostly related to above risks)

Identifiable by screening:
- Anemia
- Periodontal disease
- TVU CL <25 mm (especially <30 weeks)
- fFN positive (>50 ng/mL)

Usually symptomatic:
- Uterine contractions

Not spontaneous (indicated/iatrogenic):
- Fetal demise/major anomaly/compromise/ polyhydramnios
- Placenta previa
- Placental abruption
- Major maternal disease (HTN complications, DM, etc.)

PTB, preterm birth; STL, second trimester loss; D&E, dilatation and evacuation; ART, assisted reproductive technologies; DES, diethylstilbestrol; STIs, sexually transmitted infections; BMI, body mass index; DM, diabetes mellitus; HTN, hypertension; TVU CL, transvaginal ultrasound cervical length; fFN, fetal fibronectin.

Diagnoses/definitions

Gestational age (GA) determination is of great importance in prevention of preterm birth (PTB) **and management of presumed threatened PTB** (see Chapter 3 for best GA determination criteria).

Definitions regarding prematurity vary in different publications, but the following definitions are those most commonly accepted and used in trials.

Preterm birth (PTB): birth between 20 0/7 and 36 6/7 weeks:[1]

- very early preterm birth: birth between 20 0/7 and 23 6/7 weeks
- early preterm birth: birth between 24 0/7 and 31 6/7 weeks

- late preterm birth: birth between 32 0/7 and 36 6/7 weeks.

Pregnancy loss (PL): loss of pregnancy from conception to < 20 weeks. The term spontaneous abortion is equivalent, but should be avoided since women associate negative feelings with this term. Miscarriage is a lay term for PL (see also Chapter 14).

Second trimester PL (aka second trimester loss – STL): birth between 14 0/7 and 19 6/7 weeks.

Cervical insufficiency (CI): formerly called cervical incompetence, CI is **recurrent** painless dilatation leading to **second trimester** losses.[2]

Preterm labor (PTL): uterine contractions (≥ 4/20 minutes or ≥ 8/hour) and documented cervical change with intact membranes at 20–36 6/7weeks.

Premature preterm rupture of membranes (PPROM): vaginal pooling, positive nitrazine and/or ferning at 16–36 6/7weeks (see Chapter 16):

- early PPROM: PPROM between 24 and 33 6/7 weeks
- very early PPROM: PPROM between 16 and 23 6/7 weeks.

Symptoms of preterm labor

Cramps, abdominal 'tightenings', low backache, pelvic pressure, increased vaginal discharge, and spotting.

Epidemiology/incidence

Incidence of PTB < 37 weeks varies between 5 and 25% in different countries, and accounted for 12.7% of all US births in 2005. PTB < 32 weeks: 2% in the USA; ≤ 1% in most other developed countries. The increasing incidence of PTB in many developed countries may be due to ART (assisted reproductive technologies)-related multiple gestations, older and sicker mothers, earlier GA of registered births and neonatal improvements, better and earlier timing of births (related to ultrasound), worsening socioeconomic factors, and other factors.

Genetics

Although a genetic predisposition in certain ethnic groups and families has been reported, no clinical genetic studies are yet recommended for prediction/prevention of PTB, due to insufficient evidence.

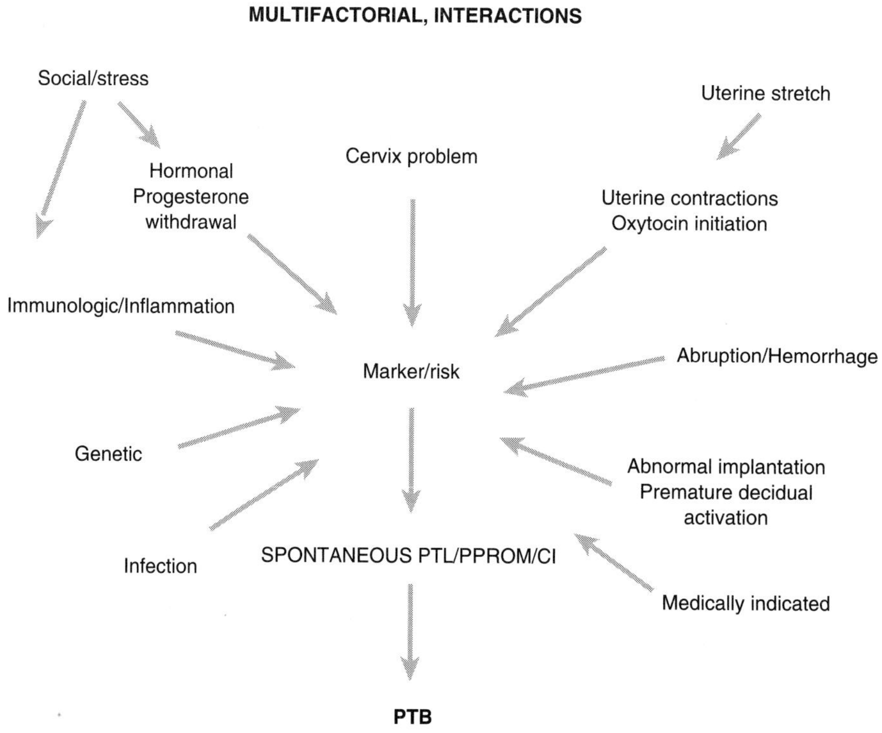

MULTIFACTORIAL, INTERACTIONS

Figure 15.1   Preterm birth is the final common pathway of many associated possible etiologies. For abbreviations, see Diagnosis/definitions section.

Etiology/basic pathophysiology

Just like coronary artery disease, PTB is a final common manifestation of a multifactorial, complex etiology. Several processes leading to PTB are shown in Figure 15.1.

Classification (pathways)

PTB can be spontaneous, and follow PTL (50%; see below), PPROM (30%; see Chapter 16) or, rarely, CI; or be iatrogenic (20%). Cervical insufficiency may constitute about 1% of spontaneous PTB and/or second trimester losses (see below). CI represents one extreme of spontaneous PTB, as PTB is a continuum.

Risk factors/associations

Most women who have a spontaneous PTB have no identifiable risk factors. Risk factors for spontaneous PTB, presenting as PTL, PPROM, or CI, are similar (Table 15.1).

Complications

PTB is the **number one cause of perinatal mortality**: 75% of perinatal mortality occurs in preterm babies; > two-thirds of perinatal mortality (60% of total) occurs in <32-week-old infants. **Mortality and morbidities are inversely associated with GA at birth.** Morbidities include respiratory distress syndrome (RDS), bronchopulmonary dysplasia (BPD), intraventricular hemorrhage (IVH), necrotizing enterocolitis (NEC), sepsis, and retinopathy.

Pregnancy management

Principles: prevention is preferable to treatment once symptoms have been identified. Primary prevention is also preferable to secondary prevention after predictive markers have been identified, or to tertiary prevention of symptomatic women with PTL or PPROM.

ASYMPTOMATIC WOMEN
Work-up

Predictive strategies usually have poor sensitivity and specificity. Prediction is a means leading to prevention and, as such, is discussed mainly under Prevention below. A screening test is only beneficial if an intervention reduces the outcome once the screening test is positive.

- All pre-pregnancy evaluations of the cervix (e.g. hysterosalpingogram, No. 8 Hegar dilator passage, catheter traction test, etc.) aimed at screening for CI have either been inadequately studied or shown not to be sufficiently predictive and therefore useful in a prevention program (no trial ever reported).
- **An accurate history and physical should be done, especially regarding risk factors for PTB, in particular obstetric–gynecological (ob-gyn) history, maternal lifestyle, and pre-pregnancy weight.**
- A Creasy's score or other similar history-based systems to predict PTB have been associated with a low (10–30%) positive predictive value (PPV) for PTB, and are not clinically useful given negative intervention trials (see below).
- **Transvaginal ultrasound (TVU) cervical length (CL) at 16–24 weeks is indicated in women with a prior PTB not receiving a history-indicated cerclage** (see below).
- Evidence does not support the use of home uterine activity monitoring or BV screening in asymptomatic low-risk women.
- There are insufficient data to support the use of salivary estriol or fetal fibronectin (fFN) in asymptomatic women (even if FFN is one of the best predictive screening tests).
- Cytokines, matrix metalloproteinases, corticotrophin-releasing hormone (CRH), salivary estriol, relaxin, human chorionic gonadotropin (HCG), prothrombin, fetal DNA and many other tests remain research tools for prediction of PTB and are not yet clinically beneficial.

Prevention

Iatrogenic/indicated PTB. Aim to keep the pregnant woman as healthy as the non-pregnant adult. Appropriate prevention and therapy of any maternal medical or fetal/congenital anomaly disorder is paramount, as is appropriate prevention and therapy for pre-eclampsia and fetal growth restriction (FGR).

Spontaneous PTB: There are three levels of prevention: primary, secondary, and tertiary. Primary should be preferred.

Primary prevention

A primary prevention strategy is aimed at all asymptomatic pregnant women at risk for PTB (i.e. aimed at all pregnant women). Unfortunately, most primary prevention interventions have been so far either insufficiently studied or found not to be effective.

Preconception/early pregnancy: family planning

There are no trials to assess interventions. Avoiding extremes of age, of interpregnancy interval (18–23 months is the optimal interval between last delivery and next conception),[3] and multiple gestations (with ART improvements) seems self-evident for efficacy in preventing PTB, when feasible.

Avoidance of lifestyle risks

There are no trials to assess interventions. Avoiding illegal drugs such as cocaine and amfetamines, physical abuse, and sexually transmitted infections (STIs) such as chlamydia, gonorrhea, syphilis, and human immunodeficiency virus (HIV) seems self-evident for efficacy in preventing PTB. There are no trials on modifying other potential risks, such as a physically-demanding job, prolonged standing, and night work.

Proper nutrition, weight gain

The available evidence is inadequate to evaluate potential effects of balanced protein/energy supplementation as provided in most trials on prevention of PTB.[4] **Balanced protein supplementation alone (i.e. without energy supplementation) does not reduce PTB,** and is unlikely to be of benefit to pregnant women or their infants. This conclusion appears to apply even to undernourished women.[5] A high-protein diet (>25% of total energy content) cannot be recommended in pregnancy.[6]

There is insufficient high-quality evidence to show that dietary **magnesium supplementation** during pregnancy is beneficial. Overall, **oral magnesium treatment** from before the 25th week of gestation is associated with a lower frequency of PTB, but in the analysis excluding the cluster randomized trial, the effects of magnesium treatment on the frequencies of PTB are not different from placebo.[7]

Supplementation with **omega-3 fatty acids** has **not been studied with a trial** for prevention of PTB **in the general population.** Supplementation has been shown to prolong pregnancy by 4–8 days in different populations.

There are no trials aiming specifically at prevention of PTB to evaluate other nutritional changes, such as vitamin supplementation (see Chapter 1), HCG, or anticytokine supplements. Pre-pregnancy weight < 120 lbs (< 50 kg) is a very significant risk factor for PTB, and should be avoided if possible. Suggested pregnancy weight gain in pregnancy is 25–35 lbs for women with normal body mass index (BMI), but there are no trials on proper pre-pregnancy weight or pregnancy weight gain.

Secondary prevention

Screen for predictive risk factor (prediction) in asymptomatic women and avoid/treat (preventive intervention) (Table 15.2).

Table 15.2 *Effective interventions for secondary prevention of preterm birth: singleton gestations*

Risk	Intervention
Smoking	Smoking cessation programs
Prior spontaneous PTB (sPTB)	17OH-progesterone caproate Omega-3 fatty acids
Prior sPTB *and* TVU CL< 25 mm between 16 and 23 6/7 weeks	Ultrasound-indicated cerclage
Prior ≥ 3 PTB/STL	History-indicated cerclage
Asymptomatic bacteriuria	Appropriate antibiotics

PTB, preterm birth; TVU, transvaginal ultrasound; CL, cervical length; STL, second trimester loss.

Risk: smoking
Intervention: smoking cessation programs

It is estimated that 10–15% of PTB may be due to smoking. Smoking in pregnancy incidence in the USA was 12% in 2003 (38% decrease since 1989 – 20% then). All interventions for promoting smoking cessation in pregnancy are associated with a 6% decrease in smoking.[8] The trials with validated **smoking cessation**, a high-intensity intervention, and a high-quality score are associated with an absolute **decrease in continued smoking in late pregnancy of 5%**. Most studies had as intervention **provision of information on risks to fetus/infant, and benefits of quitting. Use of written material** is beneficial. Often, teaching cognitive/behavioral strategies for quitting was included. The American College of Obstetricians and Gynecologists (ACOG) has recommended use of the 5A's – ask, advice, assess, assist, arrange – approach.[9] The most effective intervention for smoking cessation in pregnancy is **social support and a reward component** (23% decrease).[10,11] If the above approach is not successful, consider nicotine replacement therapy (NRT) (see Chapter 20 of *Maternal–Fetal Evidence Based Guidelines*).

Smoking cessation counseling/support programs are associated with a 16% reduction in preterm birth, and a 19% reduction in low birth weight. Other outcomes (e.g. perinatal mortality) have not been adequately evaluated.[8]

Nicotine replacement therapy is associated with a trend for benefit.[12–14] One concern about its use in pregnancy is the possibility of adverse effects of nicotine on the fetus, through alterations in uterine, placental, or blood flow, or directly on the brain. As there are still too few trials to assure safe use in pregnancy, and animal studies suggest nicotine may be toxic to the developing central nervous system, registries of women using NRT should be established to gather more outcome data. **There is insufficient evidence to assess the safety and efficacy of nicotine gum** (only two small physiology studies without recording of PTB). **No trial has been done using bupropion**, which is safe in pregnancy. Interventions to increase smoking cessation among the partners of pregnant women, with the additional aim of facilitating cessation by the women themselves, have been insufficiently studied (only 1 trial).[8] Stages of change, or feedback, do not show benefit.[8]

Ob-gyn risk factors for preterm birth
Singleton pregnancies (unless otherwise specified)
Risk: 'pregnancy high-risk for PTB' Intervention: bed rest

There is no evidence supporting bed rest to prevent PTB. **Bed rest (rest 1 hour tid) in (asymptomatic and symptomatic) 'high-risk' singleton pregnancies is not associated with prevention of PTB over no bed rest.**[15] Bed rest can be associated with an increased incidence of complications; in-hospital extended strict bed rest for PTL or PPROM is associated with an up to 1–2% incidence of thromboembolic disease. Moreover, muscle wasting, cardiovascular deconditioning, bone demineralization, impaired glucose tolerance, heartburn, constipation, failure of volume expansion, headaches, dizziness, fatigue, depression, anxiety, stress, as well as lost wages, lost domestic productivity, and other costs may be detrimental consequences of bed rest. It is true that rest decreases uterine activity, and exercise increases it, but these are small effects that do not change rates of PTB. In non-randomized studies, exercise in pregnancy has been associated with a decrease in PTB, whereas physically demanding work, prolonged standing, shift and night work, and high cumulative work fatigue score have been associated with PTB. Despite its use in about 20% of pregnancies, bed rest for prevention of PTB cannot be recommended. It should be studied in trials before clinical use. If prescribed bed rest, women should be allowed to ambulate to the bathroom a few times a day to limit complications of strict bed rest. It is possible that women at real risk of PTB from the above or other risk factors have not been studied adequately with this intervention of bed rest.

Risk: 'pregnancy high-risk for PTB' Intervention: support

Programs of additional support during at-risk pregnancy (varying definitions) usually by a professional (social worker, midwife, or nurse) **do not reduce PTB or low birth weight.**[16] 'Additional support' was defined as some form of emotional support (e.g. counseling, reassurance, sympathetic listening) with or without additional information/ advice, occurring during home visits, clinic appointments, and/or by telephone; most of the times these were intensive programs lasting from the first or second trimesters to the end of pregnancy. Significant outcomes are that anxiety is decreased, satisfaction with care is increased, termination of pregnancy is increased, and cesarean delivery is decreased.[16]

Risk: 'pregnancy high-risk for PTB' Intervention: weekly manual exams, education

A program of weekly manual cervical exams in addition to education for women at high risk for PTB ($\geq$ 10 on Creasy score) **does not reduce PTB.**[17–19]

Risk: 'pregnancy high-risk for PTB' Intervention: antibiotics

See below under: Risk: prior PTB Intervention: antibiotics.

Risk: 'pregnancy high-risk for PTB' Intervention: cerclage

Different clinical scenarios have been studied for possible benefit of cerclage.

A history-indicated cerclage is placed based solely on prior obstetric or gynecological history (often called a prophylactic or elective cerclage). **A history-indicated cerclage prevents PTB in women with three or more second trimester losses or PTBs.**[20] Trials on women at lower risk for PTB based on prior obstetrical history have not shown benefit from history-indicated cerclage.[21,22] The other clinical indication might include CI (defined as prior painless cervical dilatation leading to recurrent second trimester losses). Unfortunately, no trial has been done to confirm the efficacy of history-indicated cerclage in reducing PTB in women with a diagnosis of CI. Other indications such as prior cone biopsy, Müllerian anomaly, diethylstibestrol (DES) exposure, prior PTB not associated with CI, and Ehlers–Danlos syndrome have occasionally been used clinically, but have not been confirmed by any trial as indications that benefit from history-indicated cerclage. History-indicated cerclage is usually performed at 12–15 weeks' gestation, and its techniques have been well described.[23]

Transabdominal (TA) cerclage has been associated with less recurrent PTB compared with controls receiving transvaginal cerclage in women with a **history of a failed (sPTB < 33 weeks despite cerclage) transvaginal history-indicated cerclage** in a case-control study.[24] There is no trial on TA cerclage. It should be noted that in this study antibiotics and progesterone were uniformly given to the TA women. The efficacy of TA cerclage for other clinical scenarios such as a cervix with no intravaginal portion has not been adequately studied. TA cerclage is usually performed prophylactically at around 10–12 weeks, and its technique has been well described.[23,24]

For efficacy of ultrasound-indicated cerclage, physical-exam-indicated cerclage, as well as cerclage in twins, see below.

Risk: prior PTB Intervention: omega-3 fatty acids

Omega-3 fatty acids (fish oil, Pikasol: 32% eicosapentaenoic acid (EPA), 23% docosahexaenoic acid (DHA), and 2 mg tocopherol/ml; 4 capsules/day: 1.3 g EPA and 0.9 g DHA, total 2.7 g/day; started at about 29–30 weeks) **reduce PTB < 37 weeks by 46% and PTB < 34 weeks by 68% in women with a prior PTB < 37 weeks and a singleton gestation.**[25] The same omega-3 fatty acid regimen does not reduce PTB in women with twins.[25] **Low-risk women without a prior PTB do not have a reduction in PTB < 37 weeks when given a lower dose of DHA** (12 eggs with 133 mg DHA vs with 33 mg DHA per week) starting at 24–28 weeks.[26] Natural sources of omega 3 fatty acids such as shark, swordfish, king mackerel, or tilefish contain high levels of mercury, and should be eaten infrequently ($\leq$ 1/week) in pregnancy. Canned light tuna, salmon, pollock, grouper, mussels, scallops, shrimp, and catfish are common fish low in mercury, and two portions (6 ounces = 1 portion) of these per week can be eaten. Albacore ('white') tuna has more mercury, and should be consumed up to 6 ounces per week. In general, for other fish, smaller fish have less mercury than larger ones. More information on fish and mercury intake in pregnancy is available at www.cfsan.fda.gov; and www.epa.gov/ost/fish. PrimaCare vitamin supplement contains 150 mg of omega-3 fatty acids, and has not been evaluated in a trial. The possible beneficial effects of omega-3 fatty acids to later fetal/neonatal/infant cognition remain not fully proven.

Risk: prior PTB Intervention: antibiotics

Clindamycin cream 2% for 7 days at 26–32 weeks does not reduce PTB < 37 weeks in women with a prior PTB 24–36 weeks, but may increase PTB < 34 weeks, especially in women without bacterial vaginosis (BV), so that antibiotics in this setting may actually be detrimental.[27]

Cefetamet pivoxil (not available in the USA) 2 g×1 at 28–32 weeks in women in Nairobi **with prior PTB**, fetal death, or LBW (low birth weight) **did not affect gestational age at delivery** (PTB was not reported).[28]

Metronidazole 250 mg three times a day×7 days **and erythromycin base 333 mg three times a day×14 days in women with a prior PTB or pre-pregnancy weight < 50 kg do not prevent PTB < 37 weeks, but may increase PTB < 34 weeks.**[29,30]

In conclusion, antibiotics are not effective in preventing PTB in women with prior PTB.

Risk: prior PTB
Intervention: progesterone

17α-Hydroxyprogesterone caproate 250 mg intramuscular (IM) every week, **starting at 16–20 weeks until 36 weeks, reduces PTB** by about 35% **in women with singleton gestations with a prior sPTB 20–36 6/7 weeks.**[31,32] Other doses, preparations (e.g. vaginal suppositories), or populations (e.g. other risk factors or multiple gestations) are either not or poorly studied, and therefore progesterone use in the second trimester to reduce PTB cannot be recommended outside of the specific condition of prior spontaneous PTB 20–36 weeks. The mechanism of action is also unknown, but probably involves an anti-inflammatory action. Safety for the fetus/neonate has not yet been proven with 100% certainty, but progesterone is known not to be a teratogen, and long-term detrimental effects have not been shown.

Risk: ≥ 3 PTB/STL
Intervention: cerclage

Cerclage decreases the incidence of PTB < 37 weeks from 53% (with no cerclage) to 32%, and the incidence of PTB < 32 weeks from 32% (with no cerclage) to 15% in women with 3 or more prior PTB or STL.[20]

Risk: cervical insufficiency
Intervention: cerclage

No intervention has been specifically studied in this population. There is insufficient evidence to recommend a history-indicated cerclage in women with < 3 prior PTB or second trimester losses. **A policy of TVU CL screening with ultrasound-indicated cerclage if CL shortens to < 25 mm at < 24 weeks has been shown to be equivalent** to a policy of universal history-indicated cerclage in women with a prior STL or PTB.[23,33]

Risk: IVF ART
Intervention: progesterone

17α-hydroxyprogesterone caproate or human chorionic gonadatropin (hCG) supplementation in the first trimester increases the incidences of fetal heart activity on ultrasound by 238%, and of pregnancy ≥ 24 weeks by 380% compared with placebo.[34]

Risk: amniocentesis
Intervention: progesterone

Natural progesterone 200 mg IM every day for 3 days post-amniocentesis followed by 17α-hydroxyprogesterone caproate 340 mg IM twice a week until the second week after the amniocentesis **did not reduce PTB < 25 weeks in women undergoing amniocentesis.**[35]

Risk: uterine contractions detected by home uterine activity monitoring
Intervention: varied, per obstetrician

Uterine contractions have been associated with PTB, but their predictive value is poor. Home uterine activity monitoring (HUAM) usually consists in trials of 1 hour of tocomonitoring twice daily at 24–36 weeks. **HUAM with or without nursing contact and education is associated with no prevention of PTB.** Some studies show earlier (at lower cervical dilatation) detection of PTL. The lack of benefit in prevention of PTB might have been secondary to lack of effective intervention (usually tocolysis) once PTL was diagnosed. Three different populations of women at high-risk for PTB have been studied:

- singleton gestations with risk factors for PTB (e.g. prior PTB)
- twin gestations
- women status–post an episode of PTL.

Unfortunately there is no published meta-analysis of all the trials, and most trials do not report results for each population specifically, and also report differing outcomes. My meta-analysis of published data shows no decrease in PTB < 37 weeks in any of these three subgroups – mostly singletons at high risk (9 trials; $n = 3613$):[36–45] relative risk (RR) = 1.01, 95% CI 0.91–1.11; twins (5 trials; $n = 998$):[39,42,44–46] RR = 0.91, 95% CI 0.80–1.04; or women status–post PTL episode (4 trials; $n = 218$):[42,47–49] RR = 1.21, 95% CI 0.92–1.60. The largest study[45] showed more unscheduled visits and prophylactic tocolytic use in the HUAM group compared with controls. Therefore, HUAM should not be routinely provided for prevention of PTB.

Risk: short cervix on ultrasound
Intervention: cerclage (ultrasound-indicated cerclage)

An ultrasound-indicated cerclage involves first screening of high-risk pregnancies with TVU of the cervix to determine during pregnancy the risk of PTB. The majority ($\approx 60\%$) of women at high risk by obstetric risk factors for PTB do not develop a short CL and deliver at term even without intervention. A short CL (<25 mm) on TVU in the second trimester (between 14–23 6/7 weeks) significantly increases the risk of PTB in all populations studied.[23] Ultrasound-indicated cerclage is defined as a cerclage performed because a short CL has been detected on TVU during pregnancy, usually in the second trimester. This cerclage has also been called therapeutic, salvage, or rescue cerclage. Ultrasound-indicated cerclage has differing effects in different populations. **In singleton gestations, especially those with a prior PTB or STL, it is associated with a significant (about 40%) reduction in PTB,[50]** but this should be confirmed by a large trial specific for this population. Efficacy is similar for CL <25 mm or ≤ 15 mm. **In twins, it has been associated with an increase in PTB, and should not be offered.[50]** There is insufficient evidence to recommend ultrasound-indicated cerclage in other populations, or after 23 weeks.

Risk: cervical dilatation
Intervention: cerclage
(physical exam-indicated cerclage)

Physical exam-indicated cerclage (aka emergency, or urgent) is the cerclage placed because of changes in the cervix (dilatation, effacement, etc.) detected by physical (manual) examination. Since about 50% of women with asymptomatic cervical dilatation ≥ 2 cm in the second trimester have microbial invasion of the amniotic cavity, an amniocentesis should be considered before offering physical exam-indicated cerclage. **There are insufficient data to assess efficacy of physical exam-indicated cerclage in women with cervical dilatation in the second trimester,** as only one small trial has been reported. In women with membranes at or beyond the external os at around 20–24 weeks, physical exam-indicated cerclage (and indomethacin) is associated with a delay in delivery of about 4 weeks compared with controls (30 vs 26 weeks).[51] The major limitations of this study are the small sample size and the inclusion of twins. Over 25 retrospective observational series, mostly with no controls, have claimed benefit of physical exam-indicated cerclage. Clearly, a large, well-designed prospective randomized trial is needed to confirm benefit.

Risk: positive fFN
Intervention: antibiotics

Fetal-fibronectin (fFN) is a basement membrane protein present between the decidua/uterus and fetal membranes/placenta and produced by the trophoblast. Its presence (>50 ng/ml) at ≥ 22 weeks in the cervicovaginal canal has been associated with an increased risk for PTB. In fact, fFN is one of the best predictors of PTB in all populations, including asymptomatic low- and high-risk women, twins, and women in PTL. Even at 13–22 weeks, higher (using 90th percentile) fFN levels are associated with a 2–3-fold increased risk in subsequent sPTB. **In women found to be fFN positive at 21–25 weeks, treatment with metronidazole 250 mg tid and erythromycin 250 mg qid$\times$10 days is associated with similar incidences of PTB <37 weeks compared to placebo. Among women with a prior PTB, this antibiotic regimen is associated with a higher incidence of PTB <37 weeks than the placebo group.[52]**

Risk: periodontal disease
Intervention: dental therapy

Periodontal disease has been associated with increased risk of PTB in several observational studies. **Periodontal treatment has been associated with a 50% decrease in PTB in women with periodontal disease.[53,54]** Scaling and root planing as treatment of periodontitis in pregnancy in one pilot trial have been associated with a non-significant decrease in PTB <35 weeks from 4.9% in the placebo to 0.8% in the treatment group.[53] Scaling, plaque control, and daily rinsing with 0.12% chlorhexidine at <28 weeks in women with gingivitis are associated with a decrease in PTB <37 weeks from 6.7% in the control group to 2.1% in the treatment group.[54]

Infections

Risk: asymptomatic bacteriuria
Intervention: antibiotics

Asymptomatic bacteriuria occurs in 2–10% of pregnancies, can lead to pyelonephritis, and is associated with an increased risk of PTB. **Screening for asymptomatic bacteriuria and treating for urine colony count of $>100\,000$ bacteria/ml reduces the incidence of PTB by 40%.[55]** The optimal time to perform the urine culture is unknown; it seems reasonable to perform the urine culture and treat, as done in most studies, at the first prenatal visit. Quantitative urine culture of a midstream or clean catch urine is the gold standard for detecting asymptomatic bacteriuria in pregnancy. The choices of nitrofurantoin, a penicillin, or a sulfonamide or sulfonamide-containing combination, based on the results of susceptibility testing, are appropriate regimens for the management of asymptomatic bacteriuria. A short (3–7 days) course of therapy for asymptomatic bacteriuria has become accepted practice, and is as effective as longer therapy. Single-day therapy has not been studied sufficiently.[56] Although it is recommended that a urine culture be done following treatment, with retreatment as necessary, the evidence is insufficient to specifically evaluate the effectiveness of this strategy. Treatment of asymptomatic pregnant women with lower colony counts is not currently recommended, but further study of appropriate strategies to best manage these women is warranted. **Asymptomatic women with even low (100 CFU (colony-forming units)) of group B streptococcus (GBS) in the urine culture at 27–31 weeks have decreased PTB < 37 weeks when treated with penicillin (PCN) 1 million IU three times per day for 6 days compared with placebo.**[57]

Antibiotic treatment compared with placebo or no treatment is effective in clearing asymptomatic bacteriuria. The incidence of pyelonephritis is reduced. Antibiotic treatment of asymptomatic bacteriuria is then clinically indicated to reduce the risk of pyelonephritis in pregnancy. If untreated, the overall incidence of pyelonephritis is about 19%. Overall, the number of women needed to treat to prevent one episode of pyelonephritis is 7, and treatment of asymptomatic bacteriuria will lead to an approximately 75% reduction in the incidence of pyelonephritis. The apparent reduction in PTB is consistent with current theories about the role of infection as a cause of PTB. Prevention of pyelonephritis, which in early studies prior to the availability of effective antimicrobial therapy was associated with PTB, may be a factor, but treatment of bacteriuria with antibiotics may also eradicate organisms colonizing the cervix and vagina that are associated with adverse pregnancy outcomes. The use of tetracycline is contraindicated in pregnancy. Insufficient data are available to determine the effectiveness of treatment to prevent recurrent bacteriuria during pregnancy. There is a need to define the appropriate frequency of follow-up cultures and retreatment strategies.[55]

Risk: bacterial vaginosis
Intervention: antibiotics

Bacterial vaginosis (BV) is a massive overgrowth of organisms such as anaerobic, *Gardnerella, Mycoplasma,* and others in the vagina. Most of these organisms are normally present in the vagina, but are at higher concentrations in BV, whereas predominant normal flora such as lactobacilli is decreased.

The diagnosis of BV is usually made clinically with at least 3 out of 4 of these (Amsel's) criteria: pH > 4.5 (most important), clue cells, thin homogeneous discharge, and 'amine' test, whereas in many studies Nugent's criteria (≥ 7 on Gram stain) are used for diagnosis. All these screening tests are not very accurate in predicting PTB (PPV 6–49%, depending on PTB prevalence and patient population) in both asymptomatic and symptomatic women. **Antibiotic therapy is effective at decreasing the presence of BV during pregnancy. In non-selected women, antibiotic treatment is not effective in reducing the incidence of PTB < 37 weeks, PTB < 34 weeks, PTB < 32 weeks, or PPROM.**[58] In women with a previous PTB, treatment did not affect the

risk of subsequent PTB, with a 17–25% non-significant trend for benefit.[58,59] It may decrease the risk of PPROM and low birth weight. Subgroup analysis of treatment with metronidazole or clindamycin does not alter incidence of PTB < 37 weeks.[59]

Risk: Trichomonas vaginalis
Intervention: antibiotics

Antibiotics (metronidazole only one tested) **do not prevent PTB** in women with *Trichomonas vaginalis* (TV) infection.[59–63] In fact, metronidazole is associated with a 78% higher incidence of PTB < 37 weeks,[62] and similar incidences of PTB < 32 weeks and perinatal mortality.[59] Even in women with a prior PTB, metronidazole is associated with an 84% higher risk of PTB.[59] Metronidazole does eradicate TV in > 90% of pregnant women with TV. Therefore, at least for the purpose of decreasing PTB, asymptomatic women should not be screened for TV. Symptomatic women with TV should still be adequately treated.

Risk: GBS cervicovaginal colonization
Intervention: antibiotics

GBS colonization of the cervicovaginal tract is common in pregnancy (10–20%), and has been associated with a slight (odds ratio [OR] = 1.5–3, usually) increased risk of PTB. Antibiotic therapy (with erythromycin) does not prevent PTB in women with GBS colonization, or affect stillbirths. Subanalysis by heavy colonization did not change results.[64]

Risk: *Ureaplasma/Mycoplasma*
cervicovaginal colonization
Intervention: antibiotics

Ureaplasma urealiticum and/or *Mycoplasma hominis* colonization of the cervicovaginal tract is common in pregnancy, and has been associated with a possible increased risk of PTB. **There is insufficient evidence to show whether giving antibiotics to women with *Ureaplasma* or *Mycoplasma* in the vagina prevents PTB.** The only trial did not report data on PTB.[65] Compared with placebo, erythromycin is associated with a non-significant 30% decrease in incidence of low birth weight < 2500 g (RR = 0.70, 95% CI 0.46–1.07). Although some studies appeared to meet the inclusion criteria for this review, in most studies *Ureaplasma/Mycoplasma* was not an essential entry criterion or reported just as a post hoc subgroup analysis of *Ureaplasma/Mycoplasma.*

There is insufficient information at this time to evaluate other interventions such as pessary, etc. Therefore, they cannot be recommended for clinical use, unless in a research trial.

Therapies aimed at asymptomatic or symptomatic multiple gestations

Bed rest

In uncomplicated twin pregnancies, **prophylactic bed rest in the hospital does not reduce PTB, perinatal mortality, low birth weight,** and other complications of pregnancy.[66] In fact, **the incidence of PTB < 34 weeks is significantly increased by 84%.**[67–71]

In twin pregnancies with cervical dilatation, bed rest in the hospital does not decrease PTB in women in Zimbabwe.[72] In the trial in which it was recorded, only 6% of women appreciated in-hospital bed rest. For complications, see above under bed rest (singleton pregnancies, page 120).

Reduction

There is no trial to assess the effect of multifetal reduction to prevent PTB. Compared with triplets/higher-order multiples, triplets/higher-order multiples reduced to twins have a higher incidence of loss < 24 weeks, but a lower incidence of PTB < 32 weeks and better neonatal outcome of the remaining twins after reduction in case-control studies (see Chapter 38 of *Maternal–Fetal Evidence Based Guidelines*).

Cerclage

History-indicated cerclage does not prevent PTB in twin gestations.[73] Ultrasound-indicated cerclage for pregnancies with twin gestations and TVU CL < 25 mm does not prevent PTB.[50]

SYMPTOMATIC WOMEN

Work-up (and document)

- History: assess risk factors (see Table 15.1); ensure correctness of GA estimation.
- Physical exam: vital signs; frequency of uterine contractions; test for PPROM (nitrazine, pooling, ferning); fFN; TVU CL; (if PPROM) assess cervical exam visually;[74] (if no PPROM) manual cervical exam (dilatation, CL, effacement, station, presentation).
- Laboratory tests: rectovaginal GBS culture; gonorrhea and *Chlamydia*; urinalysis and urine culture.

Management

- **Consider referral** to tertiary care center if neonatal intensive care unit (NICU) not adequate for GA of potential neonate.
- **Counseling** regarding morbidity and mortality for preterm infant, using latest, possibly internal data.

Current (2007) survival at our institution goes from 0% at 21 weeks to 75% at 25 weeks to > 95% at 29 weeks, whereas intact survival at 18 months is about 50% after 25 weeks. Disabilities in mental and psychomotor development, neuromotor function (including cerebral palsy), or sensory and communication function are present in at least 50% of fetuses born ≤ 25 weeks' gestation.[75] Neonatal consult at 22–34 weeks is indicated for counseling regarding prognosis and neonatal management.

Principles of management of preterm labor

Before treatment is ever considered, the diagnosis of PTL (see above, page 117) must be established.

There is insufficient evidence to justify the use of steroids for fetal lung maturity (FLM) and tocolysis before 23 weeks and after 33 6/7 weeks.

Women with PTL but negative fFN and TVU CL ≥ 30 mm have a ≤ 2% chance of delivering within 1 week, and a > 95% chance of delivering ≥ 35 weeks without therapy, and should therefore not receive any treatment.[76] 70–80% of women diagnosed with PTL do not deliver preterm. **Knowledge of fFN and TVU CL decreases time of triage and incidence of PTB.**[77] Women without cervical change do not have PTL and should not receive tocolysis. Women with multiple gestations should not be treated differently than those with singletons, except that their risk of pulmonary edema is greater when exposed to β-mimetics or magnesium sulfate.[78]

Amniocentesis may be considered to assess intra-amniotic infection (IAI) (incidence about 5–15%) and fetal lung maturity (especially between 33 and 35 weeks). IAI (documented by amniotic fluid culture) rates can be estimated by pregnancy status (Table 15.3). IAI rates can also be estimated by TVU CL.[79]

Tertiary prevention

Tertiary prevention is treatment after diagnosis of PTL in symptomatic women.

Prophylaxis to prevent neonatal morbidity/mortality from PTB (fetal maturation)

Corticosteroids

Betamethasone, dexamethasone (only two corticosteroids which cross the placenta reliably).

Dose: One course – Betamethasone 12 mg IM every 24 hours × 2 doses, or dexamethasone 6 mg IM every

Table 15.3 *Estimated incidences of intra-amniotic infection in women in different clinical scenarios*

Condition	Percent
• GA < 37 weeks	
Asymptomatic (second trimester)	0.5
PTL (intact membranes)	13
PPROM, no labor	25
PPROM, labor	39
Cervix ≥ 2 cm/80% in second trimester	50
• GA ≥ 37 weeks	
Labor	19
PROM	34

GA, gestational age; PTL, preterm labor; PPROM, premature preterm rupture of membranes; PROM, premature rupture of membranes.

6 hours × 4 doses. (Betamethasone, if available, should be preferred to dexamethasone – see below).

Mechanism of action: Enhanced maturational changes in lung architecture and induction of lung enzymes, resulting in biochemical maturation.

Evidence for effectiveness: **Corticosteroids given prior to PTB (either spontaneous or indicated) are effective in preventing RDS, IVH, and neonatal mortality.**[80] Antenatal administration of 24 mg of betamethasone (12 mg IM every 24 hours), or of 24 mg of dexamethasone (6 mg IM every 6 hours), to women expected to give birth preterm is associated with a significant (40%) reduction in mortality, 47% reduction in RDS, and 52% reduction in IVH in preterm infants. There is a trend for a 41% reduction in NEC (OR = 0.59, 95% CI 0.32–1.09). There are also decreased needs for surfactant, oxygen, and mechanical ventilation in the neonatal period. These benefits apply to GA of at least 24–33 6/7 weeks, and are not limited by gender or race. There are insufficient data (no trial) to assess effect before or after these gestational ages. The effects are significant mostly at 48 hours to 7 days from the first dose, but treatment should not be withheld even if delivery appears imminent. Such steroids should therefore be administered to any woman at these gestational ages at significant PTB risk upon identification of the risk. Higher doses do not increase the benefits. Oral dexamethasone is less effective than IM dexamethasone.[81] Betamethasone and dexamethasone have not been compared in a trial. Betamethasone has been associated with less cystic periventricular leukomalacia, and possibly more substantial reduction in complications mentioned above, but this has not been confirmed by any trial. Hydrocortisone was not effective in a small trial.[80] The results are in most part from singleton gestations, with insufficient data on multiple gestations.

Repeat doses of corticosteroids: There is not enough evidence to evaluate the use of repeated doses of corticosteroids in women who remain undelivered, but who are at continued risk of PTB.[80,82] **Fewer** (by 36%) infants in the repeat dose(s) of corticosteroids group had **severe lung disease** (including RDS) compared with infants in the placebo group.[83,84] No statistically significant differences were seen for any of the other primary outcomes that included other measures of respiratory morbidity, small-for-GA at birth, perinatal death, intraventricular hemorrhage (IVH), periventricular leukomalacia, and maternal infectious morbidity. Fewer (by 36%) infants in the repeat dose(s) of the corticosteroids group received surfactant compared with infants in the placebo group.[82] There is insufficient evidence on the benefits and risks to recommend repeat dose(s) of prenatal corticosteroids for women at risk of PTB for the prevention of neonatal respiratory disease. **Rescue (one extra course) therapy should only be considered if multiple weeks have elapsed since the initial course of corticosteroids and a new episode of PTL or PPROM, or impeding risk of PTB, presents again at an early (e.g. 28–30 weeks) gestational age.**[83] More than two courses of corticosteroids for fetal maturity should be avoided pending results of further trials.

Contraindications: None.

Side effects: When used for only 1 course, no significant side effects, except for **transient maternal hyperglycemia** for 12 hours to about 5–7 days after the dose, resulting in false-positive glucose screening tests or difficulty in managing diabetes. There is no significant increase in maternal or fetal/neonatal infection. If ≥ 4 courses are used, there is a possible association with birth weight < 10th percentile and probably not with small (< 10th percentile) neonatal head circumference, with evidence of some later 'catch-up'.[82,84] No adverse consequences of a single course of prophylactic corticosteroids for preterm birth in either the mothers or, most importantly, the infants, even at 10 + years follow-up, have been identified, but long-term follow-up is limited so far.

Thyrotropin-releasing hormone (in addition to corticosteroids)

Prenatal thyrotropin-releasing hormone (TRH), in addition to corticosteroids, given to women at risk of very preterm birth, does not improve infant outcomes and can cause maternal side effects.[85] Overall, prenatal TRH, in addition to corticosteroids, does not reduce the risk of neonatal respiratory disease or chronic oxygen dependence, and does not improve any of the fetal, neonatal, or childhood outcomes. Indeed, prenatal TRH does have adverse effects for women and their infants. Side effects are more likely to occur in women receiving TRH. In the infants, prenatal TRH increases by 16% the risk of needing ventilation, by 48% having a low Apgar score at 5 minutes, and, for the two trials providing data, was associated with poorer outcomes at childhood follow-up.[85]

Phenobarbital

The use of prophylactic maternal phenobarbital administration prior to preterm delivery does not prevent IVH or protect from neurological disability in preterm infants.[86]

Prenatal maternal phenobarbital is associated with a significant (35%) reduction in the rates of all grades of IVH and 59% reduction in severe grades of IVH (3 and 4) in the infants. These results are influenced by trials of poor quality which contribute excessive weight in the analysis due to their higher rates of severe IVH. When only the two higher-quality trials were included,[87,88] phenobarbital was not associated with any beneficial effects, including similar incidences of all grades of IVH and severe grades of IVH to placebo. No difference was found in the incidence of neurodevelopmental abnormalities at pediatric follow-up assessed between 18 and 36 months of age. Maternal sedation is more likely in women receiving phenobarbital.[85]

Vitamin K

Vitamin K administered to women prior to very preterm birth has **not been shown to significantly prevent IVH in preterm infants.** Antenatal vitamin K is associated with no reduction in all grades of IVH or in severe IVH (grades 3 and 4) for babies receiving prenatal vitamin K compared with control babies.[89] Information on neurodevelopment was only given for a small sample of children in one trial, with discrepancy in results given in the two reports.

Non-tocolytic interventions in preterm labor

Bed rest

Bed rest has never been tested in singleton gestations complicated by PTL or PPROM. In twin pregnancies with cervical dilatation, bed rest in the hospital **did not decrease** PTB in one trial in Zimbabwe.[90]

Hydration

There is **no advantage** of hydration compared with bed rest alone. Intravenous hydration does not seem to be beneficial, even during the period of evaluation soon after admission, in women with PTL. Women with evidence of dehydration may, however, benefit from the intervention.

Compared with bed rest alone, hydration is associated with similar incidences of PTB < 37 weeks, < 34 weeks, or < 32 weeks, and of admission to an NICU.[91] Cost of treatment is slightly higher (US$39) in the hydration group for hospital costs during a visit of less than 24 hours. Women studied were at low risk, as about 30% of women required tocolysis, and < 30% had PTB. No studies evaluated oral hydration.[91]

Antibiotics

There is **no clear overall benefit** or detriment from prophylactic antibiotic treatment for PTL with intact membranes on neonatal outcomes.[92,93] PTB < 36 or 37 weeks is similar in antibiotics and placebo groups. There is a trend for a 52% increase in neonatal mortality for those who received antibiotics (RR = 1.52, 95% CI 0.99–2.34), with similar overall perinatal mortality (RR = 1.22, 95% CI 0.88–1.70).[92] The only benefit is a 26% reduction in maternal infection with the use of prophylactic antibiotics. Of the different antibiotics or combinations studied so far (macrolide antibiotics, β-lactam antibiotics, a combination of β-lactam and macrolide antibiotics, and antibiotics active against anaerobes), antibiotics active against anaerobes (clindamycin[94] and ampicillin–metronidazole[95,96]) show a 10-day increase in the interval from randomization to delivery, a 38% reduction in the number of women giving birth within 7 days of enrollment, and 37% fewer admissions to an NICU in small trials. Given these data, antibiotics should not be used routinely in women with PTL and intact membranes.

Tocolysis (preterm labor)
Contraindications

Maternal
- Chorioamnionitis
- Severe vaginal bleeding/abruptio
- Pre-eclampsia
- Medical contraindications to specific tocolytic agent (see below)
- Other maternal medical condition that makes continuing the pregnancy inadvisable

Fetal
- Fetal death
- Major (especially if lethal) fetal anomaly or chromosome abnormality
- Other fetal conditions in which prolongation of pregnancy is inadvisable
- Documented fetal maturity

Principles

At 24–33 6/7weeks, steroids for fetal lung maturity (FLM) should always be given if tocolysis is initiated. Tocolysis is usually used for ≤48 hours to allow steroid effect. Given the side effects, consider stopping tocolytic therapy at ≤48 hours after steroids, if PTL is under control.

Primary tocolysis – single agent
Beta-mimetics: ritodrine, terbutaline

Dose: Ritodrine: 50–100 µg/min IV initial dose, increase 50 µg/min every 10 minutes (max 350 µg/min). [po, 1–20 mg po every 2–4 hours]. Terbutaline: 0.25 mg SQ every 20 minutes at first, then 2–3 hours; or 5–10 µg/min IV, max 80 µg/min; or 2.5–5 mg po every 2–4 hours (hold if maternal HR > 120/min).

Mechanism of action: Stimulate B_2 receptor through cyclic AMP, so no free calcium for myometrial contraction.

Evidence for effectiveness (Table 15.4): **Beta-mimetics decrease the number of women in PTL giving birth within 48 hours compared with placebo, and decrease** the number of births **within 7 days.**[97] There is a trend for a small reduction of PTB < 37 weeks' gestation. No benefit is demonstrated for beta-mimetics on perinatal death, or neonatal death. No significant effect is demonstrated for RDS. A few trials reported the following outcomes, with no difference detected: cerebral palsy, infant death, and NEC. Beta-mimetics are significantly associated with the following side effects (see below, also): withdrawal from treatment due to adverse effects; chest pain; dyspnea; tachycardia; palpitation; tremor; headaches; hypokalemia; hyperglycemia; nausea/vomiting; nasal stuffiness; and fetal tachycardia.[97] There is insufficient evidence to assess which of the studied beta-mimetics is most effective and/or associated with less side effects, with most data reported for ritodrine. For comparison with other tocolytics, see below.

Specific contraindications: Cardiac arrhythmia or other significant cardiac disease; diabetes mellitus; poorly controlled thyroid disease (for ritodrine).

Side effects:

Maternal: Hyperglycemia (glucose 140–200 mg/dl in 20–50% – mechanism: decreased peripheral insulin sensitivity and increased endogenous glucose production); hyperinsulinemia; hypokalemia (potassium < 3 mEq/L in 50%); tremors, nervousness, shortness of breath (10%); chest pain (5–10%), tachycardia/palpitations, arrhythmia (3%); electrocardiogram (EKG) changes (2–3%); hypotension (2–3%); pulmonary edema (< 1–5%; mechanism: reduced sodium excretion – sodium and therefore fluid retention). Ritodrine: altered thyroid function, antidiuresis.

Fetal/neonatal: Ritodrine: neonatal tachycardia, hypoglycemia, hypocalcemia, hyperbilirubinemia, hypotension, IVH. Terbutaline: tachycardia, hyperinsulinemia, hyperglycemia, myocardial and septal hypertrophy, myocardial ischemia.

Calcium channel blockers (CCB): nifedipine, nicardipine

Dose: Nifedipine 20–30 mg × 1, then 10–20 mg every 4–8 hours (max 90 mg/day) [nicardipine similar dosing].

Mechanism of action: Impair calcium channels, so inhibit influx of calcium into cell, and therefore prevent myometrial contraction.

Evidence for effectiveness: (See Table 15.4.) There are no studies of CCB compared with placebo for PTB prevention.

When compared with any other tocolytic agent (mainly beta-mimetics, 9/12 trials), calcium channel blockers reduce by 24% the number of women giving birth within 7 days of receiving treatment and by 17% prior to 34 weeks' gestation.[98] CCB show a trend to reduce PTB within 48 hours of initiation of treatment (RR = 0.80; 95% CI 0.61–1.05), and PTB < 37 weeks' gestation (RR = 0.95; 95% CI 0.83–1.09). **CCB also reduce by 37% the frequency of neonatal RDS, by 79% NEC, by 41% IVH, and by 27% neonatal jaundice. CCB also reduce the requirement for women to have treatment ceased for adverse drug reaction.** There are insufficient data regarding the effects of different dosage regimens and formulations of CCB on maternal and neonatal outcomes; the most studied is nifedipine, at the dosage shown above. **CCB should be preferred to beta-mimetics for tocolysis.**

Specific contraindications: Cardiac disease; hypotension (<90/50 mmHg); concomitant use of magnesium; caution in renal disease.

Side effects:

Maternal: Flushing, headache, dizziness, nausea, transient hypotension. Caution in women with hypotension and renal disease, as well as women on magnesium (cardiovascular collapse).

Fetal/neonatal: None.

Table 15.4	*Summary of the evidence for tocolytic therapy*				
Tocolytics	48 hours	7 days	PTB < 32 weeks	PTB < 37 weeks	Perinatal mortality
PRIMARY – SINGLE AGENT VS PLACEBO					
Beta-mimetics	**0.63 (0.53–0.75)**[*] [n=1209]	**0.78 (0.68–0.90)** [n=911]	N/A	0.95 (0.88–1.03) [n=1212]	1.00 (0.48–2.09) [n=1174] (neonatal)
CCB	No RCT	No RCT	No RCT	No RCT	No RCT
COX	**0.19 (0.08–0.45)** [n=70][a]	**0.43 (0.27–0.69)** [n=70][a]	NC	**0.21 (0.07–0.62)** [n=36]	0.80 (0.25–2.58) [n=106]
Mg	0.57 (0.28–1.15) [n=190]	NC	NC	0.92 (0.41–2.07) [n=29]	1.74 (0.63–4.77) [n=192]
ORA	**0.77 (0.61–0.97)** 86/302 vs 115/311 [n=613]	**0.74 (0.61–0.91)** 93/246 vs 129/254 [n=302][a]	1.33 (0.84–2.14) 35/153 vs 23/134 [n=287][a]	1.17 (0.99–1.37) [n=501]	2.25 (0.79–6.40) [n=583]
NOD	3.06 (0.74–12.63) [n=33]	NC	NC	NC	0.94 (0.05–16.37) [n=33] (neonatal)
Progesterone	N/A	N/A	N/A	N/A	N/A
COMPARISONS					
CCB vs beta-mimetic	**0.72 (0.53–0.97)** [n=470]	**0.76 (0.59–0.99)** [n=242]	**0.79 (0.65–0.96)** [n=328] (<34 weeks)	0.89 (0.76–1.05) [n=389]	1.20 (0.49-2.94) [n=529]
COX vs beta-mimetic	**0.27 (0.08–0.96)** [n=100]	0.88 (0.52–1.46) [n=146]	NC	**0.53 (0.28–0.99)** [n=80]	0.99 (0.27–3.57) [n=237]
COX vs CCB	No RCT	No RCT	No RCT	No RCT	No RCT
COX vs Mg	0.75 (0.40–1.40) [n=315]	NC	NC	0.55 (0.17–1.73) [n=88]	2.31 (0.54–9.90) [n=423]
Mg vs beta-mimetic	1.08 (0.72–1.63) [n=349]	NC	NC	0.85 (0.66–1.10) [n=147]	1.19 (0.08–17.51) [n=166]
Mg vs CCB	1.20 (0.60–2.39) [n=154]	NC	0.82 (0.45-1.50) [n=80] (<34 weeks)	1.04 (0.75–1.44) [n=148]	0.19 (0.01–3.85) [n=80]
Mg vs COX	1.51 (0.53–4.30) [n=101]	NC	NC	NC	0.98 (0.06–15.35) [n=117]
ORA vs beta-mimetic	0.98 (0.68–1.41) [n=1033]	0.91 (0.69–1.20) [n=731]	NC	0.90 (0.71–1.13) [n=244]	0.66 (0.24–1.83) [n=836]
ORA vs CCB	No RCT	No RCT	No RCT	No RCT	No RCT
ORA vs COX	No RCT	No RCT	No RCT	No RCT	No RCT
ORA vs Mg	No RCT	No RCT	No RCT	No RCT	No RCT
NOD vs β-mimetic	1.43 (0.47–4.37) [n=132]	1.10 (0.67–1.80) [n=391]	1.00 (0.49–2.06) [n=233]	**0.53 (0.35–0.81)** [n=391]	1.03 (0.18–6.02) [n=191]
NOD vs Mg	N/A	N/A	N/A	N/A	N/A

(Continued)

Table 15.4 *(Continued)*

Tocolytics	48 hours	7 days	PTB < 32 weeks	PTB < 37 weeks	Perinatal mortality
PRIMARY – MULTIPLE AGENTS					
Indo vs placebos (all on MgSO$_4$)	N/A	N/A	N/A	1.35 (0.86–2.14)[a] 23/43 vs 17/43	∞ (0.51–∞)[a] 2/47 vs 0/45
Progesterone vs placebo (all on ritodrine)	N/A	N/A	N/A	0.48 (0.14–1.44)	N/A
REFRACTORY					
Indo vs sulindac	1.50 (0.32–7.17)[a] 3/18 vs 2/18	0.88 (0.40–1.88)[a] 7/18 vs 8/18	N/A	N/A	Not calculable[a] 0/18 vs 0/18
MAINTENANCE VS PLACEBO					
Beta-mimetic (oral)	NC	NC	NC	NC	NC
Beta-mimetic (terb pump) (vs saline pump)	NC	NC	0.97 (0.51–1.84) [*n*=52] (< 34 weeks)	1.17 (0.79–1.73) [*n*=52]	NC
CCB (vs no therapy)	NC	NC	NC	1.00 (0.73–1.37) [*n*=74]	NC
COX	NC	NC	NC	NC	NC
Mg	NC	NC	NC	0.85 (0.47–1.51) [*n*=50]	5.00 (0.25–99.17) [*n*=50]
ORA	N/A	N/A	0.85 (0.47–1.54)[a] 19/158 vs 18/127	0.89 (0.71–1.12)[a] 90/267 vs 92/243	0.80 (0.23–2.72)[a] 4/252 vs 5/251 (neonatal)
COMPARISONS					
Terb pump vs po terb	NC	NC	NC	NC	NC

*All data are presented as relative risks, and (in parenthesis) 95% confidence intervals. N/A, not available in reports of studies; NC, not calculable from the available reports; no RCT, no randomized controlled trial reports on this comparison; terb, terbutaline; CCB, calcium channel blockers; COX, cyclo-oxygenase inhibitor; ORA, oxytocin receptor antagonists; Indo, indomethacin; NOD, nitric oxide donor.
[a]Author's unpublished meta-analysis

Cyclo-oxygenase (COX) inhibitors

Non-selective COX inhibitors: indomethacin (Indocin), ketorolac. Selective COX inhibitors (preferential COX-2 inhibitor): sulindac; rofecoxib (Vioxx); celecoxib; nimesulide.

Dose: Indomethacin: 50–100 mg loading dose (rectal or vaginal route preferred, oral otherwise), then 25–50 mg every 6 hours **for 48 hours max, and always < 32 weeks.** Sulindac: 200 mg po every 12 hours × 48 hours. Ketorolac: 60 mg IM, then 30 mg IM every 6 hours × 48 hours.

Mechanism of action: Cyclo-oxygenase (COX) inhibitors, so inhibit prostaglandin synthesis; therefore, inhibit myometrial contraction.

Evidence for effectiveness: (See Table 15.4.) (The non-selective COX inhibitor indomethacin was used in 10/13 trials).

When compared with placebo, COX inhibition (indomethacin only) results in a **79% significant reduction in PTB < 37 weeks' gestation** in a small trial, **an increase in GA of 3.5 weeks and a > 700 g increase in birth weight.**[99] There is a significant **reduction in delivery within 48 hours of initiation of treatment and within 7 days.** No differences were detected in any other reported outcomes including perinatal mortality, RDS, etc.

Used for 48 hours only, the **intravaginal** route (100 mg every 12 hours) decreases delivery at 48 hours and at < 7 days compared to rectal/oral (100 mg rectally, followed by 25 mg po), with some improvement in neonatal morbidities in a small trial.[100]

Compared with any other tocolytic, COX inhibition resulted in a 47% reduction in PTB < 37 weeks' gestation and a reduction in maternal drug reaction requiring cessation of treatment.[99] No differences were detected in the fetal or neonatal outcomes such as perinatal mortality; RDS; IVH; NEC; premature closure of the ductus; or persistent pulmonary hypertension of the newborn (PPHN).

Compared with **beta-mimetics**, COX inhibitors are associated with a **significant** 73% **reduction in the number of women delivering within 48 hours of initiation of treatment.**[99]

Compared with **magnesium sulfate**, COX inhibitors are associated with trends for lower number of women delivering within 48 hours and lower PTB < 37 weeks.[99]

Comparisons of non-selective (indomethacin and sulindac) COX inhibitors vs selective (rofecoxib and nimesulide) COX-2 inhibitors do not demonstrate any differences in maternal or neonatal outcomes.[101,102] Because of the small numbers, all estimates of effect are imprecise and need to be interpreted with caution.

Specific contraindications: Renal or hepatic disease, active peptic ulcer disease, poorly controlled hypertension, non-steroidal anti-inflammatory drug (NSAID)-sensitive asthma, and coagulation disorders/thrombocytopenia.

Side effects: When used for only 48 hours, no serious maternal and fetal/neonatal side effects occur, and fetal survellaince is not indicated. Usually COX inhibitors are better tolerated by the mother than other tocolytics such as magnesium and beta-mimetics.

Maternal: As with any NSAIDs, mild gastrointestinal (GI) upset – nausea, heartburn (take with some food/milk) (COX-1). GI bleeding (COX-1), coagulation and platelet abnormalities (COX-1), asthma if ASA-sensitive. May obscure elevation in temperature. Long-term rofecoxib (Vioxx) use in adults has been associated with stroke, so this drug is now not available in many countries.

Fetal/neonatal: In trials, 403 women received short-term tocolysis (up to 48 hours) with COX inhibitors (mainly indomethacin) and there was only one case (2.5/1000) of antenatal **closure of the ductus arteriosus**. There was no increase in the incidence of patent ductus arteriosus (PDA) postnatally (8 treated with COX inhibitors vs 8 treated with placebo or other tocolytics).[99] No difference in incidences of IVH, BPD, PDA, NEC, or perinatal mortality was noted in a review of trials aimed at evaluating safety.[103] Use for **> 48 hours**, especially ≥ 32 weeks, is associated with significant fetal effects such as constriction of the ductus arteriosus, which can lead to hydrops, pulmonary hypertension, and death, as well as **renal insufficiency**, manifested in utero by oligohydramnios. Other effects with prolonged use such as hyperbilirubinemia, NEC, and IVH have not been shown with < 72 hours use. Selective COX-2 inhibitors have not been shown

consistently to be any safer for the fetus/neonate than non-selective COX inhibitors such as indomethacin. Therefore, **continuous use of COX inhibitors for > 48 hours and ≥ 32 weeks is contraindicated.**

Magnesium sulfate (MgSO$_4$)

Dose: MgSO$_4$ 40 g in 1 L d51/2NS (5% dextrose and 1/2 normal saline solution). Initial: 4–6 g/30 min, then: 2–4 g/h. A dose of 5 g/h has not been shown to be beneficial in perinatal outcome compared with a dose of 2 g/h, and is associated with significant side effects.[104] Weaning MgSO$_4$ tocolysis has no benefits and a few harmful side effects compared with stopping MgSO$_4$ abruptly.[105]

Mechanism of action: Intracellular calcium antagonist.

Evidence for effectiveness: (See Table 15.4.) Compared with placebo, there is **insufficient evidence** to show if magnesium sulfate reduces the incidence of PTB or perinatal morbidity and mortality.[106]

Compared with all controls (including other tocolytics), MgSO$_4$ does not prevent PTB at 48 hours, PTB < 37 weeks or PTB < 32 weeks. Perinatal death is higher (only 2 perinatal deaths), whereas perinatal morbidities are similar. The dose of magnesium does not affect efficacy. Given these results, there is **no convincing evidence for recommending magnesium for tocolysis.**

Specific contraindications: Myasthenia gravis.

Management: Aim for 4–7 MgSO$_4$ level. MgSO$_4$ blood levels are usually not necessary, as long as kidney function and reflexes are monitored. Monitor urinary output. Follow deep tendon reflexes: ↓ at level ≥ 8, absent ≥ 10. At level ≥ 10, risk of respiratory depression; ≥ 15, risk of cardiac arrest.

Side effects:

Maternal: Flushing, lethargy, headache, muscle weakness, diplopia, dry mouth, pulmonary edema (1%; increased with intravenous overhydration), cardiac arrest.

Fetal/neonatal: Lethargy, hypotonia, hypocalcemia, respiratory depression. Prolonged use: demineralization.

Oxytocin receptor antagonists (ORA): atosiban (Tractocile in Europe)

Dose: Atosiban 6.75 mg bolus, then 300 μg/min IV × 3 hours, then 100 μg/min (max 45 hours).

Mechanism of action: Competitive inhibitor of oxytocin via blockade of oxytocin receptor.

Evidence for effectiveness: (See Table 15.4). Compared with placebo, atosiban does not reduce incidence of PTB <37 weeks **or improve neonatal outcome,**[107] but may prevent PTB within 48 hours or 7 days. In one trial, atosiban was associated with an increase in infant deaths at 12 months of age compared with placebo.[108] However, this trial randomized significantly more women to atosiban before 26 weeks' gestation. This is one of the reasons why atosiban is not available in the USA (not FDA-approved). Compared with placebo, use of atosiban results in about 140 g lower infant birth weight and more mild maternal adverse drug reactions.[107] Compared with beta-mimetics, atosiban is associated with similar incidences of PTB or perinatal morbidity/mortality, and with fewer maternal drug reactions requiring treatment cessation.[107]

Side effects: Minimal to none.

Nitric oxide donors (NOD): nitroglycerin

Dose: Nitroglycerin transdermal patch 0.4 mg/h.

Mechanism of action: Direct relaxation of uterine muscle.

Evidence for effectiveness: (See Table 15.4.) There is currently **insufficient evidence** to support the routine administration of NOD for prevention of PTB in women with PTL.[109] Compared with placebo, NOD do not prevent PTB or improve perinatal morbidity and mortality in a small trial.[110] Compared with beta-mimetics, NOD are associated with a decrease in PTB to <37 weeks. Incidences of PTB and perinatal mortality were not reported in the only trial comparing NOD with $MgSO_4$. Although headaches are more common in women receiving NOD compared with controls, other side effects are less common compared with other tocolytics. Nitroglycerin has been the only NOD used in trials.

Progesterone

The only trial to assess safety and efficacy of any type of progesterone as primary tocolysis (compared with beta-mimetic) did not report PTB outcomes.[111]

Primary tocolysis – multiple agents simultaneously

Indomethacin and magnesium vs magnesium alone

Compared with placebos, indomethacin and ampicillin sulbactam does not prevent PTB in women in PTL already receiving $MgSO_4$ tocolysis.[112]

Primary tocolysis – additional agents vs one agent only

Progesterone vs placebo, in addition to ritodrine

Compared with placebo, in women receiving ritodrine tocolysis, the addition of progesterone is not associated with a significant reduction in PTB <37 weeks (16% vs 33% in placebo) in a very small trial.[113]

Refractory tocolysis – primary agent is failing

Indomethacin vs Sulindac

Indomethacin is similar to sulindac in prevention of PTB in women failing primary $MgSO_4$ tocolysis in a small trial.[114]

Maintenance tocolysis – after successful primary tocolysis

Beta-mimetics: oral

Dose: Ritodrine: 1–20 mg po every 2–4 hours. Terbutaline: 2.5–5 mg po every 2–4 hours. Oral beta-mimetic therapy for maintenance tocolysis **does not prevent PTB, recurrent PTL, recurrent hospitalizations, or perinatal morbidity and mortality compared with placebo.**[115] Some adverse effects such as tachycardia are more frequent in the beta-mimetics group. Given this ample evidence from 11 trials, there is **absolutely no evidence** to support the use of oral beta-mimetics after PTL has resolved.

Beta-mimetics: terbutaline pump

Dose: 0.05 mg/h. Compared with **placebo**, terbutaline pump does not prevent PTB or improve perinatal morbidity and mortality. Side effects and costs associated with this therapy further **advise against its use.**[116]

Calcium channel blockers

There is insufficient evidence for efficacy of CCB maintenance therapy after successful tocolysis. Incidence of PTB <37 weeks is similar to **placebo** in one trial.[117]

COX inhibitors

Compared with **placebo**, after successful tocolysis, oral sulindac either 200 mg every 12 hours×7 days or 100 mg every 12 hours until 34 weeks does not reduce PTB.[118,119] Given the association with fetal/neonatal complications with COX inhibitor use for >48 hours, COX inhibitors should not be used for maintenance tocolysis.

Compared with oral **terbutaline,** oral indomethacin is associated with a similar incidence of PTB when used for maintenance tocolysis after successful IV tocolysis, but indomethacin is associated with significant constriction of ductus arteriosus and oligohydramnios when used for >48 hours.[120] Therefore, indomethacin should never be used for maintenance tocolysis.

Magnesium sulfate

Compared with **placebo, no treatment** or **other maintenance tocolytics,** magnesium oral maintenance therapy **does not** prevent PTB or affect perinatal morbidity and mortality in three small trials.[121]

Oxytocin receptor antagonists

Compared with **placebo,** ORA (atosiban) maintenance therapy (30 µg/min) via pump up to 36 weeks does not prevent PTB or affect perinatal morbidity and mortality, with a 5 days (32.6 vs 27.6, $p=0.02$) longer interval to delivery in one trial.[122] There are no side effects compared with placebo except for injection-site reactions. ORA are not available in oral form for maintenance.

Progesterone

Compared with identical placebo, progesterone injections did not prevent PTB in women discharged home after an episode of PTL in one old study.[123]

PTL resolved: home vs in hospital care

After PTL has resolved (and cervical dilatation has not progressed ≥4 cm), **home management is associated with similar incidences of reaching ≥36 weeks compared with hospital management.**[124,125] Hospitalization may increase maternal stress, vaginal examinations, time in recumbent position (and its consequences), and decreased plasma volume. For the many women with arrested PTL, continued hospitalization after steroids administration seems unnecessary.

Preconception counseling

Given its frequency, it is important to review risk factors for PTB in every woman planning a pregnancy. In the women with a risk factor (e.g. prior PTB), it is important to review prognosis, possible complications, and management of a future pregnancy.

Prenatal care

Preconception counseling as above, if not already done. Management should follow risk-specific recommendations mentioned above.

Antepartum testing

No specific fetal testing indicated. HUAM, discussed above, is not effective in preventing any complication.

Mode of delivery

There is **insufficient evidence** to evaluate the use of a policy for uniform *elective cesarean delivery* (CD) compared with *expectant management and selective CD* for preterm (about 24–36 weeks) babies.[126] Mothers in the elective CD group have more morbidity. Babies in the elective CD group show no statistical differences compared with expectant management, but tend to have less RDS, less neonatal seizures, and fewer deaths, although they were more likely to have a low cord pH immediately after delivery in the small trials that reported on these outcomes.[126] Differentiation of data between breech and vertex presentations is difficult, with numbers too small for definite conclusions.

Anesthesia

No specific changes.

Postpartum/breastfeeding

As in other pregnancies, breastfeeding is encouraged as tolerated by the preterm infant. Extensive counseling should be provided regarding rate of recurrence of PTB, and future management in pregnancy (see above). Treatment with antibiotics before pregnancy does not prevent recurrent PTB. **In women with a prior spontaneous PTB <34 weeks, oral azithromycin and metronidazole every 4 months after the PTB and before the next conception does not significantly reduce subsequent PTB, but is in fact associated with trends for earlier GA at delivery and lower birth weight.**[127]

REFERENCES

1. American College of Obstetricians and Gynecologists. Assessment of risk factors for preterm birth. ACOG Practice Bulletin, No. 31, 2001. [review]
2. American College of Obstetricians and Gynecologists. Cervical insufficiency. ACOG Practice Bulletin, No. 48, 2003. [review]

3. Zhu B-P, Rolfs RT, Nangle BE, Horan JM. Effect of the interval between pregnancies on perinatal outcome N Engl J Med 1999; 340: 589–94. [II-2]

4. Kramer, MS. Kakuma, R. Energy and protein intake in pregnancy. Cochrane Database Syst Rev 2007; 1. [meta-analysis: 13 RCTs, n = 4665]

5. Kramer MS. Isocaloric balanced protein supplementation in pregnancy. Database Syst Rev 2007; 1. [meta-analysis: 3 RCTs, n = 996]

6. Kramer MS. High protein supplementation in pregnancy. Cochrane Database Syst Rev 2007; 1. [meta-analysis: 2 RCTs, n = 1076]

7. Makrides M, Crowther CA. Magnesium supplementation in pregnancy. Cochrane Database Syst Rev 2007; 1.[meta-analysis: 7 RCTs, n = 2689]

8. Lumley J, Oliver SS, Chamberlain C, Oakley L. Interventions for promoting smoking cessation during pregnancy. Cochrane Database Syst Rev 2007; 1. [meta-analysis: 64 RCTs, over 20 000 women]

9. Smoking cessation during pregnancy. ACOG Educational Bulletin 260, 2000. www.acog.org [review]

10. Sexton M, Hebel JR. A clinical trial of change in maternal smoking and its effect on birth weight. JAMA 1984; 251: 911–15. [RCT, n = 935]

11. Donatelle RJ, Prows SL, Champeau D, Hudson D. Randomised controlled trial using social support and financial incentives for high risk pregnant smokers: Significant Other Supporter (SOS) program. Tobacco Control 2000; 9(Suppl 3):iii67–9. [RCT, n = 120]

12. Wisborg K, Henriksen TB, Secher NJ. A prospective intervention study of stopping smoking in pregnancy in a routine antenatal care setting. Br J Obstet Gynaecol 1998; 105: 1171–6. [RCT, n = 5156]

13. Kapur B, Hackman R, Selby P, Klein J, Koren G. Randomized, double blind, placebo-controlled trial of nicotine replacement therapy in pregnancy. Curr Ther Res 2001; 62(4): 274–8. [RCT, n = 20]

14. Hegaard H, Hjaergaard H, Moller L, Wachmann H, Ottesen B. Multimodel intervention raises smoking cessation rate during pregnancy. Acta Obstetr Gynecol Scand 2003; 82: 813–19. [RCT, n = 647]

15. Hobel CJ, Ross MG, Bemis RL et al. The West Los Angeles preterm birth prevention project. I. Program impact on high-risk women. Am J Obstet Gynecol 1994; 170: 54–62. [RCT, n => 1500]

16. Hodnett ED, Fredericks S. Support during pregnancy for women at increased risk of low birthweight babies. Cochrane Database Syst Rev 2007; 1. [meta-analysis: 16 RCTs, > 16 000 women]

17. Mueller-Heubach E, Reddick D, Barnett B, Bente R. Preterm birth prevention: evaluation of a prospective controlled trial. Am J Obstet Gynecol 1989; 160: 1172–8. [RCT, n = 800]

18. Main DM, Richardson DK, Hadley CB, Gabbe SG. Controlled trial of a preterm labor detection program: efficacy and costs. Obstet Gynecol 1989; 74: 873–7. [RCT, n = 376]

19. Collaborative group on preterm birth prevention. Multicenter randomized controlled trial of a preterm birth prevention program. Am J Obstet Gynecol 1993; 169: 352–66. [RCT, n = 2395 – includes Goldenberg RL, Davis RO, Copper RL, et al. The Alabama preterm birth prevention trial. Obstet Gynecol 1990; 75: 933–9 [RCT; n = about 1000])

20. MRC/RCOG Working Party on Cervical Cerclage. Final report of the Medical Research Council/Royal College of Obstetricians and Gynaecologists multicentre randomized trial of cervical cerclage. Br J Obstet Gynecol 1993; 100: 516–23. [RCT, n = 1292]

21. Rush RW, Isaacs S, McPherson K et al. A randomized controlled trial of cervical cerclage in women at high risk of preterm delivery. Br J Obstet Gynecol 1984; 91: 724–30. [RCT, n = 194]

22. Lazar P, Gueguen S, Dreyfus J, et al. Multicentre controlled trial of cervical cerclage in women at moderate risk of preterm delivery. Br J Obstet Gynecol 1984; 91: 731–5. [RCT, n = 506]

23. Berghella V, Baxter J, Berghella M. Cervical insufficiency. In: Apuzzio JJ, Vintzileos AM, Iffy, L eds. Operative Obstetrics, 3rd edn. Taylor and Francis; London: 2006: 157–72. [Review]

24. Davis G, Berghella V, Talucci M, Wapner RJ. Patients with a prior failed transvaginal cerclage: a comparison of obstetric outcomes with either transabdominal or transvaginal cerclage. Am J Obstet Gynecol 2000; 183: 836–9. [II-2]

25. Olsen SF, Secher NJ, Tabor A et al. Randomized clinical trials of fish oil supplementation in high risk pregnancies. Br J Obstet Gynecol 2000; 107: 382–95.[RCT, n = 232 for singletons, n = 569 for twins]

26. Smuts CM, Huang M, Mundy D et al. A randomized trial of docosahexaenoic acid supplementation during the third trimester of pregnancy. Obstet Gynecol 2003; 101: 469–79. [RCT, n = 291]

27. Vermeulen GM, Bruinse HW. Prophylactic administration of clindamycin 2% vaginal cream to reduce the incidence of spontaneous preterm birth in women with an increased recurrence risk: a randomized placebo-controlled double-blind trial. Br J Obstet Gynecol 1999; 106: 652–7. [RCT, n = 168]

28. Gichangi PB, Ndinya-Achola JO, Ombete J, Nagelkerke NJ, Temmerman M. Antimicrobial prophylaxis in pregnancy: a randomized, placebo-controlled trial with cefetamet-pivoxil in pregnant women with poor obstetrical history. Am J Obstet Gynecol 1997; 177: 680–4. [RCT, n = 253]

29. Hauth JC, Goldenberg RL, Andrews WW, DuBard MB, Copper RL. Reduced incidence of preterm delivery with metronidazole and erythromycin in women with bacterial vaginosis. N Eng J Med 1995; 333: 1732–6. [RCT, n = 358 women with prior PTB or prepregnancy weight < 50 kg, and without BV; treatment metronidazole and erythromycin]

30. Thinkhamrop J, Hofmeyr GJ, Adetoro O, Lumbiganon P. Prophylactic antibiotic administration in pregnancy to prevent infectious morbidity and mortality. Cochrane Database Syst Rev 2007; 1. [meta-analysis: 6 RCTs, n = 2189, both low- (see Chapter 1) and high-risk women]

31. Dodd JM, Flenady V, Cincotta R, Crowther CA. Prenatal administration of progesterone for preventing preterm birth. Cochrane Database Syst Rev 2007; 1. [meta-analysis: 6 RCTs, n = 988]

32. Meis PJ, Klebanoff M, Thom E et al. Prevention of recurrent preterm delivery by 17 alpha-hydroxyprogesterone caproate. N Engl J Med 2003; 348: 2379–85. [RCT, n = 463; largest trial included in meta-analysis]

33. Althuisius SM, Dekker GA, van Geijn HP, Bekedam DJ, Hummel P. Cervical incompetence prevention randomized cerclage trial (CIPRACT): study design and preliminary results. Am J Obstet Gynecol 2000; 183: 823–9. [RCT, n = 67]

34. Pritts EA, Atwood AK. Luteal phase support in infertility treatment: a meta-analysis of the randomized trials. Hum Reprod 2002; 17: 2287–99. [meta-analysis: n = about 200]

35. Corrado F, Dugo C, Cannata ML, et al. A randomized trial of progesterone prophylaxis after midtrimester amniocentesis. Eur J Obstet Gynecol Reprod Biol 2002; 188: 196–8. [RCT, n = 584]

36. Morrison JC, Martin JN, Martin RW, Gookin KS, Wiser WL. Prevention of preterm birth by ambulatory assessment of uterine activity: a randomized study. Am J Obstet Gynecol 1987; 156: 536–43. [RCT, n = 67; (18 twins) cannot differentiate populations]

37. Iams JD, Johnson FF, O'Shaunessy RW. A prospective random trial of home uterine activity monitoring in pregnancies at increased risk of preterm labor. Am J Obstet Gynecol 1987; 157: 638–43. [RCT, n = 142 (40 twins); cannot differentiate; Iams JD, Johnson FF, O'Shaunessy RW. A prospective random trial of home uterine activity monitoring in pregnancies at increased risk of preterm labor. Part II. Am J Obstet Gynecol 1988; 159: 595–603. [RCT, n = 142]]

38. Hill WC, Fleming WC, Martin RW et al. Home uterine activity monitoring is associated with a reduction in preterm birth. Obstet Gynecol 1990; 76: 13–18s [RCT, n = 245; ?twins].

39. Dyson DC, Crites YM, Ray DA, Armstrong MA. Prevention of preterm birth in high-risk patients: a role of education and provider contact versus home uterine monitoring. Am J Obstet Gynecol 1991; 164: 756–62. [RCT, n = 247 (109 twins); CAN differentiate populations].

40. Mou SM, Sunderji SG, Gall S et al. Multicenter randomized clinical trial of home uterine activity monitoring for detection of preterm labor. Am J Obstet Gynecol 1991; 165: 858–66. [RCT; first report – see Corwin et al., reference 41]

41. Corwin MJ, Mou SM, Sunderji SG et al. Multicenter randomized clinical trial of home uterine activity monitoring: pregnancy outcomes for all women randomized. Am J Obstet Gynecol 1996; 175: 1281–5. [RCT; reports PTB outcomes of Mou et al 1991 RCT–same RCT, n=339; no twins]

42. Blondel B, Breart G, Berthoux Y et al. Home uterine activity monitoring in France; a randomized, controlled trial. Am J Obstet Gynecol 1992; 167: 424–9. [RCT, n=52; cannot distinguish populations of high-risk singletons vs twins vs PTL patients]

43. Wapner RJ, Cotton DB, Artal R, Librizzi RJ, Ross MG. A randomized multicenter trial assessing a home uterine activity monitoring devise used in the absence of daily nursing contact. Am J Obstet Gynecol 1995; 172: 1026–34. [RCT, n=187; ?twins – PTB outcomes not reported]

44. The Collaborative Home Uterine Monitoring Study Group. A multicenter randomized trial of home uterine monitoring: active versus sham device. Am J Obstet Gynecol 1995; 173: 1120–7. [RCT (Devoe PI), n=about 1125; about 215 twins. Cannot differentiate populations]

45. Dyson DC, Danbe KH, Bamner JA et al. Monitoring women at risk for preterm labor. N Engl J Med 1998; 338; 15–19. [RCT, n=2422 (844 twins) can differentiate populations; data reported in %, not actual #]

46. Knuppel RA, Lake MF, Watson DL, et al. Preventing preterm birth in twin gestation: home uterine activity monitoring and perinatal nursing support. Obstet Gynecol 1990; 76(Suppl):24s–27s; 1990; 76(Suppl): 13s–18s. [RCT, n=45]

47. Watson DL, Welch RA, Mariona FG, et al. Management of preterm labor patients at home: does daily uterine activity monitoring and nursing support make a difference? Obstet Gynecol 1990; 76(Suppl): 32s–35s [RCT, n=67]

48. Nagey DA, Bailey-Jones C, Herman AA. Randomized comparison of home uterine activity monitoring and routine care in patients discharged after treatment for preterm labor. Obstet Gynecol 1993; 82: 319–23. [RCT, n=56]

49. Brown HL, Britton KA, Brizendine EJ et al. A randomized comparison of home uterine activity monitoring in the outpatient management of women treated for preterm labor. Am J Obstet Gynecol 1999; 180: 798–805 [RCT, n=162]

50. Berghella V, Obido AO, To MS, Rust OA, Althiusism SM. Cerclage for short cervix on ultrasound: meta-analysis of trials using individual patient-level data. Obstet Gynecol 2005; 106: 181–9. [meta-analysis: 4 RCTs, n=607]

51. Althuisius SM, Dekker GA, Hummel P, van Geijn HP. Cervical incompetence prevention randomized cerclage trial: Emergency cerclage with bed rest versus bed rest alone. Am J Obstet Gynecol 2003; 189: 907. [RCT, n=23]

52. Andrews WW, Sibai BM, Thom EA et al. Randomized clinical trial of metronidazole plus erythromycin to prevent spontaneous preterm delivery in fetal fibronectin-positive women. Obstet Gynecol 2003; 101: 847–55. [RCT, n=403]

53. Jeffcoat MK, Hauth JC, Geurs NC et al. Periodontal disease and preterm birth: results of a pilot intervention study. J Periodontol 2003; 74: 1214–18. [RCT, n=366. Screened and treated at 21–25 weeks. 3 intervention groups: dental prophylaxis; SRP; SRP and metronidazole (placebo controlled)]

54. Lopez NJ, Da Silva I, Ipinza J, Gutierrez J. Periodontal therapy reduces the rate of preterm low birth weight in women with pregnancy-associated gingivitis. J Periodontol 2005; 76: 2144–53. [RCT, n=834]

55. Smaill F. Antibiotics for asymptomatic bacteriuria in pregnancy. Cochrane Database Syst Rev 2007; 1. [meta-analysis: 14 RCTs, n=>2000]

56. Villar J, Widmer M, Lydon-Rochelle MT, Gulmezoglu AM, Roganti, A. Duration of treatment for asymptomatic bacteriuria during pregnancy. Cochrane Database Syst Rev 2007; 1. [meta-analysis: 10 RCTs, n=568]

57. Thompsen AC, Morup L, Hansen KB. Antibiotic elimination of group-B streptococci in urine in prevention of preterm labour. Lancet 1987; 1: 591–3. [RCT, n=69]

58. McDonald H, Brocklehurst P, Parsons J. Antibiotics for treating bacterial vaginosis in pregnancy. Cochrane Database Syst Rev 2007; 1. [meta-analysis: 13 RCTs, n=5300]

59. Okun N, Gronau KA, Hannah ME. Antibiotics for bacterial vaginosis or Trichomonas vaginalis in pregnancy: a systematic review. Obstet Gynecol 2005; 105: 857–68. [meta-analysis: 14 RCTs on BV; n=>5500. 2 RCTs on TV, n=842]

60. Gulmezoglu AM. Interventions for trichomoniasis in pregnancy. Cochrane Database Syst Rev 2007; 1. [meta-analysis: 2 RCTs, n=842]

61. Ross SM, Van Middelkoop A. Trichomonas infection in pregnancy: does it affect outcome? S Afr Med J 1983; 63: 566–7. [RCT, n=225. 2 g metronidazole×1 to women and their partners]

62. Klebanoff MA, Carey JC, Hauth JC et al. Failure of metronidazole to prevent preterm delivery among pregnant women with asymptomatic Trichomonas vaginalis infection. N Engl J Med 2001; 345: 487–93. [RCT, n=617. 2 g metronidazole every 48 hours×2 doses]

63. Kigozi GG, Brahmbhatt H, Wabwire-Mangen F et al. Treatment of Trichomonas in pregnancy and adverse outcomes of pregnancy: a subanalysis of a randomized trial in Rakai, Uganda. Am J Obstet Gynecol 2003; 189: 1398–400. [RCT, n=206 with TV (PTB <37 weeks: RR=1.28, 95% CI 0.81–2.02) – subanalysis of larger trial]

64. Klebanoff MA, Regan JA, Rao AV et al. Outcome of the vaginal infections and prematurity study: results of a clinical trial of erythromycin among pregnant women colonized with group B streptococci. Am J Obstet Gynecol 1995; 172: 1540–5 [RCT, n=938; vaginal-cervical GBS at 23–26 weeks: Erythromycin 333 mg tid or placebo for 10 weeks or up to 35 6/7 weeks, whichever came first]

65. McCormack WM, Rosner B, Lee Y-H et al. Effect of birth weight of erythromycin treatment of pregnant women. Obstet Gynecol 1987; 69: 202–7. [RCT, n=1071. 22–32 weeks vaginal culture Mycoplasma hominis and/or Ureaplasma urealyticum. RCT erythromycin estolate, clindamycin hydrochloride or placebo. Treatment was changed approximately halfway through the study (in 1975). Erythromycin estolate and clindamycin hydrochloride were stopped and patients were from then randomized to receive 250 mg erythromycin stearate or placebo]

66. Crowther CA. Hospitalization and bed rest for multiple pregnancies. Cochrane Database Syst Rev 2007; 1. [meta-analysis: 4 RCTs, >1000 women. Mostly in Harare, Zimbabwe]

67. Crowther CA, Verkuyl DAA, Neilson JP, Bannerman C, Ashurst HM. The effects of hospitalization for rest on fetal growth, neonatal morbidity and length of gestation in twin pregnancy. Br J Obstet Gynaecol 1990; 97: 872–7. [RCT, n=118]

68. Crowther CA, Verkuyl D, Ashworth M, Bannerman C, Ashurst H. The effects of hospitalisation for bed rest on duration of gestation, fetal growth and neonatal morbidity in triplet pregnancy. Acta Genet Med Gemellol (ROMA) 1991; 40: 63–8. [RCT, n=19]

69. Hartikainen-Sorri AL, Jouppila P. Is routine hospitalization needed in antenatal care of twin pregnancy? J Perinat Med 1984; 12: 31–4. [RCT, n=73]

70. MacLennan AH, Green RC, O'Shea R, Brookes C, Morris D. Routine hospital admission in twin pregnancy between 26 and 30 weeks' gestation. Lancet 1990; 335: 267–9. [RCT, n=141]

71. Saunders MC, Dick JS, Brown IM, McPherson K, Chalmers I. The effects of hospital admission for bed rest on the duration of twin pregnancy: a randomised trial. Lancet 1985; 2: 793–5 [RCT, n=212]

72. Crowther CA, Neilson JP, Verkuyl DAA, Bannerman C, Ashurst HM. Preterm labour in twin pregnancies: can it be prevented by

hospital admission? Br J Obstet Gynaecol 1989; 96: 850–3. [RCT, n = 139]

73. Dor J, Shalev J, Mashiach S, Blankstein J, Serr DM. Elective cervical suture of twin pregnancies diagnosed ultrasonically in the first trimester following induced ovulation. Gynecol Obstet Invest 1982; 13: 55–60. [RCT, n = 100]

74. Pereira L, Gould R, Pelham J, Goldberg J. Correlation between visual examination of the cervix and digital examination. J Matern Fetal Neonatal Med 2005; 17: 223–7. [II-2]

75. Perinatal care at the threshold of viability. ACOG Practice Bulletin, No. #38, 2002.[review]

76. Gomez R, Romero R, Medina L, et al. Cervicovaginal fibronectin improves the prediction of preterm delivery based on sonographic cervical length in patients with preterm uterine contractions and intact membranes. Am J Obstet Gynecol 2005; 192: 350–9. [II-3]

77. Ness A, Visintine J, Ricci E, Boyle K, Berghella V. Use of fetal fibronectin and transvaginal ultrasound cervical length to triage women with suspected preterm labor. A randomized trial. Am J Obstet Gynecol 2006; 195: s67. [RCT, n = 100]

78. Management of preterm labor. ACOG Practice Bulletin, No. #43, 2003. [review]

79. Gomez R, Romero R, Nien JK, et al. A short cervix in women with preterm labor and intact membranes: a risk factor for microbial invasion of the amniotic cavity. Am J Obstet Gynecol 2005; 192: 678–89. [II-3]

80. Crowley P. Prophylactic corticosteroids for preterm birth. Cochrane Database Syst Rev 2007; 1. [meta-analysis: 18 RCTs, n > 3,700]

81. Egerman RS, Maercer BM, Doss JL, Sibai BM. A randomized controlled trial of oral and intramuscular dexamethasone in the prevention of neonatal respiratory distress syndrome. Am J Obstet Gynecol 1998; 179: 1120–6. [RCT, n = 170]

82. Crowther CA, Harding J. Repeat doses of prenatal corticosteroids for women at risk of preterm birth for preventing neonatal respiratory disease. Cochrane Database Syst Rev 2007; 1. [meta-analysis: 3 RCTs, n = 551]

83. Guinn DA, Atkinson MW, Sullivan L et al. Single vs weekly courses of antenatal corticosteroids for women at risk of preterm delivery: a randomized trial. JAMA 2001; 286: 1581. [RCT, n = 502]

84. Wapner RJ, Sorokin Y, Thom EA et al. Single versus weekly courses of antenatal corticosteroids: evaluation of safety and efficacy. Am J Obstet Gynecol 2006; 195(3): 633–42. [RCT, n = 495]

85. Crowther CA, Alfirevic Z, Haslam RR. Thyrotropin-releasing hormone added to corticosteroids for women at risk of preterm birth for preventing neonatal respiratory disease. Cochrane Database Syst Rev 2007; 1. [meta-analysis: 13 RCTs, n = > 1300]

86. Crowther CA, Henderson-Smart DJ. Phenobarbital prior to preterm birth for preventing neonatal periventricular haemorrhage. Cochrane Database Syst Rev 2007; 1. [meta-analysis: 9 RCTs; n = 1750]

87. Shankaran S, Papile L, Wright L et al. The effect of antenatal phenobarbital therapy on neonatal intracranial hemorrhage in preterm infants. N Engl J Med 1997; 337: 466–71. [RCT, n = 610]

88. Thorp JA, Ferrette-Smith D, Gaston L et al. Antenatal vitamin K (VK) and phenobarbital (PH) for preventing intracrancial hemorrhage (ICH) in the premature newborn: a randomized double blinded placebo controlled trial. Am J Obstet and Gynecol 1995; 172: 253. [RCT, n = 353]

89. Crowther CA, Henderson-Smart DJ. Vitamin K prior to preterm birth for preventing neonatal periventricular haemorrhage. Cochrane Database Syst Rev 2007; 1. [meta-analysis: 5 RCTs, n = 520]

90. Crowther CA, Neilson JP, Verkuyl DAA, Bannerman C, Ashurst HM. Preterm labour in twin pregnancies: can it be prevented by hospital admission? Br J Obstet and Gynaecol 1989; 96: 850–3. [RCT, n = 139]

91. Stan C, Boulvain M, Hirsbrunner-Amagbaly P, Pfister R. Hydration for treatment of preterm labour. Cochrane Database Syst Rev 2007; 1. [2 RCTs, n = 228]

92. King J, Flenady V. Prophylactic antibiotics for inhibiting preterm labour with intact membranes. Cochrane Database Syst Rev 2007; 1 [11 RCTs, n = 7428]

93. Kenyon SL, Taylor DJ, Tarnow-Mordi W. Broad-spectrum antibiotics for spontaneous preterm labour: the ORACLE II randomised trial. Lancet 2001; 357: 991–6. [RCT, n = 6295. 1: 325 mg co-amoxiclav plus 250 mg erythromycin; 2. 325 mg co-amoxiclav plus erythromycin placebo; 3. 250 mg erythromycin plus co-amoxiclav placebo; 4. co-amoxiclav placebo plus erythromycin placebo. All study medications were given orally every 6 hours for 10 days or until delivery]

94. McGregor JA, French JI, Seo K. Adjunctive clindamycin therapy for preterm labor: results of a double-blind, placebo-controlled trial. Am J Obstet and Gynecol 1991; 165(4): 867–75. [RCT, n = 117. IV clindamycin 900 mg every 8 hours × 9 doses or identical placebo. IV therapy was followed by oral clindamycin 300 mg every 6 hours × 4 days vs identical placebo]

95. Norman K, Pattinson RC, de Souza et al. Ampicillin and metronidazole treatment in preterm labour: a multicentre, randomised controlled trial. Br J Obstet and Gynaecol 1994; 101: 404–8. [RCT, n = 82. IV ampicillin 1 g every 6 hours × 4 doses followed by oral amoxicillin 500 mg every 8 hours × 5 days, plus metronidazole 1 g stat then 400 mg orally every 8 hours for 5 days, or corresponding placebos]

96. Svare J, Langhoff-Roos J, Andersen LF et al. Ampicillin-metronidazole treatment in idiopathic preterm labour: a randomised controlled multicentre trial. Br J Obstet and Gynaecol 1997; 104: 892–7. [RCT, n = 112. IV ampicillin 2 g every 6 hours for 24 hours, followed by pivampicin 500 mg orally for 7 days, plus IV metronidazole 500 mg every 8 hours for 24 hours, followed by metronidazole 400mg orally every 8 hours for 7 days, or identical placebo]

97. Anotayananonth S, Subhedar NV, Garner P, Neilson JP, Harigopal S. Betamimetics for inhibiting preterm labour. Cochrane Database Syst Rev 2007; 1. [meta-analysis: 11 RCTs, n = 1332]

98. King JF, Flenady VJ, Papatsonis DNM, Dekker GA Carbonne, B. Calcium channel blockers for inhibiting preterm labour. Cochrane Database Syst Rev 2007; 1. [meta-analysis: 10 RCTs, n = 1029]

99. King J, Flenady V, Cole S, Thornton S. Cyclo-oxygenase (COX) inhibitors for treating preterm labour. Cochrane Database Syst Rev 2007; 1. [meta-analysis: 13 RCTs, n = 713]

100. Abramov Y, Nadjari M, Weinstein D et al. Indomethacin for preterm labor: a randomized comparison of vaginal and rectal-oral routes. Obstet Gynecol 2000; 95: 482–6. [RCT, n = 46]

101. Sawdy RJ, Lye S, Fisk NM, Bennett PR. A double-blind randomized study of fetal side effects during and after the short-term maternal administration of indomethacin, sulindac, and nimesulide for the treatment of preterm labor. Am J Obstet Gynecol 2003; 188: 1046–51. [RCT, n = 30. Sulindac 200 mg orally and a placebo suppository every 12 hours; vs nimesulide 200 mg rectally and a placebo capsule orally every 12 hours; vs indomethacin 100 mg rectally and a placebo capsule orally every 12 hours]

102. Stika CS, Gross GA, Leguizamon G et al. A prospective randomized safety trial of celecoxib for treatment of preterm labor. Am J Obstet Gynecol 2002; 187(3): 653–60. [RCT, n = 24. Indomethacin suppository 100 mg then 50 mg po every 6 hours for 48 hours plus oral placebo vs celecoxib po 100 mg initially then 100 mg every 12 hours for 48 hours plus rectal and oral placebo]

103. Loe SM, Sanchez-Ramos L, Kaunitz A. Assessing the neonatal safety of indomethacon tocolysis: a systematic review with meta-analysis. Obstet Gynecol 2005; 106: 173–9. [meta-analysis of safety of indomethacin; n = 1621 fetuses exposed to indomethacin in RCTs and observational studies]

104. Terrone DA, Rinehart BK, Kimmel ES et al. A prospective randomized controlled trial of high and low maintenance doses of magnesium sulfate for acute tocolysis. Am J Obstet Gynecol 2000; 182: 1477–82 [RCT, n = 160. All MgSO$_4$ 4 g load; then RCT to 2 g vs 5 g/h]

105. Lewis DF, Bergstedt S, Edwards MS et al. Successful magnesium sulfate tocolysis: is "weaning" the drug necessary? Am J Obstet Gynecol 1997; 177: 742–5 [RCT, n = 140. Stop MgSO$_4$ abruptly vs wean approx. 1 g every 4 hours]

106. Crowther CA, Hiller JE, Doyle LW. Magnesium sulfate for preventing preterm birth in threatened preterm labour. Cochrane Database Syst Rev 2007; 1. [meta-analysis: 23 RCTs, n => 2000]

107. Papatsonis D, Flenady V, Cole S, Liley H. Oxytocin receptor antagonists for inhibiting preterm labour. Cochrane Database Syst Rev 2007; 1. [Meta-analysis: 6 RCTs, n = 1695]

108. Romero R, Sibai BM, Sanchez-Ramos L et al. An oxytocin receptor antagonist (atosiban) in the treatment of preterm labor: a randomized, double-blind, placebo-controlled trial with tocolytic rescue. Am J Obstet and Gynecol 2000; 182(5): 1173–83. [RCT, n=531. Atosiban group: initial bolus of 6.75 mg atosiban administered over 1 minute. Followed by an infusion of 300 μg/min for 3 hours followed by an infusion of 100 μg/min atosiban for 45 hours. When uterine quiescence was achieved, maintenance therapy was continued subcutaneously with either atosiban or placebo until the end of the 36th week of gestation. Control: initial bolus or placebo administered over 1 minute. Followed by an infusion of placebo for 48 hours. Maintenance therapy with subcutaneous placebo until 36 weeks]

109. Durckitt K, Thornton S. Nitric oxide donors for the treatment of preterm labour. Cochrane Database Syst Rev 2007; 1. [meta-analysis: 5 RCTs, n = 466]

110. Smith GN, Walker MC, McGrath MJ. Randomized double-blind, placebo controlled trial assessing nitroglycerin as a tocolytic. Br J Obstet and Gynaecol 1999; 106: 736–9 [RCT, n = 33. GTN transdermal patch 9.6 mg/24 hours for 48 hours vs placebo]

111. Erny R, Pigne A, Prouvost C et al. The effects of oral administration of progesterone for premature labor. Am J Obstet Gynecol 1986; 154: 525–9. [RCT, n= 57]

112. Newton ER, Shields L, Rigway LE, Berkus MD, Elliott BD. Combination antibiotics and indomethacin in idiopathic preterm labor: a randomized double-blind study. Am J Obstet Gynecol 1991; 165: 1753–9. [RCT, n=86]

113. Noblot G, Audra P, Dargent D, Faguer B, Mellier G. The use of micronized progesterone in the treatment of menace of preterm delivery. Eur J Obstet Gynecol Reprod Biol 1991; 40: 203–9. [RCT, n = 40 singletons]

114. Carlan S, O'Brien WF, O'Leary TD, Mastrogiannis D. Randomized comparative trial of indomethacin and sulindac for the treatment of refractory preterm labor. Obstet Gynecol 1992; 79: 223–8. [RCT, n=36]

115. Dodd JM, Crowther CA, Dare MR, Middleton P. Oral betamimetics for maintenance therapy after threatened preterm labour. Cochrane Database Syst Rev 2007; 1. [meta-analysis: 11 RCTs, n => 700]

116. Nanda K, Cook LA, Gallo MF, Grimes DA. Terbutaline pump maintenance therapy after threatened preterm labour for preventing preterm birth. Cochrane Database Syst Rev 2007; 1. [meta-analysis: 2 RCTs, n = 94]

117. Carr DB, Clark AL, Kernek K, Spinnato JA. Maintenance oral nifedipine for preterm labor: a randomized clinical trial. Am J Obstet and Gynecol 1999; 181: 822-7. [RCT; n = 74]

118. Carlan SJ, O'Brien WF, Jones MH, O'Leary TD, Roth L. Outpatient oral sulindac to prevent recurrence of preterm labor. Obstet Gynecol 1995; 85: 769–74. [RCT, n=69; sulindac 200 mg × 7 days vs placebo]

119. Humphrey RG, Bartfield MC, Carlan SJ, O'Brien WF, O'Leary TD, Triana T. Sulindac to prevent recurrent preterm labor: a randomized controlled trial. Obstet Gynecol 2001; 98: 555–62. [RCT, n = 95. Sulindac 100 mg until 34 weeks vs placebo]

120. Bivins HA, Newman RB, Fyfe DA, Campbell BA, Stramm SL. Randomized trial of oral indomethacin and terbutaline for the long-term suppression of preterm labor. Am J Obstet Gynecol 1993; 169: 1065–70. [RCT, n=71]

121. Crowther CA, Moore V. Magnesium maintenance therapy for preventing preterm birth after threatened preterm labor. Cochrane Database Syst Rev 2007; 1. [3 RCTs, n = 303]

122. Valenzuela GJ, Sanchez-Ramos L, Romero R et al. Maintenance treatment of preterm labor with the oxytocin antagonist atosiban. Am J Obstet Gynecol 2000; 182: 1184–90. [RCT, n = 503]

123. Fuchs F, Stakeman G. Treatment of threatened premature labor with large doses of progesterone. Am J Obstet Gynecol 1960; 79: 172–6. [RCT, n = 126]

124. Yost NP, Bloom SL, McIntire DD, Leveno KJ. Hospitalization for women with arrested preterm labor. Obstet Gynecol 2005; 106: 14–8. [RCT, n = 101]

125. Goulet C, Gevry H, Lemay M et al. A randomized clinical trial of care for women with preterm labour: home management versus hospital management. CMAJ 2001; 164: 985–91. [RCT, n = 250]

126. Grant A, Glazener CMA. Elective caesarean section versus expectant management for delivery of the small baby. Cochrane Database Syst Rev 2007; 1. [meta-analysis: 6 RCTs, n = 122]

127. Andrews WW, Goldenberg RL, Hauth JC et al. Interconceptional antibiotics to prevent spontaneous preterm birth: a randomized clinical trial. Am J Obstet Gynecol 2006; 194: 617–23. [RCT, n = 241]

16

Preterm premature rupture of membranes (PPROM)

Anna Locatelli, Marianna Andreani and Patrizia Vergani

KEY POINTS

- Definite diagnosis is by direct visualization of fluid ('**pooling**'), with **nitrazine** cervicovaginal swab and **ferning** as usual confirmatory tests.
- **Complications** of preterm premature rupture of membranes (PPROM) include **premature labor/delivery** with related complications of prematurity such as **respiratory distress syndrome (RDS), intraventricular hemorrhage (IVH) and periventricular leukomalacia (PVL)**, infection and **necrotizing enterocolitis (NEC)**; maternal or neonatal infections (**chorioamnionitis, endometritis, and sepsis**); **abruptio placentae, cord prolapse**, and, especially for PPROM <24 weeks, **perinatal death, pulmonary hypoplasia, compression deformities, long-term infant morbidities, increased need for cesarean delivery**, and **retained placenta**.
- If intrauterine infection, labor, or non-reassuring fetal heart tracing (NRFHT) is present, delivery is indicated.
- **Corticosteroids** should be administered in women with PPROM at 24–32 weeks, as this intervention is associated with **lower** incidences of **RDS, IVH, NEC**, and a trend for a lower **neonatal death rate.**
- **Antibiotics** (in particular **ampicillin and erythromycin** or **erythromycin**) are associated with less **chorioamnionitis, preterm birth (PTB) within 48 hours, PTB within 7 days, neonatal infection, surfactant, oxygen therapy**, and **abnormal cerebral ultrasound scan** (including IVH). RDS and NEC are also decreased with ampicillin and erythromycin treatment.
- **Tocolysis in the presence of preterm labor may be used** for ≤48 hours to allow administration of corticosteroids; such a regimen should always be accompanied by antibiotic prophylaxis.
- At ≥32 weeks, **cerclage** should be immediately removed. Management of PPROM in the presence of a cerclage between 24 and 31 weeks is controversial. It can be left in place for about 48 hours to allow steroid therapy.

- Before 32 weeks, conservative management is indicated if possible.
- **There is no role of expectant management in women ≥34 weeks or with proven fetal maturity.**
- There are no trials published to assess the benefit of interventions for PPROM <24 weeks.

Definition

Preterm premature rupture of membranes (PPROM) refers to chorioamniotic membrane rupture before the onset of labor in pregnancies at less than 37 weeks of gestation.

Diagnosis

Definite diagnosis is by direct visualization of fluid ('**pooling**') in the posterior vaginal fornix at sterile speculum examination. Confirmatory tests commonly done are **nitrazine** test on a cervicovaginal swab and the presence of arborization (**ferning**). History of persistent leakage of fluid and ultrasonographic diagnosis of oligohydramnios are two other confirmatory but not diagnostic findings. A negative fetal fibronectin assay after 21 weeks of gestation has a negative predictive value of only 81–99%, and is not recommended. Although promising at preliminary studies, there is insufficient evidence to assess if placental alpha microglobulin-1 rapid immunoassay (AmniSure) significantly improves the accuracy provided by pooling, nitrazine, and ferning tests.

Symptoms

Over 90% of women with PPROM report a history of 'gush of fluid'.

Incidence

PPROM occurs < 1% at < 24 weeks, about 2–5% at 24–33 weeks, 3–8% at 34–36 weeks, compared with about 8–10% for PROM at term. PPROM is responsible for 25–30% of all preterm births (PTB).

Etiology/basic pathophysiology

Etiology is complex and multifactorial (see Chapter 15). Possible mechanisms leading to PPROM are choriodecidual infection, collagen degradation, decreased membrane collagen content, localized membrane defects, uterine overdistention, and programmed amniotic cell death.[1] Evidence that supports a causal association between PPROM and infection is vast, and includes the fact that microorganisms in the amniotic fluid are more frequently present and the rate of histological chorioamnionitis is higher in PPROM than in intact membranes at preterm delivery and the frequency of PPROM is significantly higher in women with lower genital tract infections (e.g. group B streptococcus [GBS], bacterial vaginosis). Microorganisms that colonize the lower genital tract produce phospholipases, which can stimulate the production of prostaglandins and lead to uterine contractions; the immune response in endocervix and/or fetal membranes leads to the production of multiple inflammatory mediators (particularly matrix metalloproteinases) that can weaken membranes and result in PPROM.[1]

Classification

PPROM can be classified in **PPROM < 24 weeks** (usually 16–23 6/7 weeks, and called also previable or midtrimester or very early PPROM – see also end of this chapter), and PPROM 24 0/7–36 6/7 weeks. PPROM at 24–36 weeks can be further subdivided into **PPROM 24–33 6/7 weeks** (early PPROM) and **PPROM 34–36 6/7** weeks (near-term PPROM – for management, see also Chapter 18).

Risk factors

See Chapter 15. Transvaginal ultrasound **cervical length < 25 mm** is associated with a high rate of PPROM–compared with preterm labor (PTL)–related PTB.

Complications

Complications are inversely correlated with gestational age (GA) at PPROM.

- **Premature labor/delivery:** in 50% of PPROM, labor occurs within 24 hours, and in 80–90% within 7 days. **Preterm delivery** and complications of prematurity are the most important causes of **perinatal mortality** and morbidity; complications decrease with advancing GA.
  - Most common neonatal morbidities are respiratory distress syndrome (RDS), **intraventricular hemorrhage (IVH)**, and **periventricular leukomalacia (PVL)**, infection and necrotizing enterocolitis (NEC).
- **Infections: mother** is at risk of **chorioamnionitis, endometritis, and sepsis.** Serious maternal consequences are uncommon. Mean incidence of chorioamnionitis is about 3–15%. Major **neonatal infections** occur in 5% of PPROM, and 15–20% of cases develop chorioamnionitis. Fetal infection can precede clinically evident chorioamnionitis, resulting in neonatal pulmonary and cerebral morbidities.
- Other complications such as **abruptio placentae, cord prolapse, perinatal death, pulmonary hypoplasia, compression syndrome, long-term infant morbidities, increased need for cesarean delivery,** and **retained placenta** are most common with early and very early PPROM, and are discussed more in detail for PPROM < 24 weeks.

Management (Figure 16.1)

Prevention

See Chapter 15.

Preconception counseling

See Chapter 15. Women with prior PPROM have a 20–30% chance of PTB, including a 15–20% chance of recurrent PPROM in the next pregnancy. These incidences are inversely correlated with GA at PPROM.

Prenatal counseling

Counseling regarding prognosis, possible complications, management, and expectations for neonatal outcome should be provided. Prognosis depends most on GA at PPROM, latency (interval between PPROM and delivery), and GA at delivery. Latency is inversely correlated with GA at PPROM (Table 16.1), and can be prolonged by some therapies (see below).

Latency does not seem to differ for twin vs singleton gestations before 30 weeks, but seems to be shorter for twins after 30 weeks. Fetal maturity depends on GA, and is probably not enhanced or delayed by PPROM.

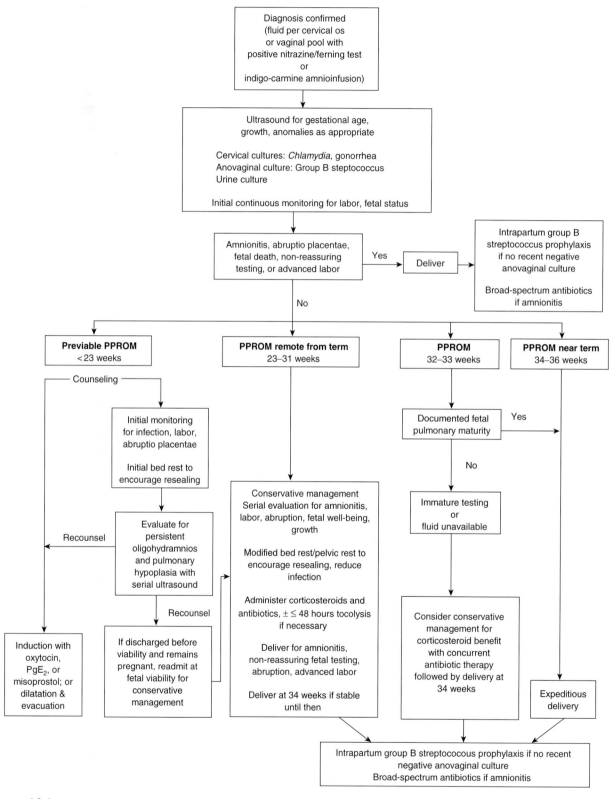

Figure 16.1
Management of preterm premature rupture of membranes (PPROM). (Adapted from Mercer.[4]) PgE$_2$, prostaglandin E$_2$

Table 16.1	*Latency depending on gestational age (GA) at preterm premature rupture of membranes (PPROM)*			
		Delivery		
GA at PPROM (weeks)	Mean latency	< 48 hours	< 7 days	< 14 days
< 24	7 days	20%	40–50%	70%
24–33 6/7	3–6 days	40–50%	70–80%	90%
34–36 6/7	24 hours	70–80%	90%	> 95%

Work up (see also Chapter 15)

Speculum examination is necessary to confirm the diagnosis (see above), for direct visualization of leakage; ferning; and nitrazine tests. The nitrazine test can be falsely positive with blood or seminal fluid, and has been associated with a 25% false-positive rate. Ferning can be falsely positive with highly estrogenized cervical mucus or extraneous saline, and falsely negative at very early GA. Testing for gonorrhea and *Chlamydia* is indicated, especially in high-risk groups. GBS culture should be sent from anorectal and vaginal areas.

Avoid manual/digital examination of the cervix once PPROM is diagnosed by speculum examination. Digital examination is associated with shorter latency and higher incidences of infection.

Ultrasound should evaluate at least presentation, biometry for gestational age, anatomy, placenta and cord location, and amniotic fluid. The lower is the amniotic fluid volume (usually measured by deepest vertical pocket [DVP] or amniotic fluid index [AFI] in most studies), the higher is the incidence of perinatal infection and the shorter the latency period.

Infection precautions

Women with active herpes simplex virus (HSV) infection or human immunodeficiency virus (HIV) with viral loads > 1000 are **not** in general expectantly managed, especially if PPROM has occurred ≥ 32 weeks (see Chapters 31 and 44 in *Maternal–Fetal Evidence Based Guidelines*). Management needs to be individualized with PPROM 24–32 weeks in the presence of these infections.

Amniocentesis

Amniocentesis can be of use for the evaluation of:

- The **diagnosis**. If diagnosis is in doubt, 1 ml of indigo carmine in 9 ml of normal saline can be injected into the amniotic cavity under continuous ultrasound guidance. Presence of blue on a pad worn on the perineum for 2–4 hours confirms the diagnosis.

- The **infectious** state of the amniotic cavity. Send amniotic fluid glucose (< 15 mg/dl associated with positive culture), Gram stain, and culture.
- The fetal **lung maturity**. Results of similar accuracy to amniocentesis can be obtained non-invasively by collecting vaginal fluid using a bedpan.

Despite oligohydramnios, there is a 90% rate of success for transabdominal amniocentesis in PROM.

There are insufficient data to assess the effect of amniocentesis on outcomes in PPROM. A small trial reported a **lower rate of non-reassuring heart rate tracing (NRHRT)** in labor, **shorter neonatal stay**, and otherwise similar maternal and neonatal outcomes in a group randomized to amniocentesis compared with one expectantly managed.[2]

Fetal pulmonary maturity assessment

It can be obtained from amniotic fluid by amniocentesis or from the vaginal pool (see Chapter 52 of *Maternal–Fetal Evidence Based Guidelines*). The predictive value of lung maturity tests are not modified by PPROM. Phosphatidylglycerol (PG), surfactant/albumin ratio (TDx/FLM), and lamellar body counts (LBC) are accurate when tested in the vaginal pool. PG is not accurate in the presence of meconium or blood, LBC is not accurate in the presence of meconium, while the **TDx/FLM is accurate with blood and/or meconium in the vaginal pool**, yielding results similar to those observed with samples obtained with amniocentesis.

Hospitalization

There is **insufficient evidence** to compare hospital vs home management for PPROM. Home management can be offered only to consenting, reliable patients with: absence of infection, dependable transportation, living near hospital, evaluation in hospital before discharge, vertex presentation, vertical pocket of amniotic fluid > 2 cm, home bed rest, recording of temperature and pulse every 6 hours, fetal movements count, twice-weekly non-stress tests (NST) and complete blood count, and weekly ultrasound. Only 18% of patients with

PPROM meet these criteria,[3] so that most are managed in the hospital. In a small trial of women with PPROM at 24–36 weeks and the above characteristics, expectant management at home or in the hospital was associated with no differences in maternal or neonatal outcomes between groups, with the home group having lower maternal costs but 11% delivering unexpectedly at outside hospitals.[3] We manage all women with PPROM ≥ 24 weeks in the hospital until delivery.

Maternal surveillance

All women with PPROM should be monitored for signs and symptoms of infection by assessment of clinical parameters (e.g. fever, maternal/fetal tachycardia, uterine tenderness, purulent vaginal discharge). A diagnosis of chorioamnionitis is usually made by the presence of ≥ 2 of these criteria. The presence of a fever of unknown origin in the presence of PPROM is highly suspicious for chorioamnionitis, so that an amniocentesis should be considered if expectant management is still being considered.

Fetal surveillance (antepartum testing)

The two most common types of fetal surveillance are NST and biophysical profile (BPP).[4] Abnormalities of these tests can be somewhat predictive of fetal infection and umbilical cord compression related to oligohydramnios. There is insufficient evidence to assess the optimal type or frequency of testing. The NST or BPP performed daily have poor sensitivity (39 and 25%, respectively) and similar predictive values for predicting infection.[5] No improvement in perinatal outcome has been reported in one trial.[5] Given lower cost, the NST is usually suggested for daily to twice a week fetal surveillance. Monitoring may be more frequent with oligohydramnios, with a preference for BPP as a back-up if the NST is non-reassuring.[4]

Amnioinfusion for prolonging latency

Compared with no amnioinfusion, **transabdominal** amnioinfusion with a 20G needle for an average of 250 ml of isotonic sodium chloride solution enough to restore a normal AFI in women with PPROM at 24–32 6/7 weeks is associated with **increase in latency** from 9 to 21 days and a decrease in delivery within 7 days from 64 to 11% in a small trial.[6] This benefit is supported by case-control studies performed at lower GA.[7]

Corticosteroids for fetal/neonatal maturation and benefit (see also Chapter 15)

Antenatal steroid therapy should be administered in women with PPROM at 24–32 weeks, as this intervention is associated with **lower** neonatal complications: 44% less **RDS**, 53% less **IVH**, 79% less **NEC**, and a trend for a 32% lower incidence in **neonatal death**, without any increase in maternal or neonatal infection.[8] Antenatal steroid therapy (24 mg of betamethasone – 12 mg intramuscularly [IM] every 24 hours – or 24 mg of dexamethasone – 6 mg IM every 6 hours) should not be repeated routinely in patients with PPROM, since weekly courses improve severe RDS, resulting in less composite neonatal morbidity among neonates delivered at 24–27 weeks, but are associated with shorter latency, higher risks of chorioamnionitis and neonatal sepsis, and no improvement in overall composite neonatal morbidity.[9] Rescue therapy can be considered if several weeks have elapsed since the initial course of antenatal corticosteroids (ACS) therapy and the delivery seems imminent with GA below 28–30 weeks.

The National Institutes of Health (NIH) consensus conference recommended steroid therapy PPROM at < 32 weeks of gestation without clinical chorioamnionitis.[10] For patients admitted with PPROM at 32–34 weeks of gestation, if fetal lung maturity cannot be confirmed, a course of corticosteroids should be administered.[4,8]

Antibiotics for prolongation of latency and fetal/neonatal benefit

Compared with placebo, antibiotics for women with PPROM are associated with **benefits** for both women and neonates, and should be routinely given.[11–13] Benefits of maternal antibiotic therapy when there is PPROM are:

- Maternal: 43% less **chorioamnionitis.**
- Fetal/neonatal: prolongation of pregnancy; 29% reduction in **PTB within 48 hours**; 20% reduction in **PTB within 7 days**; 32% reduction in **neonatal infection**, 17% in use of **surfactant**, 12% in **oxygen therapy**, and 18% in **abnormal cerebral ultrasound scan** (including IVH) prior to discharge from hospital. There is a trend for a 10% decrease in perinatal mortality (RR = 0.90, 95% CI 0.74–1.10).[11] **RDS** and **NEC** are also decreased with ampicillin and erythromycin treatment (see below).[11,12]

Type

There is scant evidence on the optimal antibiotic type (and regimen) in women with PPROM. **Ampicillin and erythromycin**[12] or **erythromycin**[13] are associated with significant benefits in neonatal outcomes, and should be used routinely in women with PPROM 24–34 weeks.[11] A combination of ampicillin and erythromycin – e.g. ampicillin 2 g and erythromycin 250 mg both intravenously (IV) every 6 hours for 48 hours, followed by amoxicillin 250 mg and erythromycin base 333 mg both orally (po) every 8 hours for 5 days, for a total of 7 days – in women with PPROM with no concomitant steroids use showed an improvement in neonatal health by significantly reducing the rates of infants with one or more major infant morbidity (composite morbidity: death, RDS, early sepsis, severe IVH, severe NEC) from 53% to 44%.[12] Compared with placebo, erythromycin 250 mg po four times a day for 10 days is associated with decreases in neonatal death, chronic lung disease, major cerebral abnormalities, and prolongation of pregnancy in women with PPROM < 37 weeks who received steroids in >75% of cases.[13]

In a large trial, amoxicillin/clavulanate was associated with an increased risk of neonatal NEC, although there is no consistent trend towards a positive or negative effect of broad-spectrum antibiotics for NEC in the literature.[4,13] Possible antibiotic regimens are listed in Table 16.2.

Detection of specific cervicovaginal pathogens should be appropriately treated (see Chapters 28–37 of *Maternal–Fetal Evidence Based Guidelines*).

Clinical chorioamnionitis requires therapeutic antibiotics, for example ampicillin (2 g IV every 6 hours) plus gentamicin (1.5 mg/kg IV every 8 hours or 7 mg/kg ideal body weight every 24 hours).

If cesarean delivery is performed, prophylactic antibiotics are indicated (see Chapter 12).

Intrapartum GBS prophylaxis should be given until culture results are available, and to carriers. There are insufficient data to assess the need for this intervention in women with PPROM in whom GBS is sensitive to antibiotics already given for PPROM, or if there has been no time for culture results. The suggested regimen is penicillin (5 million units IV, and then 2.5 million units every 4 hours), or (if unavailable) ampicillin (2 g intravenously, then 1 g every 4 hours).

Tocolysis for prolongation of latency and fetal/neonatal benefit

There is insufficient evidence to assess the effect of tocolytic therapy in women with PPROM, as the trials are small.[14–21]

Tocolysis may be used for ≤48 hours with concurrent administration of antibiotic and corticosteroids for prolongation of pregnancy and achieving fetal maturity before 32 weeks in the presence of contractions and in the absence of contraindications to expectant management.

Prophylactic therapy with oral ritodrine in cases not in labor demonstrated a brief prolongation of pregnancy without any difference in maternal or fetal risks in 2 small trials.[14,15]

Intravenous tocolysis in women with PPROM presenting also with some uterine contractions is associated with some prolongation of pregnancy in most trials,[14,16,17,19] significant in one.[17] Steroids were used only in one study,[19] and prophylactic antibiotics were used only in one study.[17] No differences in maternal or perinatal complication were observed in the individual studies, probably due to small numbers, with no meta-analysis available or beneficial, given the heterogeneity of these trials.

Compared with short-term tocolysis to allow steroid effect, **long-term tocolysis >48 hours** is associated with a non-significant prolongation of pregnancy, no differences in neonatal complications, but increases in chorioamnionitis and postpartum endometritis. It **should** therefore **be avoided**.[20]

Cerclage removal (Figure 16.2)

There is no trial to assess if cerclage should be removed or left in place in a woman with PPROM and cerclage in place. The prognosis of pregnancies with PPROM and immediate cerclage removal compared with those of PPROM without cerclage in place are similar.[22,23] While leaving the cerclage in place is associated with a slightly longer latency, expectant management of PPROM, especially with cerclage in place, is associated with increased maternal and fetal/neonatal infection risks.[24–26]

If intrauterine infection, labor, or NRFHT is present, delivery is indicated. At ≥32 weeks, cerclage should be

Table 16.2	*Possible antibiotic regimens for PPROM*
Antibiotic	Dose
Ampicillin	2 g IV every 6 hours and
Erythromycin	250 mg IV every 6 hours for 48 hours followed by
Amoxicillin	250 mg po every 8 hours and
Erythromycin	333 mg po every 8 hours for 5 days
Ampicillin	1 or 2 g IV every 6 hours for 24 hours, then 500 mg po every 6 hours for 6 days
Erythromycin base	333 mg po every 8 hours for 7 days

IV, intravenously; po, orally.

immediately removed. At < 32 weeks, it might be reasonable to administer steroids and antibiotics and remove the cerclage after 48 hours to allow the benefit of these interventions (see Figure 16.2).

Vitamin C and E

There is **insufficient evidence** to assess the effect of vitamin supplementation in women with PPROM. In one small trial, compared with placebo, vitamin C 500 mg and vitamin E 400 IU daily in women with PPROM at 26–34 weeks was associated with 7-day prolongation in latency, but no other effects on maternal or neonatal morbidity and mortality.[27]

Delivery
Timing (Figure 16.1)

Delivery before 32 weeks is associated with risk of neonatal complications, including severe morbidity and death. Conservative management is indicated if possible.

The latency with PPROM ≥ 30 weeks is usually only 2–4 days at most. All trials comparing immediate delivery to expectant management did not use steroids for fetal maturity, or tocolytics or antibiotics for pregnancy prolongation.[28–31]

There is no role of expectant management in any women ≥ 34 weeks or with proven fetal maturity[28,29,31] since there are no fetal/neonatal benefits, whereas in all studies **maternal infection is increased with expectant management.**

Between 32.0 and 33.6 weeks, delivery is indicated if a mature fetal lung test is available. If there is no amniotic fluid available for test or the test is negative, expectant management with corticosteroids and antibiotic therapy is suggested.

Amnioinfusion for preventing NRFHT

There is insufficient evidence to assess the effect of routine amnioinfusion in all women with PPROM. Compared with no amnioinfusion, amnioinfusion (warmed saline at 10 ml/min for 1 hour, then 3 ml/min – total volume infused mean 1160 ml) at the time of labor for women with PPROM at 26–35 weeks is associated with statistically similar but **favorable** incidences of cesarean delivery, low Apgar scores, and neonatal death in one small trial.[32] In the amnioinfusion group, the number of severe fetal heart rate decelerations per hour during the first stage of labor was reduced by just about one in this small trial. These outcomes are consistent with the benefits found for amnioinfusion for cord compression, but insufficient for a recommendation.

Mode

Mode of delivery should not be altered solely for the presence of PPROM. Malpresentation is more common with PTB (see Chapter 20).

Site

Delivery should occur in a facility and by personnel capable of providing all the necessary support to the mother and fetus/neonate born preterm.

Anesthesia

No specific precautions.

Postpartum

See Chapter 15. Women with PPROM are at high risk of recurrence in subsequent pregnancies, with an association between GA at the time of PPROM, latency period, interval between pregnancies, and PPROM recurrence. Patients with a history of cervical insufficiency and fetal loss/miscarriage should be considered at increased risk of midtrimester PPROM in the following pregnancy.

PPROM < 24 weeks
Definition

PROM < 24 weeks or 'previable PPROM' (arbitrary definition that varies among investigators and from year to year because of advances in neonatal intensive care) is a relevant and unique nosological entity because of its significant association with severe fetal and neonatal morbidity and mortality.

Incidence

The incidence is about 0.6% of pregnancies.

Etiology/basic pathophysiology

There are two different categories: spontaneous and iatrogenic. **Risk factors for spontaneous PPROM < 24 weeks are similar to those for PTL and for PPROM later in pregnancy.** Fluid leakage or PPROM occur in about 1% of genetic amniocenteses,[33] 3–5% of diagnostic fetoscopies,[34] and 10% of invasive fetoscopies.[35]

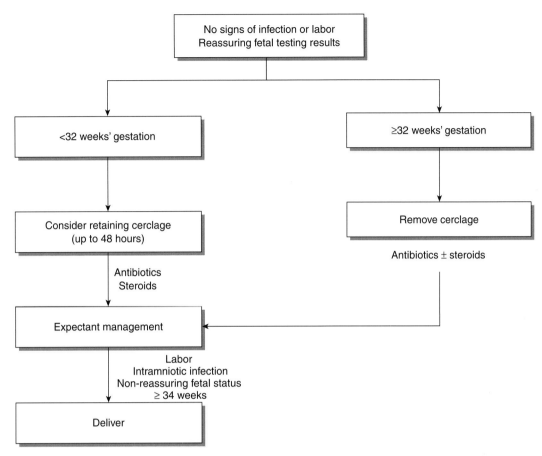

Figure 16.2
Timing of cerclage removal based upon gestational age. (Adapted from Jenkins et al.[25])

Complications

Incidences of most complications are **inversely proportional to GA at PPROM, latency, residual amniotic fluid volume, and GA at delivery.**

Fetal/neonatal

Neonatal death: Previable (< 23 weeks) delivery in PPROM is lethal. Neonatal death rates vary widely, depending on populations and range of GA studied, averaging for PROM < 24 weeks approximately **60–70% or higher.**[36–40] The mortality rate may be underestimated by including only patients continuing pregnancy or who have experienced initial PROM latency several days long. A recent study reports a perinatal survival of 47% in PROM < 24 weeks routinely managed mostly with antibiotics, antenatal steroids, postnatal surfactant and high-frequency ventilation.[39] Neonatal mortality is comparable to that in preterm deliveries matched for GA without PPROM.

Chorioamnionitis: Antenatal infection is the major complication limiting the latency interval. **If clinical intramniotic** infection occurs at any time during the latency period, delivery is indicated. Chorioamnionitis complicates 24–77% of midtrimester PPROM, with an average of **40%** in most studies.[38] Differences are mainly due to variability in criteria for infection diagnosis and antibiotic prophylaxis use. The occurrence of chorioamnionitis is higher early in the latency period; **more than 50% of cases occur within the first 7 days after rupture,**[41] with the maximum clinical occurrence on days 2–5.[41,42] After the first week of latency, the incidence falls, suggesting that subclinical uterine or chorioamniotic infection that weakens membranes and causes rupture infection was probably present prior to membrane rupture, whereas bacteria migration is a less-important component. The risk of chorioamnionitis is inversely proportional to residual amniotic fluid volume.[43]

Placental abruption: Abruptio placentae is more frequent in pregnancies with midtrimester PPROM, occurring in up to **44%** of cases compared with 0.8% of the general obstetric population.[44] The risk is highest with lower GA at PPROM and with vaginal bleeding occurring prior to or after membrane rupture.[44,45]

Table1 6.3 *Phases of lung development*		
Gestational age (weeks)	Stage of lung development	Description
4–6	Embryonic	Lung bud arises
7–16	Pseudoglandular	Non-respiratory bronchi and bronchioles develop
17–24	Canalicular	First gas exchanging acini and pulmonary capillaries are forming
25–37	Terminal sac	Subsaccules and alveoli develop with extensive capillary invasion and expansion of the alveolar blood barrier surface area
38 to age 3 years	Alveolar	Subsaccules become alveoli

Cord prolapse: The incidence of cord prolapse is about 2%.[46]

Fetal death: Fetal demise is primarily related to abruption, cord prolapse and compression, or infection. The average risk of fetal death after midtrimester PPROM is about 10%, and is inversely related to GA at PPROM and residual amniotic fluid volume.[47]

Pulmonary hypoplasia (PH): PH is a decrease in the number of lung cells, airways, and alveoli, mainly due in PPROM to alterations of normal amniotic fluid pressure and egress of lung fluid during the canalicular stage of lung development (ending at nearly 25 weeks) (Table 16.3). The gold standard for the diagnosis of PH is lung weight by autopsy. The incidence of PH resulting from midtrimester PROM varies from 13 to 28%.[36,38,45,48,49] The mortality rate in neonates with this condition is 70–95%.[45,47–50]

The main independent reported risk factors for development of PH are:

- Early GA at membrane rupture;[36,47–49] a risk of 50–60% was reported when PROM occurs at 20 weeks or less.
- Low residual amniotic fluid volume;[36,38,39,49] PH is more common among pregnancies with maximum pocket < 2 cm or AFI < 5, after controlling for GA at rupture.[48,50] Incidences of PH with severe, moderate, and absent to mild oligohydramnios are 43, 19, and 7%, respectively.[36]
- Latency.

Tests proposed to identify PH prenatally are ultrasound measurement of amniotic fluid, fetal breathing movements, fetal chest circumference, lung length, lung volume, Doppler studies of pulmonary vessels, and O$_2$ tests. In general, the predictive accuracy is poor, and may be improved by combining tests.[38]

Fetal compression syndrome: In early PPROM, asymmetric intrauterine pressure and restriction in fetal movement can lead to limb position deformities and craniofacial defects of variable severity, originally described in the context of renal agenesis. The mean frequency of skeletal deformities is 7%. Duration of latency and severity of oligohydramnios independently increase the risk of skeletal abnormalities and act synergistically.[49] The gestational age at PPROM is not a significant determinant due to the progressive and continuous development of the axial skeleton. Increased likelihood of skeletal deformities observed among infants diagnosed with PH suggests that the two disorders share common risk factors. Surgical correction is not generally required as they resolve with postnatal growth and physiotherapy.

Other morbidities: Other neonatal morbidities are similar to those in PTB, and are related to GA at PPROM. These include RDS, bronchopulmonary dysplasia (BPD), IVH, NEC, sepsis, and retinopathy of prematurity. The incidence of neonatal IVH and cystic PVL increases in cases complicated by clinical chorioamnionitis.[51] Since midtrimester PROM is associated with early delivery and infections, it constitutes a potential risk factor for long-term neurological morbidities. There may be a higher risk of PVL in infants born after early prolonged PROM compared with other types of prematurity.[52,53] Prolonged latency in midtrimester PROM patients is not associated with an increasing frequency of abnormal neonatal cranial ultrasound examination.[42]

Long-term morbidities: About 63–84% of survivors after midtrimester PROM will be neurologically intact.[38]

Maternal

Cesarean delivery (CD): The CD rate increases secondary to more common fetal heart rate abnormalities (related to oligohydramnios and chorioamnionitis) and abruptio. A classical uterine incision may be required to reduce uterine artery lacerations and fetal trauma at early GA (oligohydramnios, fetal malpresentation, and lower uterine segment characteristics constitute a risk factor).

Retained placenta: The risk of undergoing either uterine exploration or curettage is **9–18%** and more likely if PPROM occurs prior to 20 weeks of gestation.

Postpartum endometritis: This condition occurs in about **13%** of cases. Postpartum maternal **sepsis** (about 0.8%) and **death** (about 1/1000) are uncommon. The risk of maternal infection is inversely proportional to the latency period.

Management

Counseling

Parents should be counseled regarding the prognosis, complications, and management of PPROM < 24 weeks. The **options** are **expectant management** or **delivery**. The impact of immediate delivery on neonatal outcome, and potential benefits and risks of conservative management, should be reviewed. PPROM related to genetic amniocentesis is associated with favorable outcomes even with expectant management (91–99% perinatal survival), which is very different than the prognosis with spontaneous PPROM < 25 weeks.

Incidences of most complications are inversely proportional to **GA at PPROM, latency, residual amniotic fluid volume,** and **GA at delivery.**

The **latency** period between membrane rupture and delivery is critical in determining perinatal outcome. Latency is indirectly correlated with GA at PPROM (Table 16.1).[46] While the mean latency is about 7 days, the median latency may be up to about 10–21 days because of the few pregnancies which gain a lot more than 14 days. **Up to 14%** of women with midtrimester PROM **stop amniotic fluid loss,** presumably due to resealing of membranes.[41,54] This subgroup of cases has outcomes similar to pregnancies uncomplicated by membrane rupture. In 10–20% of patients, amniotic fluid loss continues, but a partial reaccumulation during expectant management is observed.[43,47]

Oligohydramnios (AFI < 5 or deepest vertical pocket < 2 cm) on admission, during latency period, or at the last ultrasonographic examination is associated with shorter latency, occurrence of pulmonary hypoplasia, chorioamnionitis, and perinatal mortality.[7,50,55] Conversely, adequate residual amniotic fluid volume identifies cases with elevated odds of perinatal survival (85–93%) and better long-term neurological outcomes.[7,45]

Work-up

See above.

Therapy

(See Figure 16.1.)

Delivery in previable PROM is **indicated in** the presence of:

- **intrauterine death**
- spontaneous onset of **labor**
- evidence of **maternal and/or or fetal infections**
- any other obstetric **medical condition necessitating delivery** (e.g. abruptio placentae, pre-eclampsia)
- **pregnancy termination request.**

Delivery (termination) can be carried out usually by induction, or by dilatation and evacuation (D&E) by experienced operators, with no trials comparing these two modalities.

For management of women who elect **expectant management,** unfortunately there **are no trials on any interventions for PPROM < 24 weeks.** There are therefore **insufficient data to assess the effect of any of the interventions studied for PPROM ≥ 24 weeks, such as hospitalization, steroids, antibiotics, tocolysis, or others.** Data for any benefit of these interventions is available only for PPROM diagnosed at ≥ 24 weeks, so these interventions should be used with caution before this GA, with the patients understanding these limitations in medical knowledge. If pregnancy continues, patients need to be counseled on clinical variables and complications that may affect outcome and treatment serially at diagnosis, during the latency period, and at delivery. Given the high incidence of infection, cerclage should be removed in women with cerclage in place at the time of PPROM < 24 weeks. Use of intracervical tissue sealants with fibrin or a gelatin sponge,[56,57] intra-amniotic injection of platelets and cryoprecipitate (i.e. amniopatch),[35] and serial amnioinfusions[7] have not been tested in any trials and should not be used in clinical practice outside of trials.

Proposed management (see Figure 16.1): Hospital bed rest during the first week awaits possible membranes resealing; consider administering an initial course of broad-spectrum antibiotic prophylaxis (7 days or until cultures resulting). Take **urinary and anovaginal cultures on admission** and every 2 weeks (plus treatment of positive results for potentially pathogenic bacteria). **Avoid vaginal examination until labor or delivery.** During expectant management, monitor for the onset of infective complications, observing temperature, maternal or fetal tachycardia, uterine contractions or tenderness, purulent vaginal discharge, white blood cell counts, and C-reactive protein (CRP). After 7 days, discharge on bed rest. Instruct to maintain bed rest, avoid intercourse, check temperature, and refer to hospital for vaginal bleeding and contractions. **At 24 weeks, (re)admission to the hospital** and active expectant management, including administration of one course of steroids.

References

1. Canavan TP, Simhan HN, Caritis S. An evidence-based approach to the evaluation and treatment of premature rupture of membranes: part I. Obstet Gynecol Surv 2004; 59: 669–77.[review]

2. Cotton DB, Gonik B, Bottoms SF. Conservative versus aggressive management of preterm rupture of membranes: a randomized trial of amniocentesis. Am J Perinatol 1984; 1: 322–4. [RCT, n=47]

3. Carlan SJ, O'Brien WF, Parsons MT, Lense JJ. Preterm premature rupture of membranes: a randomized study of home versus hospital management. Obstet Gynecol 1993; 81: 61–4. [RCT, n=67]

4. Mercer BM. Preterm premature rupture of membranes. Obstet Gynecol 2003; 101: 178–93. [review]

5. Lewis DF, Adair CD, Weeks JW et al. A randomized clinical trial of daily nonstress testing versus biophysical profile in the management of preterm premature rupture of membranes. Am J Obstet Gynecol 1999; 181: 1495–9. [RCT, n=135]

6. Tranquilli AL, Giannubilo SR, Bezzeccheri V, Scagnoli. Transabdominal amnioinfusion in preterm premature rupture of membranes: a randomized controlled trial. Br J Obstet Gynaecol 2005; 112: 759–63 [RCT, n=34]

7. Locatelli A, Vergani P, Di Pirro G et al. Role of amnioinfusion in the management of premature preterm rupture of membranes at < 26 weeks gestation. Am J Obstet Gynecol 2000; 183: 878–82. [II–2]

8. Harding JE, Pang JM, Knight DB, Liggins GC. Do antenatal corticosteroids help in the setting of preterm rupture of membranes? Am J Obstet Gynecol 2001; 184: 131–9. [meta-analysis: 15 RCTs, n=>1400]

9. Lee MJ, Davies J, Guinn D et al. Single versus weekly courses of antenatal corticosteroids in preterm premature rupture of membranes. Obstet Gynecol 2004; 103: 274–81. [RCT, n=161 with PPROM]

10. Report on the Consensus Development Conference on the Effect of Corticosteroids for Fetal Maturation on Perinatal Outcomes. US Department of Health and Human Services, Public Health Service, NIH Pub No. 95–3784, November 1994. [review]

11. Kenyon S, Boulvain M. Neilson, J. Antibiotics for preterm rupture of membranes. Cochrane Database Syst Rev 2007; 1. [meta-analysis: 22 RCTs, n=>6000]

12. Mercer BM, Miodovnik M, Thurnau GR et al. Antibiotic therapy for reduction of infant morbidity after preterm premature rupture of the membranes: a randomized controlled trial. JAMA 1997; 278: 989–95. [RCT, n=614]

13. Kenyon SL, Taylor DJ, Tarnow-Mordi W, ORACLE Collaborative Group. Broad-spectrum antibiotics for preterm, prelabour rupture of fetal membranes: the ORACLE I randomised trial. Lancet 2001; 357: 979–88. [RCT, n=4826]

14. Christensen KK, Ingermarsson I, Leideman T, Solum H, Svenningsen N. Effect of ritodrine on labor after premature rupture of the membranes. Obstet Gynecol 1980; 55: 187–90. [RCT, n=30]

15. Levy DL, Warsof SL. Oral ritodrine and preterm premature rupture of membranes. Obstet Gynecol 1985; 66: 621–3. [RCT, n=41]

16. Garite TJ, Keegan KA, Freeman RK, Nageotte MP. A randomized trial of ritodrine tocolysis in patients with preterm premature rupture of membranes. Am J Obstet Gynecol 1987; 157: 388–93. [RCT, n=79]

17. Dunlop P, Crowley PA, Lamont RF, Hawkins DF. Preterm ruptured membranes, no contractions. J Obstet Gynecol 1988; 159: 216. [RCT, n=48]

18. Weiner CP, Renk K, Klugman M. The therapeutic efficacy and cost-effectiveness of aggressive tocolysis for premature labor associated with premature rupture of the membranes. Am J Obstet Gynecol 1988; 159: 216–22. [RCT, n=75]

19. Matsuda Y, Ikenoue T, Hokanishi H. Premature rupture of membranes. Aggressive versus conservative approach: effect of tocolysis and antibiotic therapy. Gynecol Obstet Invest 1993; 36: 102–7. [RCT, n=81]

20. Decavalas G, Mastrogiannis D, Papadopoulos U, Tzingounis V. Short-term versus long-term prophylactic tocolysis in patient with preterm premature rupture of membranes. Eur J Obstet Gynecol Reprod Biol 1995; 59: 143–7. [RCT, n=241]

21. How HY, Cook CR, Cook VD, Miles DE, Spinnato J. Preterm premature rupture of membranes: aggressive tocolysis versus expectant management. J Matern Fetal Med 1998; 7: 8–12. [RCT, n=145]

22. Yeast JD, Garite TR. The role of cervical cerclage in the management of preterm premature rupture of membranes. Am J Obstet Gynecol 1988; 158: 106–10. [II–2]

23. Blickstein I, Katz Z, Lancet M, Molgilner BM. The outcome of pregnancies complicated by preterm rupture of the membranes with and without cerclage. Int J Gynaecol Obstet 1989; 28: 237–42. [II–2]

24. Ludmir J, Bader T, Chen L, Lindenbaum C, Wong G. Poor perinatal outcome associated with retained cerclage in patients with premature rupture of membranes. Obstet Gynecol 1994; 84: 823–6. [II–2, n=30]

25. Jenkins TM, Berghella V, Shlossman PA et al. Timing of cerclage removal after preterm premature rupture of membranes: maternal and neonatal outcomes. Am J Obstet Gynecol 2000; 183: 847–52. [II–2, n=62]

26. McElrath TF, Norwitz ER, Lieberman ES, Heffner LJ. Management of cervical cerclage and preterm premature rupture of the membranes: should the stitch be removed? Am J Obstet Gynecol 2000; 183: 840–6. [II–2, n=81]

27. Borna S, Borna H, Daneshbodie B. Vitamins C and E in the latency period in women with preterm premature rupture of membranes. Int J Gynaecol Obstet 2005; 90: 16–20. [RCT, n=60]

28. Spinnato JA, Shaver DC, Bray EM, Lipshitz J. Preterm premature rupture of the membranes with fetal pulmonary maturity present: a prospective study [RCT, n=47. PPROM at 25–36 weeks with L/S > 2 or foam stability index > 46. Tocolytics, steroids, or antibiotics were not used]

29. Mercer BM, Crocker LG, Boe NM, Sibai BM. Induction versus expectant management in premature rupture of the membranes with mature amniotic fluid at 32 to 36 weeks: a randomized trial. Am J Obstet Gynecol 1993; 169: 775. [RCT, n=93 women with PPROM at 32–36 6/7 weeks of gestation and a mature fetal lung profile. Tocolytics, steroids, or antibiotics were not used]

30. Cox SM, Leveno KJ. Intentional delivery versus expectant management with preterm ruptured membranes at 30–34 weeks' gestation. Obstet Gynecol 1995; 86: 875. [RCT, n=129 women with PPROM at 30–34 weeks of gestation. Tocolytics, steroids, or antibiotics were not used. 3/62 (5%) neonatal deaths in intentional delivery, vs 1/69 (1.4%) fetal death in induction groups]

31. Naef RW 3rd, Allbert JR, Ross EL et al. Premature rupture of membranes at 34 to 37 weeks' gestation: aggressive versus conservative management. Am J Obstet Gynecol 1998; 178: 126. [RCT, n=120 women with PPROM at 34–36 weeks of gestation: chorioamnionitis 2% in induction vs 16% in expectantly managed group. Tocolytics, steroids were not used; penicillin to all women for GBS prophylaxis]

32. Nageotte MP, Freeman RK, Garite TJ, Dorchester W. Prophylactic intrapartum amnioinfusion in patients with preterm premature rupture of membranes. Am J Obstet Gynecol 1985; 153: 557–62.[RCT, n=61]

33. Borgida AF, Mills AA, Feldman DM et al. Outcome of pregnancies complicated by ruptured membranes after genetic amniocentesis. Am J Obstet Gynecol 2000; 183: 937–9. [II–3]

34. Rodeck CH. Fetoscopy guided by real-time ultrasound for pure fetal blood samples, fetal skin samples, and examination of the fetus in utero. Br J Obstet Gynaecol 1980; 87: 449–56. [II–3]

35. Quintero RA, Morales WJ, Allen M et al. Treatment of iatrogenic previable premature rupture of membranes with intra-amniotic injection of platelets and cryoprecipitate (amniopatch): preliminary experience. Am J Obstet Gynecol 1999; 181: 744–9. [III]

36. Kilbride HW, Yeast J, Thibeault DW. Defining limits of survival: lethal pulmonary hypoplasia after midtrimester premature rupture of membranes. Am J Obstet Gynecol 1996; 175: 675–81. [II–2]

37. Falk SJ, Campbell LJ, Lee-Parritz A et al. Expectant management in spontaneous preterm premature rupture of membranes between 14 and 24 weeks' gestation. J Perinatol 2004; 24: 611–16. [II–3]

38. Canavan TP, Simhan HN, Caritis S. An evidence based approach to the evaluation and treatment of premature rupture of membranes: Part II. Obstet Gynecol Surv 2004; 59: 678–89. [review]

39. Dinsmoor MJ, Bachman R, Haney EI et al. Outcomes after expectant management of extremely preterm premature rupture of the membranes. Am J Obstet Gynecol 2004; 190: 183–7. [II–3]

40. Carroll SG, Blott M, Nicolaides KH. Preterm prelabor amniorrhexis: outcome of live births. Obstet Gynecol 1995; 86: 18–25. [II–3]

41. Beydoun SN, Yasin SY. Premature rupture of the membranes before 28 weeks: conservative management. Am J Obstet Gynecol 1986; 155: 471–9. [II–3]

42. McElrath TF, Allred EN, Leviton A. Prolonged latency after preterm premature rupture of membranes: an evaluation of histologic condition and intracranial ultrasonic abnormality in the neonate born at <28 weeks of gestation. Am J Obstet Gynecol 2003; 189: 794–8. [II–2]

43. Hadi HA, Hodson CA, Strickland D. Premature rupture of the membranes between 20 and 25 weeks' gestation: role of amniotic fluid volume in perinatal outcome. Am J Obstet Gynecol 1994; 170: 1139–44. [II–2]

44. Holmgren PA, Olofsson JI. Preterm premature rupture of membranes and the associated risk for placental abruption. Inverse correlation to gestational length. Acta Obstet Gynecol Scand 1997; 76: 743–7. [II–2]

45. Farooqi A, Holmgren PA, Engberg S et al. Survival and 2-year outcome with expectant management of second-trimester rupture of membranes. Obstet Gynecol 1998; 92: 895–901. [II–3]

46. Schucker JL, Mercer BM. Midtrimester premature rupture of the membranes. Semin Perinatol 1996; 20: 389–400. [review]

47. Winn HN, Chen M, Amon E et al. Neonatal pulmonary hypoplasia and perinatal mortality in patients with midtrimester rupture of amniotic membranes – a critical analysis. Am J Obstet Gynecol 2000; 182: 1638–44. [II–3]

48. Vergani P, Ghidini A, Locatelli A et al. Risk factors of pulmonary hypoplasia in second trimester premature rupture of membranes. Am J Obstet Gynecol 1994; 170: 1359–64. [II–2]

49. Rotschild A, Ling EW, Puterman ML et al. Neonatal outcome after prolonged preterm rupture of the membranes. Am J Obstet Gynecol 1990; 162: 46–52. [II–2]

50. Shumway JB, Al-Malt A, Amon E et al. Impact of oligohydramnios on maternal and perinatal outcomes of spontaneous premature rupture of the membranes at 18–28 weeks. J Matern Fetal Med 1999; 8: 20–3. [II–3]

51. Verma U, Tejani N, Klein S et al. Obstetric antecedents of intraventricular hemorrhage and periventricular leukomalacia in the low-birth-weight neonate. Am J Obstet Gynecol 1997; 176: 275–81. [II–2]

52. Perlman JM, Risser R, Broyles S. Bilateral cystic periventricular leukomalacia in the premature infant: associated risk factors. Pediatrics 1996; 97: 822–7. [II–2]

53. Locatelli A, Ghidini A, Paterlini G et al. Gestational age of preterm premature rupture of membranes: A risk factor for neonatal white mattes damage. Am J Obstet Gynecol 2005; 193: 947–51. [II–2]

54. Fortunato SJ, Welt SI, Eggleston MK Jr et al. Active expectant management in very early gestations complicated by premature rupture of the fetal membranes. J Reprod Med 1994; 39: 13–16. [II–3]

55. Vintzileos AM, Campbell WA, Nochimson DJ et al. Degree of oligohydramnios and pregnancy outcome in patients with premature rupture of the membranes. Obstet Gynecol 1985; 66: 162–7. [II–2]

56. O'Brien JM, Barton JR, Milligan DA. An aggressive interventional protocol for early midtrimester premature rupture of the membranes using gelatin sponge for cervical plugging. Am J Obstet Gynecol 2002; 187: 1143–6. [III]

57. Sciscione AC, Manley JS, Pollock M et al. Intracervical fibrin sealants: a potential treatment for early preterm premature rupture of the membranes. Am J Obstet Gynecol 2001; 184: 368–73. [III]

17

Induction of labor

Jeff M Denney and Anthony C Sciscione

KEY POINTS

- Complications of induction of labor at term include **prolonged first stage of labor, operative vaginal and cesarean delivery,** and their risks. Preterm induction is associated with prematurity risks.
- **An ultrasound examination** (usually < 20 weeks) determining accurate gestational age is associated with a **reduction in the rates of induction of labor for post-term pregnancy.**
- **Indications** for induction of labor include abruptio placentae, fetal demise, chorioamnionitis, premature rupture of membranes ≥ 34 weeks, prolonged pregnancy (≥ 41 weeks), non-reassuring fetal heart rate (NRFHR) testing, fetal compromise, and some maternal medical conditions.
- An induction based solely on maternal request should be designated as such (induction for maternal request), with counseling regarding the possible maternal and perinatal consequences of induction.
- **Contraindications** to induction of labor include transverse or oblique fetal lie, umbilical cord prolapse, previous classical uterine incision or transfundal uterine surgery (e.g. from myomectomy), placenta or vasa previa, and any contraindication to vaginal delivery, or indication for cesarean delivery.
- **Misoprostol should not be used for cervical ripening or labor induction in women with prior uterine incisions,** given the > 5% risk of uterine rupture. In women with prior uterine incisions, PGE_2 (prostaglandin E_2) for cervical ripening is associated with approximately 1.4–2.5% risk of rupture; oxytocin has a 1.1% risk.
- Unfavorable (< 5) Bishop scores at admission for induction of labor are associated with **two- to three-fold increased risk of cesarean delivery,** while a score of ≥ 9 is usually associated with a **probability of vaginal delivery** after labor induction **similar to that after spontaneous labor.** Transvaginal ultrasound cervical length (TVU CL) is a better predictor than any Bishop score parameter.
- Cervical ripening is not necessary with a favorable cervical examination (TVU CL < 15 mm, or Bishop score ≥ 9).
- In women with **an unfavorable** cervical examination:
  - **Cervical ripening agents (i.e. Foley catheter, prostaglandins) decrease the incidence of cesarean delivery** compared with oxytocin alone.
  - **The Foley balloon** is associated with **less hyperstimulation** with fetal heart rate (FHR) changes, but **longer induction times** than prostaglandin E_2 (PGE_2) gel.
  - **Extra-amniotic saline infusion** is associated with shorter time to reach a favorable Bishop score compared with **prostaglandin E_2.**
  - **Sweeping of membranes** at term doubles the rate of onset of labor (to about **36%**) **in the next 48 hours,** without complications.
  - **Vaginal misoprostol** in doses above 25 µg every 4 hours is more effective than other methods of labor induction but is associated with more uterine hyperstimulation. Vaginal misoprostol **25 µg every 4–6 hours** is the preferred safe dosage, as effective as PGE_2 or any other method. Oral misoprostol is less effective than vaginal misoprostol.
  - **PGE_2 tablet, gel, and pessary** appear to be as safe and efficacious as each other in terms of hyperstimulation, cesarean delivery rates, and neonatal outcomes. The PGE_2 tablet is cheaper, but the **PGE_2 insert** is associated with a **shorter induction-to-delivery interval.**
  - **Oxytocin** is as effective an induction agent as Foley or prostaglandins **only in women with premature rupture of membranes (PROM).**
  - **Other cervical ripening or induction agents** are either not sufficiently studied, unsafe, or not as effective as the agents already mentioned.
- In women with **favorable** cervical examination:
  - Oxytocin is safe and effective for induction of labor. **High-dose oxytocin** is associated with **shorter average time from admission to delivery, higher incidence of uterine hyperstimulation,** but with similar incidences of cesarean section and neonatal outcomes to low-dose oxytocin.
- There are insufficient safety data for **outpatient use of** cervical ripening or induction agents.

- Contraction pressures of ≥ 200 Montevideo units should be targeted in induction or augmentation of laboring patients to achieve **adequate labor**. A **failed induction** should not be diagnosed until after **12 hours of oxytocin after membrane rupture in the active phase**, assuming reassuring fetal heart pattern.

Definitions

Induction of labor is the stimulation of uterine contractions prior to spontaneous labor in order to achieve childbirth. **Cervical ripening** is a process that occurs prior to labor in which the cervix is softened, thinned, and dilated.

Incidence/epidemiology

Of the 4 021 726 US live births in 2002, 20.6% were the result of induced labors; this represents an induction rate more than double that of the 9.0% reported in 1989. From 1989 to 2000, induction rates increased for all gestational ages. Since 2000, the rate of reported preterm inductions has decreased while inductions after 37 weeks continue to increase.[1] One explanation for increasing induction rates is that elective inductions – those without medical or obstetric indication – are on the rise, being 25% of all inductions in a recent report.[2]

Basic pathophysiology

The cervix functions as a barrier to parturition and, thus, ensures the integrity of the pregnancy. Histologically, the cervix is composed of mostly collagen, with some smooth muscle; these components and their stability, and yet ability to become dynamic when stressed on a physical and molecular level, is what changes the cervical status. This cervical status prior to induction is predictive of induction success, as described below.[3]

Risk factors/associations

Risk factors for complications are nulliparity, no prior vaginal delivery, unfavorable cervical examination, post-term, and large fetus.

Complications

Prolonged first stage of labor (especially latent phase); **operative vaginal and cesarean delivery**.[4] Preterm induction is associated with prematurity risks.

Pregnancy considerations

The risks and complications of induction should be weighed against the possible benefits. A **successful induction** has been defined in many different ways but usually is one that achieves active phase (≥ 4 cm dilatation with regular contractions) within 24 hours, and later achieves an uncomplicated vaginal delivery. If active phase is not achieved within 24 hours, this is not a reason per se for cesarean delivery. A **failed induction** should not be diagnosed until after 12 hours of oxytocin after membrane rupture in the active phase, assuming reassuring fetal heart pattern.[5]

Management
Prevention

A routine (i.e. performed on every pregnant woman) ultrasound examination < 20 weeks is associated with a 39% reduction in the incidence of post-term pregnancies and rates of induction of labor for post-term pregnancy by allowing a more precise estimation of exact gestational age. An ultrasound performed in the first trimester (6–14 weeks) provides the best estimate of gestational age and the most benefit in terms of avoiding induction for post-term pregnancy (see also Chapter 3).[6]

General criteria for induction: work-up/counseling

Gestational age should be **documented accurately** before considering induction, both to avoid post-term inductions which are not really post-term, and to avoid unnecessary inductions of preterm pregnancies. Indications and contraindications need to be carefully reviewed. Women demanding an induction based only on their request should be particularly aware of the risks of the induction. Counseling with the patient should include discussion of specific indications, risks (possible complications), and benefits of induction. Women are prepared to spend more time in the delivery suite if this means a safer labor and better perinatal outcome.

Indications

Once a term gestation has been confirmed, **indications for induction** are shown in Table 17.1. For more specifics on the indications, see each specific guideline (e.g. Chapter 23). The term *elective* induction should be avoided, as an induction should be usually performed upon a precise and accepted indication. An induction based solely on maternal request should be designated as such (induction for maternal request).

Table 17.1 *Indications for induction of labor*

At detection:
- Abruptio placentae
- Fetal demise
- Chorioamnionitis
- Premature rupture of membranes ≥ 34 weeks
- Prolonged pregnancy (≥ 41 weeks)
- Fetal NRFHT

Various gestational ages depending on severity:
- Fetal compromise (e.g. isoimmunization, severe fetal growth restriction)
- Maternal medical conditions (e.g. chronic hypertension, diabetes mellitus, chronic pulmonary disease, or renal disease)
- Pre-eclampsia

NRFHT, non-reassuring fetal heart testing.

Table 17.2 *Contraindications to induction of labor*

- Transverse or oblique fetal lie
- Umbilical cord prolapse
- Previous classical uterine incision or transfundal uterine surgery (e.g. from myomectomy)
- Placenta or vasa previa
- Any contraindications to vaginal delivery, or indication for cesarean delivery

Contraindications

Induction of labor is **contraindicated** in the situations shown in Table 17.2. The American College of Obstetricians and Gynecologists (ACOG) suggest that the attending physician use his or her own discretion in the event of multifetal pregnancy, polyhydramnios, maternal heart disease, breech presentation, prior low-transverse cesarean delivery, severe hypertension, abnormal fetal heart rate patterns not necessitating emergent delivery, or when the presenting part is above the pelvic inlet.[7] The **risk of uterine rupture** after induction in **women with a prior cesarean delivery** deserves special attention. Misoprostol induction in women with a prior cesarean delivery is

associated with a 5.6% risk of uterine rupture in one of the largest series.[8] **Therefore, misoprostol should not be used for cervical ripening or labor induction in women with prior uterine incisions.**

According to retrospective studies, using prostaglandin E_2 (PGE_2) for cervical ripening in women who have a history of previous cesarean increases risk of uterine rupture. No trials have assessed this association.[9–12] Risk of rupture is approximately **1.4–2.5 with induction with PGE_2** (with or without oxytocin),[11,12] and about **1.1 with oxytocin alone**.[12] A patient who has a prior cesarean delivery, no previous vaginal delivery, and an unfavorable Bishop score up to 39–40 weeks has more risks (e.g. septicemia, uterine rupture, and hysterectomy) from induction; these women may elect for repeat cesarean delivery after counseling [9–12] (see also Chapter 13).

Prediction of successful induction

Bishop score: In 1964, Bishop reported that his pelvic score (Table 17.3) is inversely proportional to the time from examination to time at which spontaneous labor begins.[3] **Unfavorable (< 5) Bishop scores at admission for induction of labor are associated with a two- to threefold increased risk of cesarean delivery** when compared with spontaneous onset of labor.[3,4,13] Data show a score of ≥ 9 predicts a short time until onset of spontaneous labor and, therefore, indicates favorability for induction.[14] A Bishop score of ≥ 9 is usually associated with a **probability of vaginal delivery** after labor induction **similar to that after spontaneous labor**.[7]

TVU CL: A short cervical length (CL) (< 30 mm or < 25 mm) on transvaginal ultrasound (TVU) is associated with a short duration of labor and a higher incidence of vaginal delivery compared with longer cervix in women at term undergoing induction.[15,16] Several studies did find that **TVU CL is a better predictor than any Bishop score parameter**.[15,16] A recent randomized trial showed that the use of TVU CL instead of Bishop score for management of induction is associated with a **decreased need for intracervical prostaglandin treatment** without adverse effects on the success of the induction.[17] Fetal fibronectin does not seem to add significantly to this predictive accuracy.

Table 17.3 *Bishop score for cervical favorability*

Score	Dilation (cm)	Effacement (%)	Station	Cervical consistency	Position of cervix
0	Closed	0–30	−3	Firm	Posterior
1	1–2	40–50	−2	Medium	Midposition
2	3–4	60–70	−1, 0	Soft	Anterior
3	5–6	80	+1, +2	–	–

Modified from Bishop.[3]

Induction/ripening methods

Induction is also one of the best-studied interventions in obstetrics, with hundreds of trials reported. The two major classes of cervical ripening/induction agents are **mechanical** and **pharmacological methods**. Mechanical methods have been utilized since the days of Hippocrates, 460–360 BC. Many methods have been compared not only to placebo or no treatment, but also among themselves, in different populations and clinical settings, making for an extensive review.

Mechanical methods

Mechanical methods include hygroscopic dilators (laminaria, lamicel, or dilapan); balloon (e.g. Foley); and balloon with extra-amniotic saline infusion (EASI). Other methods reviewed under this category are membrane stripping and amniotomy. First, we'll review all the mechanical methods together.

All mechanical methods together

Compared with placebo/no treatment, there is **insufficient evidence** to assess the effectiveness of mechanical methods. Laminaria yielded similar incidence of vaginal delivery achieved in 24 hours (69 vs 77%) in one small trial. Assessing all mechanical methods, the risk of cesarean is similar to placebo/no treatment (34% for both) in 6 trials. There were no reported cases of severe neonatal and maternal morbidity.[18]

Compared to vaginal PGE$_2$, there is insufficient evidence, but higher incidence of vaginal delivery not achieved in 24 hours (73% vs 42%) in one small trial. **Compared with intracervical PGE$_2$**, there is insufficient evidence, but higher incidence of vaginal delivery not achieved in 24 hours (68% vs 40%) in one small trial. **Compared with misoprostol**, the effectiveness of mechanical methods was similar (34% vs 30%).[18]

The use of a mechanical method **reduced the risk of hyperstimulation with fetal heart rate (FHR) changes when compared with prostaglandins**: vaginal PGE$_2$ (0 vs 6%), intracervical PGE$_2$ (0 vs 1%), and misoprostol (4 vs 9%). There was no difference in the risk of cesarean section between mechanical methods and prostaglandins. Serious neonatal (three cases) and maternal morbidity (one case) were very infrequently reported.[18]

When compared with oxytocin, use of mechanical methods **reduced the risk of cesarean section** (17 vs 32%). The likelihood of vaginal delivery in 24 hours and of hyperstimulation with FHR changes was not reported. There were no reported cases of serious maternal morbidity, and severe neonatal morbidity was not reported.

These results are similar, regardless of the chosen mechanical method.

Hygroscopic (osmotic) dilators (laminaria, Lamicel, Dilapan)

Hygroscopic devices are made from either synthetic or organic material. The **laminaria** are organic hygroscopic devices made from cold water seaweed. Under direct visualization facilitated by the speculum, laminaria are placed in the cervical canal. Once in the cervix, the device attracts water from surrounding tissues, absorbs the water, and swells and increases in diameter. This swelling passively stretches, dilates, and effaces the cervix. Generally, the laminaria are left in place for 6–12 hours.

No current evidence supports using laminaria to decrease either the interval from induction to delivery or the rate of cesarean delivery. Moreover, their use may cause an increase in maternal endometritis and neonatal sepsis due to inability to ensure sterility in this organic product.[18] In an attempt to avoid problems associated with lack of sterility, polyvinyl alcohol polymer–magnesium sulfate (**Lamicel**), and polyacrylonitrile (**Dilapan**) were developed as synthetic hygroscopic devices. Like the laminaria, they are inserted in the same manner and function by attracting water from the surrounding tissue to achieve cervical softening, effacement, and dilation. However, Lamicel and Dilapan may be delivered sterile.

Compared with placebo/no treatment, laminaria are associated with a similar incidence of cesarean section.[18] Similarly, no differences were noted between lack of treatment and Dilapan in one trial.[19]

Compared with any prostaglandins (vaginal PGE$_2$, intracervical PGE$_2$, or misoprostol), laminaria are also associated with similar incidence of cesarean section, but less hyperstimulation with FHR changes. Serious maternal or perinatal morbidity is infrequent.[18]

Compared with oxytocin, laminaria are associated with a similar incidence of cesarean section.[18]

Compared with **extra-amniotic induction**, laminaria are associated with similar outcomes.[18]

Compared with prostaglandin alone, the addition of laminaria is not associated with significant benefit.[18]

Compared with **oxytocin alone**, there is insufficient evidence (one trial only) but no evidence of benefit from the addition of laminaria.[18]

Foley catheter

In 1853, Kraus first described a balloon device for preinduction cervical ripening. Much like the placement of laminaria, a speculum is most commonly utilized to insert the Foley catheter in the cervical os. Optimally, the catheter is placed at a level above the internal cervical os, often with the assistance of forceps or a clamp. Various sizes and balloon capacities have been investigated and used; these include a range from 25 to 50 ml balloons with 14F to 18F catheters.

Once placed above the internal os, the operator uses sterile saline to inflate the catheter's balloon. Correct placement is verified by gentle traction on the catheter until the inflated balloon meets the resistance of the internal os. Once the location is verified, gentle traction is applied by taping the distal end of the catheter to the patient's inner thigh. The cervix dilates as the balloon is expelled. After expulsion, a favorable Bishop score is most often achieved and induction may begin.

The Foley catheter affects cervical ripening in two ways: (1) gradual mechanical dilation and (2) separation of the decidua from the amnion, stimulating prostaglandin release. Many studies have demonstrated the Foley catheter to be an effective tool for achieving a favorable cervix.[18, 20–25]

Compared with no treatment, one trial reported Foley catheters to have no effect in risk of cesarean delivery.[18]

Compared with intracervical PGE$_2$ gel for preinduction cervical ripening, the Foley catheter yields more favorable Bishop scores following ripening, a higher change in Bishop score, **less hyperstimulation with FHR changes,** but **longer induction times** (not achieving vaginal delivery within 24 hours), and, in effect, less expensive patient care. The risk of cesarean section is similar between groups.[18]

Compared with oxytocin, the **risk of cesarean section is lower** in the balloon catheter groups.[18]

Compared with vaginal misoprostol, there is insufficient evidence, but the transcervical Foley catheter has been demonstrated to be **equivalent** for cervical ripening, with less meconium passage and uterine contractile abnormalities in one trial.[25]

Compared with prostaglandin alone, the **addition of balloon** catheter to prostaglandin increased the likelihood of vaginal delivery within 24 hours, in one trial, with a lower likelihood of observing no cervical change when a balloon catheter was used.[18]

Foley bulbs were equally effective ripening agents in both **outpatient** and inpatient settings per the results of one small trial.[26]

In women with singleton gestation who undergo term induction with a Foley catheter, **early amniotomy after expulsion of the catheter** is associated with a similar labor length but **higher incidence of cesarean delivery and cesarean delivery for dystocia** compared with oxytocin and late amniotomy.[27]

Using the Foley catheter is, however, **contraindicated** in certain instances in addition to those already cited in Table 17.2, such as **cervical infection, low-lying placenta, or third trimester bleeding.** Foley catheter use is associated with certain complications: bleeding, fever, displacement of the presenting part, and premature rupture of membranes (PROM). However, no randomized trial has shown an increase in these complications in comparison to other methods, as they are infrequent occurrences. Overall, the Foley catheter is an inexpensive, safe, well-tolerated, and easy tool for cervical dilation.[20–25]

Extra-amniotic saline infusion (EASI)

Compared with PGE$_2$, EASI with a Foley balloon was associated with **shorter time intervals to yield a favorable Bishop score,** and similar incidence of cesarean delivery.[28–30]

Compared with vaginal misoprostol, EASI with Foley balloon and oxytocin was associated with shorter induction-to-delivery interval, and less non-reassuring fetal heart testing (NRFHT), but similar incidence of cesarean delivery in one trial.[31]

Compared with laminaria, EASI with a Foley balloon was associated with **shorter induction-to-delivery interval,** and less **cesarean delivery for failed induction** in one trial.[32]

Compared with EASI, extra-amniotic PGE$_2$ infusion with a Foley balloon is associated with higher Bishop scores and lower need for oxytocin, but similar labor duration and incidence of cesarean delivery in one trial.[33]

Membrane stripping (or sweeping)

Membrane stripping is the practice of inserting a finger through the internal os as far as possible and rotating to separate the membranes from the lower uterine segment. This technique is thought to stimulate prostaglandin release as plasma prostaglandin levels have been observed to increase post-stripping. Sweeping the membranes promotes the onset of labor. Compared with no sweeping, **sweeping of the membranes,** performed as a general policy in women at term (e.g. weekly starting at 38 weeks), **is associated with reduced duration of pregnancy** and **reduced frequency of pregnancy continuing beyond 41 weeks and 42 weeks.**[34,35] To avoid one formal induction of labor, sweeping of membranes must be performed in eight women. **Risk of cesarean section and maternal or neonatal infection is similar.** Discomfort during vaginal examination and other adverse effects (bleeding, irregular contractions) are more frequently reported by women allocated to sweeping, but are not associated with complications. Studies comparing sweeping with prostaglandin administration are of limited sample size and do not provide evidence of benefit.

When used as a means for induction of labor, the reduction in the use of more formal methods of induction needs to be balanced against the woman's discomfort, bleeding, and irregular contractions, and the woman needs to be counseled that her chance of going to spontaneous labor after one sweeping at term is about **36% in the next 48 hours** vs 17% without sweeping (so doubling the rate of onset of labor).[34] Possible complications such as bleeding, infection, and ruptured membranes are not found to be increased with stripping.[34]

In nulliparas being induced with PGE$_2$ and oxytocin, the **addition of membrane sweeping** is associated with **shorter induction to delivery interval and increased vaginal delivery rates** in one trial.[36] No differences were noted in nulliparas with favorable cervices or in multiparas.

Amniotomy

Amniotomy – artificial rupture of the membranes – is another technique used in labor induction. There is **insufficient evidence** to assess the effectiveness of amniotomy alone vs no intervention, and amniotomy alone vs oxytocin alone.[37] No trials compared amniotomy alone with intracervical prostaglandins. One trial compared amniotomy alone with a single dose of vaginal prostaglandins for women with a favorable cervix, and found a significant increase in the need for oxytocin augmentation in the amniotomy alone group (44 vs 15%).[37] This should be interpreted with caution, as this was the result of a single-center trial. Furthermore, secondary intervention occurred 4 hours after amniotomy, and this time interval may not have been appropriate.

If performed without cervical ripening or achieving a favorable cervix, amniotomy may be followed by long intervals before onset of labor. Although early amniotomy may be associated with **shorter labor**, it is also associated with an **increase in non-reassuring fetal heart rate (NRFHR) patterns consistent with cord compression and chorioamnionitis**.[38]

Compared with amniotomy alone, amniotomy and intravenous (IV) oxytocin are associated with **fewer women being undelivered vaginally at 24 hours** in one small trial.[39] Compared with **placebo**, amniotomy and IV oxytocin are associated with significantly fewer instrumental vaginal deliveries than placebo. Compared with **vaginal prostaglandins**, amniotomy and intravenous oxytocin result in **more postpartum hemorrhage**, and **more dissatisfaction in women**.[39]

Pharmacological methods

Pharmacological methods include the prostaglandins (PGE_1, misoprostol; PGE_2, dinoprostone; and $PGF_{2\alpha}$), as well as mifepristone, estrogen, relaxin, and oxytocin.

Misoprostol

Misoprostol (Cytotec) is PGE_1, which is an endogenously produced hormone that acts locally on surrounding tissues. Although it is currently on the market as a $100\,\mu g$ tablet to prevent peptic ulcers, misoprostol is available and widely used in an 'off label' form for preinduction cervical ripening and induction. Through complex molecular actions, PGE_1 stimulates uterine contractions and cervical dilation in a manner akin to the onset of spontaneous labor. More specifically, PGE_1 potentiates calcium ion transport across the cellular membrane and regulates cyclic adenosine monophosphate (cAMP) within the uterine smooth muscle cells to trigger contractions. Additionally, PGE_1 facilitates cervical ripening by stimulating the pathway leading to the activation of collagenases. Collagenases, in turn, break down the structural collagen network of the cervix, yielding a softer, thinner cervix. **Misoprostol should not be used for cervical ripening or labor induction in women with prior uterine incisions** (e.g. prior cesarean delivery).[7,8] Misoprostol can be administered vaginally, orally (buccal), or sublingually.

Vaginal misoprostol

Compared with placebo, misoprostol is associated with reduced failure to achieve vaginal delivery within 24 hours, and with increased uterine hyperstimulation without FHR changes.[40]

Compared with vaginal PGE_2, intracervical PGE_2 and oxytocin, vaginal misoprostol is associated with less epidural analgesia use, **fewer failures to achieve vaginal delivery within 24 hours**, and **more uterine hyperstimulation**.

Compared with vaginal or intracervical PGE_2, oxytocin augmentation was less common with misoprostol and meconium-stained liquor more common.[40]

Vaginal misoprostol is most commonly administered by placing a tablet in the **posterior fornix of the vagina**. Several studies have focused on the dose administered. **Vaginal misoprostol in doses $>25\,\mu g$ every 4 hours is more effective** (higher success rate for vaginal delivery within 24 hours of induction, decreased need for oxytocin, and decreased induction to delivery intervals) **than conventional methods of labor induction, but with more uterine hyperstimulation. Lower doses ($25\,\mu g$) are similar to conventional methods in effectiveness and risks.**

Lower doses of misoprostol compared with higher doses were associated with more need for oxytocin augmentation and less uterine hyperstimulation, with and without FHR changes, and less meconium aspiration; therefore, $25\,\mu g$ of misoprostol (a quarter of a $100\,\mu g$ tablet) given not more frequently than every 4–6 hours is recommended.[41]

Oral misoprostol

Compared with placebo in women with PROM, oral misoprostol reduced the need for oxytocin infusion from 51% to 13% and shortened delivery time by 8.7 hours in one trial.[42]

Compared with vaginal or intracervical prostaglandins, oral misoprostol showed no beneficial or harmful effects, with limited evidence.

Compared to oxytocin in women with PROM, there were no significant differences in two small trials.[42]

Compared with vaginal misoprostol, oral misoprostol appeared to be less effective in 7 trials. More women in the oral misoprostol group did not achieve vaginal delivery within 24 hours of randomization (50%) compared with 40% in the vaginal misoprostol group.[42] The **cesarean section rate is lower in the oral misoprostol** group (16.7%) compared with 21.7% in the vaginal misoprostol group. There was **no difference in uterine hyperstimulation with**

FHR changes (8.5 vs 7.4%). There were no reported cases of severe neonatal and maternal morbidity. The data on optimal regimens and safety are lacking. It is possible that effective oral regimens may have an unacceptably high incidence of complications such as uterine hyperstimulation and possibly uterine rupture.[42]

Sublingual misoprostol

Based on only three small trials, **sublingual** misoprostol appears to be at least as effective as when the same dose is administered orally, but there are **inadequate data** to assess safety, optimal dose and side effects.[43] When the same dosage ($50\,\mu g$) is used sublingually vs orally, the sublingual route is associated with less failure to achieve vaginal delivery within 24 hours, reduced oxytocin augmentation, and reduced cesarean section in a small trial, but the differences are not statistically significant. When a smaller dose was used sublingually then orally, there were no differences in any of the outcomes.

Outpatient misoprostol

There is insufficient evidence to assess the safety of **outpatient** misoprostol for induction of labor. Although effective in decreasing the length of gestation and induction-to-delivery interval, the safety of this approach, even at low ($25\,\mu g$) doses, is still unproven in the three small trials.[44–46]

Prostaglandin E₂ (dinoprostone)

Prostaglandin E_2 (PGE_2) is an endogenously produced hormone that acts locally on surrounding tissues. PGE_2 facilitates cervical ripening by stimulating the pathway leading to the activation of collagenases. Collagenases, in turn, break down the structural collagen network of the cervix, yielding a softer, thinner cervix. Through other complex molecular actions, PGE_2 stimulates cervical dilation and uterine contractions in a manner akin to the onset of spontaneous labor. More specifically, PGE_2 potentiates calcium ion transport across the cellular membrane and regulates cAMP within the uterine smooth muscle cells to trigger contraction. Such an effect is manifested in the smooth muscle of the uterus and gastrointestinal tract.

Prostaglandin E_2 can be used for induction of labor via different routes of administration, such as vaginal, extra-amniotic, oral, and intravenous.

Vaginal PGE₂

The vaginal route is the most common route of administration of PGE_2 for labor induction. It can be given in different forms, such as tablet, gel, and insert.

All PGE₂ vaginal forms: Compared with placebo or no treatment, vaginal PGE_2 (**all forms**) is associated with a **reduction in the likelihood of vaginal delivery not being achieved within 24 hours** (18 vs 99%), no difference in cesarean section rates, and an increase in the risk of uterine hyperstimulation with FHR changes (5 vs 0.5%).[47]

PGE₂ vaginal gel (intracervical): Dinoprostone gel (Prepidil) is packaged as an 0.5 mg dose in a 2.5 ml syringe. A shielded catheter is added to the syringe end to facilitate safe injection. Under direct visualization using a speculum, the syringe contents should be injected into the endocervical canal using a sterile technique. The patient should remain supine for 30 minutes to minimize leakage from the canal. An alternative method for administering the gel is to inject into the posterior fornix or intravaginal administration. Until achieving a favorable cervix, dinoprostone 0.5 mg may be repeated every 6 hours up to a maximum dose of 1.5 mg in a 24-hour period. Once the cervix is favorable, oxytocin may be initiated for induction 6 hours after the last dose.

Compared with PGE_2 tablets, PGE_2 gel is associated with a **lower need for oxytocin.**[47] Cervical ripening with dinoprostone gel has been shown to be an effective method for preinduction cervical ripening in randomized trials.[47]

PGE₂ vaginal insert (pessary): PGE_2 vaginal insert (Cervidil) (also called slow-release pessary) is a thin, vaginal insert containing 10 mg of dinoprostone. It delivers roughly 0.3 mg of dinoprostone each hour over a 24-hour period. The insert is placed in the posterior fornix of the vagina and left in place until the desired ripening has occurred, when it is removed. Removal should occur at least 30 minutes prior to starting oxytocin. Cervidil use is indicated for cervical ripening and induction of labor in patients who have a medical indication for induction at or near term. However, it should be used with caution in the following situations: fetal malpresentation, previous uterine or cervical surgery, cephalopelvic disproportion, NHFRT, current pelvic inflammatory disease, multiple gestation, when labor has begun, patients with more than 3 term deliveries, or any other contraindication to vaginal delivery.

Compared with placebo, Cervidil use results in the following adverse effects: uterine hyperstimulation (2.8 vs 0.3%), uterine tachysystole (4.7 vs 0%), and NRFHT without uterine hyperstimulation (3.8 vs 1.2%). Other side effects such as fever, nausea, vomiting, diarrhea, and abdominal pain are reported in less than 1% of patients. In regard to neonatal status, 5-minute Apgar scores were ≥ 7 in 98.2% of mothers who received Cervidil.[47]

Compared with PGE_2 gel, PGE_2 insert is associated with **shorter induction-to-delivery interval and lower need for oxytocin** in a small trial.[48] Incidences of hyperstimulation and cesarean delivery were similar in the three trials.[47–50]

PGE_2 **tablet, gel, and pessary appear to be as efficacious as each other** in terms of hyperstimulation, cesarean delivery rates, and neonatal outcomes. Lower-dose regimens (e.g. $PGE_2 \leq 3$ mg) appear as efficacious as higher-dose regimens.[47] PGE_2 tablets are cheaper, but must be balanced vs a shorter **induction-to-delivery interval** associated with PGE_2 insert.

Cervidil started concurrently with oxytocin was associated with a shorter induction-to-delivery interval and higher incidence of vaginal deliveries than **Cervidil followed by oxytocin** within 24 hours in one small trial.[51]

Extra-amniotic prostaglandins

There is insufficient evidence to fully assess the effectiveness of extra-amniotic prostaglandins for induction of labor, with enough evidence to **discourage their use** compared with other methods. Compared with placebo, extra-amniotic prostaglandins are associated with 50% less use of oxytocin to initiate or augment labor.[52] Compared with any prostaglandin, extra-amniotic infusion with prostaglandin is associated with a higher likelihood of not achieving vaginal delivery within 24 hours (57 vs 42%), and higher risk of cesarean section (31 vs 22%), without a reduction of the risk of hyperstimulation.[52]

Oral prostaglandins

Compared with placebo or no treatment, oral PGE_2 is associated with a 54% decrease in cesarean delivery. Otherwise, there were no significant differences between PGE_2 and other interventions for this outcome.[53]

Compared with vaginal prostaglandins, there is insufficient evidence, but no gross differences in 3 small trials.[53]

Compared with all oxytocin treatments, oral PGE_2 is associated with a trend for a lower incidence of vaginal delivery not achieved within 24 hours (RR = 1.97, 95% CI 0.86–4.48).

Oral prostaglandin is associated with **vomiting** across all comparison groups. There are **no clear advantages** to oral prostaglandin over other methods of induction of labor.

Intravenous prostaglandins

Compared with oxytocin, IV prostaglandin is associated with **higher rates of uterine hyperstimulation** both with and without changes in the FHR, and a similar incidence of vaginal delivery.[54] Use of IV prostaglandins is also associated with significantly **more maternal side effects** (gastrointestinal, thrombophlebitis, and pyrexia). No significant differences emerged from subgroup analysis or from the trials comparing combination oxytocin/$PGF_{2\alpha}$ and oxytocin or extra-amniotic vs intravenous PGE_2.[54] There is insufficient information to assess a combination of $PGF_{2\alpha}$ and oxytocin compared with oxytocin alone or extra-amniotic and IV PGE_2.

Prostaglandin $F_{2\alpha}$

Compared with placebo, vaginal $PGF_{2\alpha}$ is associated with improved cervical score (60 vs 15%), reduced need for oxytocin augmentation (54 vs 89%), and similar cesarean section rates.[47] There were **insufficient data** to make meaningful conclusions for the comparison of vaginal PGE_2 and $PGF_{2\alpha}$.[47]

Mifepristone

Compared with **placebo**, mifepristone is associated with a **lower incidence of an unfavorable cervix at 48 or 96 hours, higher incidence of delivery within 48 and 96 hours, and lower incidence of cesarean section.**[55] There is **little information about fetal/neonatal outcomes**, although there is no evidence that neonatal hypoglycemia might be more common after exposure to mifepristone. Similarly, there is little information about maternal side effects, although some nausea and vomiting was reported in one trial. There are **no trials** comparing mifepristone with alternative methods of inducing labor such as prostaglandins.

Estrogen

There were **insufficient data** to draw any conclusions regarding the efficacy of estrogen as an induction agent, given small, differing trials with different controls and different outcomes reported.[56]

Relaxin

There is **insufficient evidence** to assess the safety and efficacy of relaxin as an intervention for induction of labor. There are no reported cases of uterine hyperstimulation with NRFHT in any of the 4 small trials.[57] Compared with placebo, relaxin is not associated with differences in cesarean delivery, but there is a reduction in the risk of the cervix remaining unfavorable or unchanged with induction with relaxin (22% vs 49%).[57]

Oxytocin

In 1948, the posterior pituitary extract, oxytocin, was first used for labor induction via IV drip. Oxytocin was then synthesized by du Vigneaud and associates in 1953; this accomplishment won the Nobel Prize for Chemistry in 1955. Oxytocin is now widely utilized worldwide. It is routinely used also as the drug of choice for augmentation of labor. Whereas induction of labor is the stimulation of contractions before the spontaneous onset of labor, augmentation is the stimulation of contractions in the face of inadequate contractions following the spontaneous onset of labor.

By increasing intracellular calcium concentration, oxytocin stimulates the smooth muscle cells of breast, vessels, and the uterus. Receptors for oxytocin are expressed in cells of the endometrium, liver, pancreas, and breast tissue. After the 13th week of gestation, myometrial cells express oxytocin receptors as well. Peak expression by the myometrium and endometrium occurs at term. Oxytocin increases both the amplitude and frequency of contractions, making labor effective. When continuously administered intravenously, oxytocin affects uterine response within 1 minute. Steady-state plasma concentrations are obtained within 40 minutes.

Overall, comparison of oxytocin alone with either intravaginal or intracervical PGE_2 reveals that the prostaglandin agents probably have more benefits than oxytocin alone. In women with ruptured membranes, induction can be recommended by either method, and in women with intact membranes, there is insufficient information to make firm recommendations.

Oxytocin alone reduces the rate of unsuccessful vaginal delivery within 24 hours when compared with expectant management (8.3% vs 54%), but the cesarean section rate is slightly increased (10.4% vs 8.9%).[58] This increase in cesarean section rate is not apparent in the subgroup analyses. Women are **less likely to be unsatisfied with induction rather than expectant management** (5.5% vs 13.7%) in one trial.[58]

Compared with vaginal prostaglandins, oxytocin alone is associated with an **increase in unsuccessful vaginal delivery within 24 hours** (52% vs 28%), irrespective of membrane status, but there was no difference in cesarean section rates.

Compared with intracervical PGE_2, oxytocin alone is associated with an **increase in unsuccessful vaginal delivery within 24 hours** (51% vs 35%). For all women with an unfavorable cervix, regardless of membrane status, the cesarean section rate is increased (19% vs 13%).[58]

Oxytocin seems to be as effective as prostaglandins in women with PROM.[58]

Oxytocin: high- vs low-dose regimens

Either low- or high-dose oxytocin regimens are reasonable.[7,59–63] Table 17.4 shows examples of each regimen.

Compared with low-dose oxytocin, **high-dose oxytocin** has been associated in some studies with **shorter average time from admission to delivery** and **higher incidence of uterine hyperstimulation**, but with similar incidences of cesarean section (lower incidence of cesarean delivery for failed induction) and **similar neonatal outcomes.**[59–63]

Other methods

Acupuncture

There is insufficient evidence to assess the efficacy of acupuncture for induction of labor. The only trial on this intervention did not report results as intention to treat.[64]

Breast stimulation

Breast stimulation appears beneficial in relation to the number of women not in labor after 72 hours, and reduced postpartum hemorrhage rates. Until **safety issues** have been fully evaluated it should not be used in high-risk women.[65]

Compared with **no intervention**, breast stimulation is associated with a significant **reduction in the number of women not in labor at 72 hours** (63% vs 94%). This result is not significant in women with an unfavorable cervix. The rate of postpartum hemorrhage is reduced (0.7% vs 6%). There is no significant difference in the cesarean section rate, in the rate of meconium staining, or uterine hyperstimulation. The three perinatal deaths were associated just with breast stimulation (1.8% vs 0%).[65]

Compared with **oxytocin alone**, breast stimulation is associated with a higher number of women not in labor after 72 hours (59% vs 25%), and similar cesarean section rates and meconium staining. Three of the four perinatal deaths were in high-risk women in the breast stimulation group (17.6% vs 5%).[65]

Castor oil

Castor oil **should not be used for induction of labor.**[66] Compared with no treatment, a single dose of castor oil is

Table 17.4	*Labor stimulation with oxytocin: examples of low- and high-dose oxytocin protocols*		
Regimen	Starting dose (mU/min)	Incremental increase[a] (mU/min)	Dosage interval (min)
Low-dose	0.5–1	1	30–40
	1–2	2	15
High-dose	~6	~6	15
	6	6,[a] 3, 1	20–40

[a]The incremental increase is reduced to 3 mU/min in the presence of hyperstimulation and reduced to 1 mU/min with recurrent hyperstimulation.

associated with similar cesarean section rates, meconium-stained liquor or Apgar score <7 at 5 minutes.[66] There is insufficient information on other neonatal or maternal mortality or morbidity. The number of participants was small; hence, only large differences in outcomes could have been detected. All women who ingested castor oil felt nauseous.[66]

Homeopathy

There is insufficient evidence to recommend the use of homeopathy (e.g. with Caulophyllum) as a method of induction. **No benefits** were seen in the two small, poor-quality trials.[67]

Sexual intercourse

There is insufficient evidence to assess the safety and efficacy of sexual intercourse for induction of labor, as there is only one very small trial with few important outcomes reported on this subject.[68]

There are no trials on corticosteroids, enemas, baths, or other methods for induction of labor.

Antepartum testing during cervical ripening

Fetal heart monitoring during cervical ripening depends on the agent used. There are no trials to assess the effectiveness and best modality for monitoring. In general, a non-stress test (NST) should be obtained before any induction or cervical ripening agent is used to assure fetal well-being. After administration of **PGE$_2$ gel or tablet**, the fetal heart can be monitored continuously for about 0.5–2 hours. After administration of **PGE$_2$ insert**, the fetal heart can be monitored continuously for the duration of the insertion.[69] After administration of **misoprostol**, the fetal heart should be monitored continuously, given the higher chance of contractions, and uterine hyperstimulation with related NRFHT.

Labor management with induction

The patterns by which labor progresses in spontaneous labor and electively induced labor are significantly different.[13] Latent and early active phases proceed **slower** than a spontaneous labor in induced labor in which cervical ripening was necessary. Induction non-necessitating cervical ripening may be associated with a quicker labor course from 4 to 10 cm.[13] The risk of **cesarean delivery** is increased during the first stage of labor of an induction needing cervical ripening, mainly because of dystocia. Induction without

need for cervical ripening may have no effect or only a minor effect on the risk of cesarean.[13] Applying the same standards of spontaneous labor curves (e.g. Friedman's curve) to induced patients may lead to an increased cesarean section rate with induction.[70]

When administering oxytocin, the target is to stimulate uterine activity that is sufficient to effect cervical change as well as fetal descent without compromising the fetus. Minimally effective uterine activity is usually defined as 3 contractions per 10 minutes averaging greater than 25 mmHg above baseline, with 5 contractions in 10 minutes considered adequate for the progression of labor. The Montevideo unit was created in 1957 to describe the summation of the amplitudes of all contractions in a 10-minute window. Uterine tachysystole is usually defined as >5 contractions in 10 minutes, contractions lasting in excess of 2 minutes (hypertonus), or contractions occurring within 1 minute of one another. If the tachysystole is accompanied by a NRFHR testing, then hyperstimulation is said to occur.[71] Some clinicians define **hyperstimulation** as ≥6 contractions in 10 minutes.[72] (see also Chapter 9, page 67)

During induction with oxytocin, 91% of patients delivered vaginally achieved 200 Montevideo units without neonatal morbidity in one retrospective study.[73]

Contraction pressures of ≥200 Montevideo units should be targeted in induction or augmentation of laboring patients to achieve adequate labor.[71,73]

Labor should be managed in general as for spontaneous labor (see Chapter 6–8). If the active phase is not achieved within 24 hours, this is not a reason per se for cesarean delivery. A **failed induction** should not be diagnosed until after **12 hours of oxytocin after membrane rupture in the active phase**, assuming reassuring fetal heart pattern.[5, 13]

References

1. Martin JA, Hamilton BE, Sutton PD et al. National Vital Statistics Reports, Vol. 52, No. 10, December 17, 2003. [epidemiologic data report]
2. Glantz JC. Labor induction rate variation in upstate New York: What is the difference? Birth 2003; 30(3): 168–74. [II–2]
3. Bishop EH. Pelvic scoring for elective induction. Obstet Gynecol 1964; 24: 266–8. [II–3]
4. Vrouenraets FP, Roumen FJ, Dehing CJ et al. Bishop score and risk of cesarean delivery after induction of labor in nulliparous women. Obstet Gynecol 2005; 105: 690–7. [II–2, n = 765]
5. Rouse DJ, Owen J, Hauth JC. Criteria for failed labor induction: prospective evaluation of a standardized protocol. Obstet Gynecol 2000; 96: 671–7. [II–3, n = 509]
6. Neilson JP. Ultrasound for fetal assessment in early pregnancy. Cochrane Database Syst Rev 2007; 1. [meta-analysis: 9 RCTs, n => 24 000]
7. American College of Obstetricians and Gynecologists. Induction of Labor. ACOG Practice Bulletin, Number 10, November 1999. [review]
8. Plaut MM, Schwartz ML, Lubarsky SL. Uterine rupture associated with the use of misoprostol in the gravid patient with a previous cesarean section. Am J Obstet Gynecol 1999; 180: 1535–42. [II–2, n = 512]
9. Hoffman MK, Sciscione AC, Srinivasana M et al. Uterine rupture in patients with a prior cesarean delivery: the impact of cervical ripening. Am J Perinatology 2004; 21: 217–22. [II–2, n = 972]

10. Bujold E, Blackwell SC, Hendler I et al. Modified Bishop score and induction of labor with patients with previous cesarean delivery. Am J Obstet Gynecol 2004; 191: 1644–8. [II–2; n = 685]

11. Landon MB, Hauth JC, Leveno KJ et al. Maternal and perinatal outcomes associated with a trial of labor after prior cesarean delivery. N Engl J Med 2004; 351(25): 2581–9. [II–2, prospective, n = 33 699]

12. Lyndon-Rochelle M, Holt VL, Easterling TR, Martin DP. Risk of uterine rupture during labor among women with a prior cesarean delivery. N Engl J Med 2001; 345(1): 3–8. [II–2, n = 20 095]

13. Vahration A, Zhang J, Troendle JF et al. Labor progression and risk of cesarean delivery in electively induced nulliparas. Obstet Gynecol 2005; 105: 698–704. [II–2, n = 429]

14. Williams MC, Krammer J, O'Brien WF. The value of the cervical score in predicting successful outcome of labor induction. Obstet Gynecol 1997; 90: 784–9. [prospective RCT, n = 443]

15. Ramanathan G, Yu C, Osei E, Nicolaides KH. Ultrasound examination at 37 weeks' gestation in the prediction of pregnancy outcome: the value of cervical assessment. Ultrasound Obstet Gynecol 2003; 22: 598–603. [II–2; n = 1571]

16. Gabriel R, Darnaud T, Chalot F et al. Transvaginal sonography of the uterine cervix prior to labor induction. Ultrasound Obstet Gynecol 2002; 19: 254–7. [II–2, prospective, n = 179]

17. Bartha JL, Romero-Carmona R, Martinez-Del-Fresno P, Comino-Delgado R. Bishop score and transvaginal ultrasound for preinduction cervical assessment: a randomized clinical trial. Ultrasound Obstet Gynecol 2005; 25: 155–9. [RCT, n = 80]

18. Boulvain M, Kelly A, Lohse C, Stan C, Irion O. Mechanical methods for induction of labour. Cochrane Database Syst Rev 2007; 1. [meta-analysis: 45 RCTs, n = >5000]

19. Gilson GJ, Russell DJ, Izquierdo LA, Qualls CR, Curet LB. A prospective, randomized evaluation of a hygroscopic cervical dilator, Dilapan, in the preinduction ripening of patients undergoing induction of labor. Am J Obstet Gynecol 1996; 175: 145–9. [RCT, n = 240]

20. Sciscione AC, McCullough H, Manley JS et al. A prospective, randomized comparison of Foley catheter insertion versus intracervical prostaglandin E₂ gel for preinduction cervical ripening. Am J Obstet Gynecol 1999; 180: 55–9. [RCT, n = 149]

21. Thomas IL, Chenoweth JN, Tronc GN, Johnson IR. Preparation for induction of labour of the unfavourable cervix with Foley catheter compared with vaginal prostaglandin. Aust N Z J Obstet Gynaecol 1986; 26: 30–5. [RCT, n = 57]

22. Orhue A. Induction of labour at term in primigravidae with low Bishop's score: a comparison of three methods. Eur J Obstet Gynecol Reprod Biol 1995; 58: 119–25. [RCT, n = 90]

23. St. Onge RD, Conners GT. Preinduction cervical ripening: a comparison of intracervical prostaglandin E₂ gel versus the Foley catheter. Am J Obstet Gynecol 1995; 172: 687–90. [RCT, n = 66]

24. Lieberman JR, Piura B, Choim W, Cohen A. The cervical balloon method for induction of labor. Acta Obstet Gynecol Scand 1977; 56: 499–503. [RCT, n = 194]

25. Sciscione AC, Ngyuen L, Manley J et al. A randomized comparison of transcervical Foley catheter to intravaginal misoprostol for preinduction cervical ripening. Obstet Gynecol 2001; 97: 603–7. [RCT, n = 111]

26. Sciscione AC, Muench M, Pollock M et al. Transcervical Foley catheter for preinduction cervical ripening in an outpatient versus inpatient setting. Obstet Gynecol 2001; 98: 5(1): 751–6. [RCT, n = 61]

27. Levy R, Ferber A, Ben-Arie A et al. A randomized comparison of early versus late amniotomy following cervical ripening with a Foley catheter. Br J Obstet Gynaecol 2002; 109: 168–72. [RCT, n = 168]

28. Schreyer P, Sherman DJ, Ariely S, Herman A, Caspi E. Ripening the highly unfavorable cervix with extra-amniotic saline instillation or vaginal prostaglandin E₂ application. Obstet Gynecol 1989; 73: 938–41. [RCT, n = 106]

29. Rouben D, Arias F. A randomized trial of extra-amniotic saline infusion plus intracervical Foley catheter balloon versus prostaglandin E₂ vaginal gel for ripening the cervix and inducing labor in patients with unfavorable cervices. Obstet Gynecol 1993; 82: 290–4. [RCT, n = 112]

30. Goldman JB, Wigton TR. A randomized comparison of extra-amniotic saline infusion and intracervical dinoprostone gel for cervical ripening. Obstet Gynecol 1999; 93: 271–4. [RCT, n = 52]

31. Mullin PM, House M, Paul RH, Wing DA. A comparison of vaginally administered misoprostol with extra-amniotic saline infusion for cervical ripening and labor induction. Am J Obstet Gynecol 2002; 187: 847–52. [RCT, n = 200]

32. Lin A, Kupferminc M, Dooley S. A randomized trial of extra-amniotic saline infusion versus laminaria for cervical ripening. Obstet Gynecol 1995; 86: 545–9. [RCT, n = 52]

33. Sherman DJ, Frenkel E, Pansky M et al. Balloon cervical ripening with extra-amniotic infusion of saline or prostaglandin E₂: a double-blind, randomized controlled study. Obstet Gynecol 2001; 97: 375–80. [RCT, n = 116]

34. Boulvain M, Stan C, Irion O. Membrane sweeping for induction of labour. Cochrane Database Syst Rev 2007; 1. [meta-analysis: 22 RCTs, n = 2797]

35. Berghella V, Rogers RA, Lescale K. Stripping of membranes as a safe method to reduce prolonged pregnancies. Obstet Gynecol 1996; 87(6): 927–9. [RCT, n = 142]

36. Foong LC, Vanaja K, Tan G, Chua S. Membranes sweeping in conjunction with labor induction. Obstet Gynecol 2000; 96: 539–42. [RCT, n = 248 (n = 130 nulliparas)]

37. Bricker L, Luckas M. Amniotomy alone for induction of labour. Cochrane Database Syst Rev 2007; 1. [meta-analysis: 2 RCTs, n = 310]

38. Mercer BM, McNanley T, O'Brien JM, Randa L, Sibai BM. Early versus late amniotomy for labor induction: a randomized trial. Am J Obstet Gynecol 1995; 173: 1371. [RCT, n = 209]

39. Howarth GR, Botha DJ. Amniotomy plus intravenous oxytocin for induction of labour. Cochrane Database Syst Rev 2007; 1. [meta-analysis: 17 RCTs, n = 2566]

40. Hofmeyr GJ, Gulmezoglu AM. Vaginal misoprostol for cervical ripening and induction of labour. Cochrane Database Syst Rev 2007; 1. [meta-analysis: 70 RCTs, n = >5000]

41. American College of Obstetricians and Gynecologists. Induction of Labor with Misoprostol. Committee Opinion No. 228, November 1999. [review]

42. Alfirevic Z. Oral misoprostol for induction of labour. Cochrane Database Syst Rev 2007; 1. [meta-analysis: 12 RCTs, n = >2400]

43. Muzonzini G, Hofmeyr GJ. Buccal or sublingual misoprostol for cervical ripening and induction of labour. Cochrane Database Syst Rev 2007; 1. [meta-analysis: 3 RCTs, n = 503]

44. McKenna DS, Ester JB, Proffitt M, Waddell KR. Misoprostol outpatient cervical ripening without subsequent induction of labor: a randomized trial. Obstet Gynecol 2004; 104: 579–84. [RCT, n = 33]

45. Stitely ML, Browning J, Fowler M, Gendron RT, Gherman RB. Outpatient cervical ripening with intravaginal misoprostol. Obstet Gynecol 2000; 96: 684–8. [RCT, n = 60]

46. Incerpi MH, Fassett MJ, Kjos SL, Tran SH, Wing DA. Vaginally administered misoprostol for outpatient cervical ripening in pregnancies complicated by diabetes mellitus. Am J Obstet Gynecol 2001; 185: 916–19. [RCT, n = 120]

47. Kelly AJ, Kavanagh J, Thomas J. Vaginal prostaglandin (PGE₂ and PGF₂ₐ) for induction of labour at term. Cochrane Database Syst Rev 2007; 1. [meta-analysis: 57 RCTs, n = 10 039]

48. Chyu J, Strassner HT. Prostaglandin E₂ for cervical ripening: a randomized comparison of Cervidil versus Prepidil. Am J Obstet Gynecol 1997; 177: 606–11. [RCT, n = 73]

49. Smith CV, Rayburn WF, Miller AM. Intravaginal prostaglandin E₂ for cervical ripening and initiation of labor. Comparison of a multidose gel and single, controlled-release pessary. J Reprod Med 1994; 39(5): 381–4. [RCT, n = 121]

50. Perryman D, Yeast J, Holst V. Cervical ripening: a randomized study comparing prostaglandin E$_2$ gel to prostaglandin E$_2$ suppositories. Obstet Gynecol 1992; 79: 670–2. [RCT, n = 90]

51. Christensen FC, Tehranifar M, Gonzalez JL et al. Randomized trial of concurrent oxytocin with a sustained-release dinoprostone vaginal insert for labor induction at term. Am J Obstet Gynecol 2002; 186: 61–5. [RCT, n = 71]

52. Hutton E, Mozurkewich E. Extra-amniotic prostaglandin for induction of labour. Cochrane Database Syst Rev 2007; 1. [meta-analysis: 3 RCTs, n = 170]

53. French L. Oral prostaglandin E$_2$ for induction of labour. Cochrane Database Syst Rev 2007; 1. [meta-analysis: 15 RCTs, n => 500]

54. Luckas M, Bricker L. Intravenous prostaglandin for induction of labour. Cochrane Database Syst Rev 2007; 1. [meta-analysis: 13 RCTs, n = 1165]

55. Neilson JP. Mifepristone for induction of labour. Cochrane Database Syst Rev 2007; 1. [meta-analysis: 7 RCTs, n = 594 – all trials compare to placebo or no treatment]

56. Thomas J, Kelly AJ, Kavanagh J. Oestrogens alone or with amniotomy for cervical ripening or induction of labour. Cochrane Database Syst Rev 2007; 1. [meta-analysis: 8 RCTs, n = 421]

57. Kelly AJ, Kavanagh J, Thomas J. Relaxin for cervical ripening and induction of labour. Cochrane Database Syst Rev 2007; 1. [meta-analysis: 4 RCTs, n = 267]

58. Kelly AJ, Tan B. Intravenous oxytocin alone for cervical ripening and induction of labour. Cochrane Database Syst Rev 2007; 1. [meta-analysis: 58 RCTs, n = 11 129]

59. Satin AJ, Leveno KJ, Sherman ML et al. High- versus low-dose oxytocin for labour stimulation. Obstet Gynecol 1992, 80: 111–16. [II–1, n = 1112]

60. Cummiskey KC, Dawood MY. Induction of labor with pulsatile oxytocin. Am J Obstet Gynecol 1990; 163: 1868–74. [RCT, n = 106]

61. Blakemore KJ, Qin NG, Petrie RH, Paine LL. A prospective comparison of hourly and quarter-hourly oxytocin dose increase intervals for the induction of labor at term. Obstet Gynecol 1990; 75: 757–61. RCT, n = 52]

62. Mercer B, Pilgrim P, Sibai B. Labor induction with continuous low-dose oxytocin infusion: a randomized trial. Obstet Gynecol 1991; 77: 659–63. [RCT, n = 123]

63. Muller PR, Stubbs TM, Laurent SL. A prospective randomized clinical trial comparing two oxytocin induction protocols. Am J Obstet Gynecol 1992; 167: 373–81. [RCT, n = 151]

64. Rabl M, Ahner R, Bitschnau, Zaisler H, Husslein P. Acupuncture for cervical ripening and induction of labour at term: a randomised controlled trial. Wien Klin Wochenschr 2001; 113(23–24): 942–6. [RCT, n = 56]

65. Kavanagh J, Kelly AJ, Thomas J. Breast stimulation for cervical ripening and induction of labour. Cochrane Database Syst Rev 2007; 1. [meta-analysis: 6 RCTs, n = 719]

66. Garry D, Figueroa R, Guillaume J, Cucco V. Use of castor oil in pregnancies at term. Altern Ther Health Med 2000; 6: 77–9. [RCT, n = 100]

67. Smith CA. Homoeopathy for induction of labour. Cochrane Database Syst Rev 2007; 1. [meta-analysis: 2 RCTs, n = 133]

68. Kavanagh J, Kelly AJ, Thomas J. Sexual intercourse for cervical ripening and induction of labour. Cochrane Database Syst Rev 2007; 1. [meta-analysis: 1 RCT, n = 28]

69. Monitoring during induction of labor with dinoprostone. ACOG Committee Opinion No. 209, 1998. [review]

70. Rinehart BK, Terrone DA, Hudson C et al. Lack of utility of standard labor curves in the prediction of progression during labor induction. Am J Obstet Gynecol 2000; 182: 1520–6. [retrospective chart review, II–3, n = 123]

71. American College of Obstetricians and Gynecologists. Dystocia and augmentation of labor. ACOG Practice Bulletin, No. 49, December 2003. [review]

72. National Institute of Child Health and Human Development Research Planning Workshop. Electronic fetal heart rate monitoring: research guidelines for interpretation. Am J Obstet Gynecol 1997; 177: 1385–90. [review]

73. Hauth JC, Hankins GD, Gilstrap LC III, Strickland DM. Uterine contraction pressures with oxytocin induction/augmentation. Obstet Gynecol 1986; 68: 305–9. [II–2, n = 109]

18

Premature rupture of membranes at or near term

Victoria S Myers

KEY POINTS

- **The diagnosis** of premature rupture of membranes (PROM) at term is based on **pooling, ferning**, and **nitrazine tests**.
- The main **complication** is **intrauterine infection**; this incidence increases with the duration of PROM, and, with longer latency, the risk of **neonatal infection** also increases.
- Women with PROM at term should be **hospitalized**, and **induced** with **oxytocin** within 6–12 hours of PROM. **Most women with PROM at term, if given a choice, prefer induction.** Oxytocin induction is safe, effective, and cost-effective. Misoprostol induction is an alternative just as effective, but there are insufficient data on its safety. Women with group B streptococcus (GBS) colonization should be induced immediately.
- Women with non-reassuring fetal heart rate (NRFHR) testing should be delivered promptly.

Definition

Premature rupture of membranes (PROM) prior to the onset of labor (as defined by uterine contractions causing cervical change) at term (≥ 37 weeks). This guideline also includes information on PROM near term (34–36 6/7 weeks).

Diagnosis

See also Chapter 16. Diagnosis should be made based on history and physical examination. Physical examination includes a sterile speculum examination to evaluate for **pooling** of amniotic fluid in the vaginal vault, **fern test**, and **nitrazine test**. The pH of the vagina is usually < 4.5 (3.8–4.2), whereas amniotic fluid has a pH 7.0–7.7; nitrazine paper turns blue with pH > 6.5. The sensitivity, specificity, and positive and negative predictive values of nitrazine[1] and ferning[2] tests are all $> 95\%$. Valsalva or coughing can help produce some fluid in the vagina for testing. If these tests are equivocal, an ultrasound can be performed to evaluate for amniotic fluid, but oligohydramnios is not diagnostic of PROM, since it can be associated with other etiologies, such as placental insufficiency.

Incidence

It is found that **8%** of term pregnancies will have PROM at term.[3]

Etiology

The etiology of PROM without signs of infection or bleeding is often unknown, and this should be considered a physiological, not a pathological, event.

Risk factors

Rupture of membranes at term often occurs in the absence of recognized risk factors. However, some factors that may be associated with PROM include infection, smoking, vaginal bleeding, uterine distention, and lower socioeconomic status.

Complications

The most important and common complication is **intrauterine infection**. The incidence increases with duration of PROM. With longer latency, the risk of **neonatal infection** also increases. Maternal colonization with group B streptococcus (GBS) is another risk factor for neonatal infection in women with term PROM. Incidence of cesarean delivery is not affected by management with either induction or expectant management, but depends on other risk factors (e.g. nulliparity).

Management

Principles/counseling

About 50% of women with PROM at term deliver within 6–12 hours and about 70–90% within 24 hours.[4]

Work-up

Diagnosis (see above) should be confirmed. A digital cervical examination should be avoided, as frequent cervical examinations increase the risk of infection. The cervix can be evaluated visually for dilatation and effacement.[5] Fetal presentation (using ultrasound),[3] gestational age by records (see Chapter 3), and fetal status by external monitoring should be accurately checked and documented.

Therapy

Hospitalization

Compared with management in the hospital, management of PROM at term at **home** is associated with a 52% increase in **need for maternal antibiotics** for nulliparas and 97% more **neonatal infections**.[6]

Patients with PROM at term who show signs of fetal compromise (non-reassuring fetal heart rate [**NRFHR**] testing) should be delivered immediately.[3]

If the patient has a known positive **GBS** culture, antibiotic prophylaxis should be started. If GBS status is unknown and the patient has no risk factors (previous infant with GBS sepsis, < 37 weeks, rupture of membranes > 18 hours), there is no need for GBS prophylaxis. If the patient is known to be GBS negative, antibiotic prophylaxis does not need to be started even in the presence of the risk factors listed above[7] (see also Chapter 36 of *Maternal–Fetal Evidence Based Guidelines*).

Induction (type) vs expectant management

The evidence

Compared with expectant management, **induction with oxytocin or prostaglandins** is associated with similar incidences of cesarean delivery, operative vaginal birth, and neonatal infection, but **decrease**d by 26% in **chorioamnionitis**, by 70% in **endometritis**, and by 28% in **neonatal intensive or special care admission**.[8] In a single large trial, significantly more women with planned management by induction **viewed their care more positively** than those expectantly managed.[4]

Compared with expectant management, induction of labor by **oxytocin** is associated with a 37% **decrease** in risk

of **maternal infection**, 28% in **endometritis**, and 36% in **neonatal infection**.[9] Based on one trial, women were more likely to view their care positively if labor was induced with oxytocin.[4] Cesarean delivery rates are similar between groups. Oxytocin is associated with more frequent use of pain relief and internal fetal heart rate monitoring. Perinatal mortality rates are low and not significantly different between groups, although the **trend** is towards **fewer perinatal deaths** with induction of labor by oxytocin.[9]

Compared with placebo or no treatment, **vaginal prostaglandin E_2 (PGE$_2$) or prostaglandin $F_{2\alpha}$ (PGF$_{2\alpha}$)** both reduce the likelihood of vaginal delivery not being achieved within 24 hours, with no evidence of a difference in cesarean delivery.[10] Induction of labor by prostaglandins is associated with a decrease by 23% in risk of chorioamnionitis and by 21% in admission to a neonatal intensive care unit (NICU). Induction by prostaglandins is associated with a more frequent maternal diarrhea and use of anesthesia and/or analgesia.[11] There are insufficient data to make meaningful conclusions for the comparison of vaginal PGE$_2$ and PGF$_{2\alpha}$. PGE$_2$ tablet, gel, and pessary appear to be as efficacious as each other. Lower-dose regimens appear as efficacious as higher-dose regimens.[10]

Compared with **prostaglandins**, induction with **oxytocin** is associated with **decrease** in maternal nausea and/or vomiting, numerous vaginal examinations, **chorioamnionitis** and **neonatal infections**, neonatal antibiotic therapy, and **admission to NICU**, but increase in epidural analgesia and internal fetal heart rate monitoring. Cesarean delivery, endometritis, and perinatal mortality are not significantly different between the groups.[12] Cost is less with oxytocin induction.

Vaginal **misoprostol** in doses above 25 µg every 4 hours is more effective than PGE$_2$, intracervical PGE$_2$, and oxytocin (or obviously expectant management) in achieving vaginal delivery.[13] **Compared with oxytocin, misoprostol** was associated with a decrease in cesarean delivery from 51% to 20% in a small trial in women with an unfavorable cervix and from 14% to 11% in other women.[13] If a dose of 50 µg of vaginal misoprostol is used, in 85% of cases only one dose is needed for induction with term PROM, but this is associated with a higher rate of uterine tachysystole compared with oxytocin, with similar maternal and neonatal outcomes.[14] However, the studies reviewed were not large enough to exclude the possibility of serious adverse events with misoprostol, including neonatal complications from uterine hyperstimulation. Lower doses of vaginal misoprostol were similar to other methods in effectiveness and risk. Oral misoprostol appears to be an effective means of labor induction comparable to oxytocin, but again the studies reviewed were not large enough to exclude the possibility of serious adverse events with misoprostol.[15–17]

There is no trial evaluating the efficacy of the Foley bulb or other mechanical means of induction in women with PPROM.

Women with **GBS colonization** should also be **induced immediately**, since expectant management is associated with higher rate of neonatal infections.[18]

Recommendations based on the evidence

In patients with PPROM at term, **induction of labor is recommended**. Induction should probably occur at least within 6–12 hours of PPROM, or earlier if feasible. **Oxytocin is a safe and effective** (as well as cost-effective) means of induction with PROM at term. Vaginal or oral misoprostol are also effective means of labor induction, but the data on adverse outcomes are lacking and do not exclude the possibility of adverse outcomes such as uterine hyperstimulation and uterine rupture. Given good outcomes in general with short-term expectant management, women should also be counseled regarding all the options for management, and given a chance to choose their preferred management. In the study in which it was evaluated, **most women with PROM at term, if given a choice, prefer induction**.[4]

Antibiotics

Given the low rate of maternal infection in the control population (approximately 7%), it does not seem justifiable to expose all women with term PROM to antibiotics when treatment can be restricted to those who develop clinical indications for antibiotic treatment. Compared with placebo, antibiotics are associated with a statistically significant **reduction in maternal infectious morbidity (chorioamnionitis or endometritis)**. No other benefits were detected in the 2 trials.[19–21]

References

1. Abe T. The detection of rupture of fetal membranes with the nitrazine indicator. Am J Obstet Gynecol 1940; 39: 4000. [II–3]
2. Davidson KM. Detection of premature rupture of membranes. Clin Obstet Gynecol 1991; 34: 715. [II–3]
3. ACOG Practice Bulletin. Premature rupture of membranes, No. 1, June 1998. [review]
4. Hannah ME, Ohlsson A, Farine D et al. Induction of labor compared with expectant management for prelabor rupture of the membranes at term. N Engl J Med 1996; 334: 1005–10. [RCT, n = 5041]
5. Pereira L, Gould R, Pelham J, Goldberg J. Correlation between visual examination of the cervix and digital examination. J Matern Fetal Neonatal Med 2005; 17(3): 223–7. [II–2]
6. Hannah ME, Hodnett ED, Willan A et al. Prelabor rupture of the membranes at term: expectant management at home or in the hospital? Obstet Gynecol 2000; 96: 533–8. [RCT secondary analysis, n = 1670]
7. CDC Guidelines. Prevention of perinatal group B streptococcal disease. August 16, 2002 / 51(RR11); 1–22 [guideline]
8. Dare MR, Middleton P, Crowther CA, Flenady VJ, Varatharaju B. Planned early birth versus expectant management (waiting) for prelabour rupture of membranes at term (37 weeks or more). Cochrane Database Syst Rev 2007; 1. [meta-analysis: 12 RCTs, n = 6814]
9. Tan BP, Hannah ME. Oxytocin for prelabour rupture of membranes at or near term. Cochrane Database Syst Rev 2007; 1. [meta-analysis: 18 RCTs, n => 6700]
10. Kelly AJ, Kavanagh J, Thomas J. Vaginal prostaglandin (PGE$_2$ and PGF$_{2a}$) for induction of labour at term. Cochrane Database Syst Rev 2007; 1. [meta-analysis: 57 RCTs, n = 10 039]
11. Tan BP, Hannah ME. Prostaglandins for prelabour rupture of membranes at or near term. Cochrane Database Syst Rev 2007; 1. [meta-analysis: 15 RCTs, n => 4500]
12. Tan BP, Hannah ME. Prostaglandins versus oxytocin for prelabour rupture of membranes at term. Cochrane Database Syst Rev 2007; 1. [meta-analysis: 8 RCTs, n => 2700]
13. Hofmeyr GJ, Gulmezoglu AM. Vaginal misoprostol for cervical ripening and induction of labour. Cochrane Database Syst Rev 2007; 1. [meta-analysis: 3 RCTs on misoprostol vs oxytocin for term PROM]
14. Sanchez-Ramos L, Chen AH, Kaunitz AM, Gaudier FL, Delke I. Labor induction with intravaginal misoprostol in term premature rupture of membranes: a randomized study. Obstet Gynecol 1997; 89: 909–12. [RCT, n = 141]
15. Butt KD, Bennett KA, Crane JMG, Hutchens D, Young DC. Randomized comparison of oral misoprostol and oxytocin for labor induction in term prelabor membranes rupture. Obstet Gynecol 1999; 94: 994–9. [RCT, n = 108]
16. Ngai SW, Chan YM, Lam SW, Lao TT. Labour characteristics and uterine activity: misoprostol compared to oxytocin in women at term with prelabour rupture of membranes. Br J Obstet Gynaecol 2000; 107: 222–7. [RCT, n = 80]
17. Mozurkewich E, Horrocks J, Daley S et al; MisoPROM study. The MisoPROM study: a multicenter randomized comparison of oral misoprostol and oxytocin for premature rupture of membranes at term. Am J Obstet Gynecol 2003; 189: 1026–30. [RCT, n = 305]
18. Hannah ME, Ohlsson A, Wang EE et al. Maternal colonization with group B streptococcus and prelabor rupture of membranes at term: the role of induction of labor. TermPROM Study Group. Am J Obstet Gynecol 1997; 177: 780–5. [RCT secondary analysis]
19. Flenady V, King J. Antibiotics for prelabour rupture of membranes at or near term. Cochrane Database Syst Rev 2007; 1. [meta-analysis: 2 RCTs, n = 838]
20. Cararach V, Botet F, Sentis J, Almirall R, Perez-Picanol E. Administration of antibiotics to patients with rupture of membranes at term: a prospective, randomized, multicentric study. Collaborative Group on PROM. Acta Obstet Gynecol Scand 1998; 77: 298–302. [RCT, n = 733. IV ampicillin 1 g every 6 hours and IM gentamicin 80 mg every 8 hours or IM erythromycin 500 mg every 6 hours for women with penicillin allergy]
21. Ovalle A, Gomez R, Martinez MA et al. Antibiotic treatment of patients with term premature rupture of membranes reduces the incidence of infection-related complications. Am J Obstet Gynecol 1995; 172: 301. [RCT, n = 105. IV clindamycin 600 mg every 6 hours and IV cefuroxime 750 mg every 8 hours for 48 hours, then oral cefuroxime 250 mg every 12 hours and clindamycin 300 mg every 6 hours for a further 24 hours]

19

Meconium

Sarah Poggi and Alessandro Ghidini

KEY POINTS

- Fetal passage of meconium is common (12%), usually after 34 weeks and especially post-term.
- In a minority of cases, the association of meconium with fetal hypoxia may be secondary to the fact that **fetal hypoxic stress may stimulate colonic activity, and may also stimulate fetal gasping, leading to meconium aspiration. Therefore, meconium may not be causative, but merely associated with fetal hypoxia and its complications.**
- Prevention of meconium passage and of meconium aspiration syndrome may be accomplished by reducing the rate of post-term deliveries, achievable with early ultrasound dating.
- **Amnioinfusion** for meconium is associated with a 38% decrease in meconium aspiration syndrome (MAS) and a trend for a 49% decrease in perinatal mortality, but these cumulative beneficial results stem from many small studies, while **the largest trial did not show any benefit or detriment from this intervention. Therefore, routine amnioinfusion is not indicated just for presence of meconium.**
- **Oro- and nasopharyngeal suctioning** before delivery of the shoulder **does not decrease the incidence of MAS, need for mechanical ventilation for MAS, any other associated morbidities, or neonatal mortality.**
- **Routine endotracheal intubation** at birth in meconium-stained neonates that are otherwise vigorous **does not improve neonatal outcomes over routine resuscitation.**

Historic notes

Meconium is a term derived from the Greek *mekoni*, which means poppy juice or opium. Confirming previous clinical impressions, meconium passage was formally recognized to be associated with increased perinatal morbidity and mortality in the 1975 Collaborative Study of Cerebral Palsy.

Diagnoses/definitions

Meconium is the intestinal content of the fetus and is variably composed of mucopolysacharides, blood byproducts,

hair, and squamous cells. Diagnosis of meconium-stained amniotic fluid is made clinically on the basis of appearance (greenish or brownish staining) or by histopathological examination of the placenta. Particularly in the preterm (<33 week) gestation, a clinical impression of meconium-stained fluid may be false and instead reflect staining by another mechanism (i.e. hemosiderin). The diagnosis of meconium aspiration syndrome is respiratory distress requiring supplemental oxygen usually in the first 4 hours of life in the presence of meconium in a neonate without other causes of respiratory distress, and classified as shown below.

Epidemiology/incidence

- About 17–19% of term placentas have some degree of meconium staining.
- About 12% (7–22%) of term pregnancies are complicated by meconium staining of the amniotic fluid. Meconium aspiration syndrome (MAS) occurs in about 5% of these cases, and, of these, approximately 4% die.
- Incidence increases with term/postdates pregnancies:
  - about 10% of 39–41 week gestations, 18% of >41 week gestations.

Etiology/basic pathophysiology

The fetal hormone motilin promotes peristalsis. Motilin is not present in significant quantity in the extremely preterm (i.e. midtrimester) fetus to cause in-utero defecation. In later preterm, term, and post-term fetuses, increased motilin levels leading to meconium passage may be mediated by fetal stress from hypoxia, infection, or cord compression. However, particularly in the post-term fetus, passage may simply indicate gastrointestinal maturation.[1–5] Chronic or acute asphyxia and intrauterine infection are more likely sources of respiratory compromise in the presence of meconium than meconium aspiration itself.[1] **Fetal hypoxic stress may stimulate colonic activity, and may also** stimulate fetal gasping, leading to meconium aspiration. Therefore, meconium may not be causative, but just associated with fetal hypoxia and its complications. Meconium is associated with a chemical pneumonitis in neonatal lungs, which is associated then with inhibition of surfactant function, inflammation, and obstruction, leading to MAS.

Symptoms of meconium aspiration syndrome

Symptoms of neonatal **MAS** include respiratory compromise, with tachypnea, cyanosis, and reduced pulmonary compliance. In some cases, pulmonary hypertension develops.

Classification of meconium aspiration syndrome

- Mild: < 48 hours of supplemental oxygen at < 40%.
- Moderate: ≥ 48 hours supplemental oxygen at ≥ 40%.
- Severe: need for intubation (or primary pulmonary hypertension).

Risk factors

- **Post-term pregnancy.**
- **Fetal acidemia** (association, not necessarily causative).

Complications

It is associated with **fetal acidemia, neonatal seizures, neonatal intensive care unit (NICU) admission, respiratory distress, long-term sequela of cerebral palsy** (but **not necessarily causative**).[1–5]

Pregnancy management

Meconium at genetic amniocentesis

Suspicion of meconium-stained amniotic fluid in the extreme preterm fetus (i.e. at genetic amniocentesis) should prompt **evaluation for other causes of discolored amniotic fluid** (e.g. infection and/or abruption work-up).

Meconium in later preterm and term fetus < 39 weeks

Meconium-stained amniotic fluid in the later preterm and term fetus < 39 weeks should prompt evaluation for **infection and fetal hypoxia,** as the finding may not be attributable to normal physiology alone at this gestation.

Meconium at ≥ 39 weeks

Meconium-stained amniotic fluid in the full term (≥ 39 weeks) or post-term fetus may reflect normal physiology and maturation of the gastrointestinal tract only, but the possibilities of infection or hypoxia as etiologies cannot be excluded. Progression in meconium consistency in labor from no/little meconium to presence of thicker meconium should elicit particular concern, as this may be associated with higher rates of fetal acidemia.

Prevention

Prevention of meconium passage and of MAS may be accomplished by reducing the rate of post-term deliveries. Early ultrasound dating and stripping of membranes at ≥ 38 weeks both decrease the incidence of post-term pregnancies (see Chapter 23).

Management techniques used in the setting of meconium-stained amniotic fluid

Amnioinfusion

The efficacy of amnioinfusion to 'dilute' meconium and reduce associated neonatal morbidity is controversial. Randomized trials in some settings have shown benefit in terms of meconium aspiration syndrome, NICU admission, and neonatal hypoxic-ischemic encephalopathy,[6–18] although a recent, well-powered study failed to demonstrate any benefit.[19] More trials[19–22] have been published since the last meta-analysis.[6–18] No increased maternal risk has been consistently demonstrated. Amnioinfusion is associated with improvements in perinatal outcome, particularly in settings where facilities for perinatal surveillance are limited.

In the most recent meta-analysis, under **standard perinatal surveillance,** compared with no amnioinfusion, **amnioinfusion** for meconium (usually thick) staining of amniotic fluid is associated with a **reduction in heavy meconium staining of the liquor** (97% reduction); **variable fetal heart rate deceleration** (35%); **cesarean delivery** (18%), **MAS** (56%), and **pH < 7.20** (34%).[6–18] No perinatal deaths were reported.[6–18]

In the most recent meta-analysis, under **limited perinatal surveillance,** compared with no amnioinfusion, **amnioinfusion** for meconium (usually thick) staining of amniotic fluid is associated with a reduction in **MAS** (76%); **neonatal hypoxic-ischemic encephalopathy** (93%), and **neonatal ventilation or NICU admission** (44%); there is a trend towards reduced **perinatal mortality** (RR = 0.34, 95% CI 0.11–1.06).[6–18] The trials reviewed are too small to address the possibility of rare but serious maternal adverse effects of amnioinfusion.[6–18]

Our own meta-analysis of the trials in the meta-analysis[6–18] and the most recent large trial,[19] reveals still a **38% decrease in MAS** (67/1904 vs 110/1948; RR=0.62, 95% CI 0.46–0.84) and a **trend for a 49% decrease in perinatal mortality** (9/1813 vs 17/1743; RR=0.51, 95% CI 0.23–1.12). The result of all these meta-analyses are driven by small, poor-quality studies. Since the largest and best-quality study showed no benefit,[19] **routine amnioinfusion is not indicated just for the presence of meconium.** Amnioinfusion can be considered in the presence of recurrent variable decelerations, regardless of meconium (see Chapter 9).

In general, amnioinfusion is offered at ≥ 34 weeks. There are many variations of the amnioinfusion technique, but a 'typical' protocol calls for infusion via an intrauterine pressure catheter (obviously in a woman with dilated cervix and ruptured membranes) of **500 ml of normal saline over a period of 30 minutes** (see also Chapter 9).

For amnioinfusion in presence of variable decelerations, see Chapter 9; for amnioinfusion for oligohydramnios without PPROM, see Chapter 50 of *Maternal–Fetal Evidence Based Guidelines*; for amnioinfusion for PPROM, see Chapter 16.

Oro- and nasopharyngeal suctioning

Although commonly employed, suctioning of the oro- and nasopharynx before delivery of the shoulder or the 'first cry' **does not decrease the incidence of MAS, need for mechanical ventilation for MAS, any other associated morbidities, or neonatal mortality.**[23,24]

Endotracheal intubation

A policy of routine endotracheal intubation at birth in meconium-stained babies that are otherwise vigorous **does not improve neonatal outcomes over routine resuscitation.**[25] It is likely that routine aspiration of the upper airways is beneficial and should not be discarded. For depressed or non-vigorous newborns, endotracheal intubation and suctioning may still be performed in infants born through meconium-stained amniotic fluid.[25]

References

1. Ghidini A, Spong C. Severe meconium aspiration is not caused by aspiration of meconium. Obstet Gynecol 2001; 185: 931–8. [review]
2. Locatelli A, Regalia AL, Patregnani C et al. Prognostic value of change in amniotic fluid color during labor. Fetal Diagn Ther 2005; 20(1): 5–9. [II–2]
3. Nathan L, Leveno KJ, Carmody TJ 3rd, Kelly MA, Sherman ML. Meconium: a 1990s perspective on an old obstetric hazard. Obstet Gynecol 1994; 83(3): 329–32. [review]
4. Rossi EM, Philipson EH, Williams TG, Kalhan SC. Meconium aspiration syndrome: intrapartum and neonatal attributes. Am J Obstet Gynecol 1989; 161: 1106–10. [II–3]
5. Usher RH, Boyd ME, McLean FH, Kramer MS. Assessment of fetal risk in postdate pregnancies. Am J Obstet Gynecol 1988; 158: 259. [II–2]
6. Hofmeyr GJ. Amnioinfusion for meconium-stained liquor in labour. Cochrane Database Syst Rev 2007; 1. [meta-analysis: 12 RCTs, n=1877 – Refs 7–18]
7. Adam K, Cano L, Moise KJ. The effect of intrapartum amnioinfusion on the outcome of the fetus with heavy meconium stained amniotic fluid. Proceedings of 9th Annual Meeting of the Society of Perinatal Obstetricians, New Orleans, LA; 1989: 438. [RCT]
8. Alvarez M, Puertas A, Suarez AM, Herruzo A, Miranda JA. Transcervical amnioinfusion in deliveries with meconium-stained amniotic fluid. Prog Obstet Ginecol 1999; 42: 365–72. [RCT]
9. Cialone PR, Sherer DM, Ryan RM, Sinkin RA, Abramowicz JS. Amnioinfusion during labor complicated by particulate meconium-stained amniotic fluid decreases neonatal morbidity. Am J Obstet Gynecol 1994; 170: 842–9. [RCT]
10. Eriksen N, Hostetter M, Parisi V. Prophylactic amnioinfusion in pregnancies complicated by thick meconium. Am J Obstet Gynecol 1994; 170: 344. [RCT]
11. Hofmeyr GJ, Gulmezoglu AM, Buchmann E et al. The Collaborative Randomised Amnioinfusion for Meconium Project (CRAMP): 1. South Africa. Br J Obstet Gynaecol 1998; 105: 304–8. [RCT]
12. Ilagan NB, Kazzi GM, Shankaran S et al. Transcervical amnioinfusion for the prevention of neonatal meconium aspiration. Pediatr Res 1992; 31(4): 205A. [RCT]
13. Macri CJ, Schrimmer DB, Leung A, Greenspoon JS, Paul RH. Prophylactic amnioinfusion improves outcome of pregnancy complicated by thick meconium and oligohydramnios. Am J Obstet Gynecol 1992; 67: 117–21. [RCT]
14. Mahomed K, Mulambo T, Woelk G, Hofmeyr GJ, Gulmezoglu AM. The Collaborative Randomised Amnioinfusion for Meconium Project (CRAMP): 2. Zimbabwe. Br J Obstet Gynaecol 1998; 105: 309–13. [RCT]
15. Moodley J, Matchaba P, Payne AJ. Intrapartum amnioinfusion for meconium-stained liquor in developing countries. Tropical Doctor 1998; 28: 31–4. [RCT]
16. Sadovsky Y, Amon E, Bade ME, Petrie RH. Prophylactic amnioinfusion during labor complicated by meconium: a preliminary report. Am J Obstet Gynecol 1989; 61: 613–17. [RCT]
17. Spong CY, Ogunipe OA, Ross MG. Prophylactic amnioinfusion for meconium-stained amniotic fluid. Am J Obstet Gynecol 1994; 171: 931–5. [RCT]
18. Wenstrom KD, Parsons MT. The prevention of meconium aspiration in labor using amnioinfusion. Obstet Gynecol 1989; 73: 647–51. [RCT]
19. Fraser WD, Hofmeyr J, Lede R et al; Amnioinfusion Trial Group. Amnioinfusion for the prevention of the meconium aspiration syndrome. N Engl J Med 2005; 353: 909–17. [RCT, n=1998]
20. Puertas A, Paz Carrillo M, Molto L et al; Meconium-stained amniotic fluid in labor: a randomized trial of prophylactic amnioinfusion. Eur J Obstet Gynecol Reprod Biol 2001; 99: 33–7. [RCT]
21. Rathor AM, Singh R, Ramji S, Tripathi R. Randomised trial of amnioinfusion during labour with meconium stained amniotic fluid. Br J Obstet Gynaecol 2002; 109(1): 17–20. [RCT]
22. Sood M, Charulata, Dimple D Amnioinfusion in thick meconium. Indian J Pediatrics 2004; 71: 677–81. [RCT, n=196]
23. Falciglia HS, Henderschott C, Potter P, Helmchen R. Does DeLee suction at the perineum prevent meconium aspiration syndrome? Am J Obstet Gynecol 1992; 167(5): 1243–9. [II–2]
24. Vain NE, Szyld EG, Prudent LM et al. Oropharyngeal and nasopharyngeal suctioning of meconium-stained neonates before delivery of their shoulders: multicentre, randomised controlled trial. Lancet 2004; 364: 597–602. [RCT, n=2514]
25. Halliday HL, Sweet D. Endotracheal intubation at birth for preventing morbidity and mortality in vigorous, meconium stained infants born at term. Cochrane Database Syst Rev 2007; 1. [meta-analysis: 4 RCTs, n=2884]

20

Malpresentation and malposition

Mark C Molnar

KEY POINTS

- **Malpresentation is associated** with **uterine anomalies, fibroids, placenta previa, grandmultiparty, contracted maternal pelvis, pelvic tumors, prematurity** (the earlier the gestational age, the higher the incidence of malpresentation), **multiple gestation, polyhydramnios, short umbilical cord, fetal anomalies** (e.g. anencephaly, hydrocephalus), **abnormal fetal motor ability, and prior breech delivery.**

- **Complications** of breech presentation are **congenital anomalies, preterm birth, birth trauma, low Apgar scores, and lower pH,** mostly regardless of mode of delivery. **Cord prolapse, head hyperextension, and head or arm entrapment** are more common with vaginal breech delivery.

- **External cephalic version** (ECV) is a safe and effective intervention. **Urgent cesarean delivery** for non-reassuring fetal heart rate (NRFHR) testing and placental **abruption** occur in <1% of ECV.

- ECV should be avoided with **any contraindications to vaginal delivery** such as placenta **previa,** or **prior classical uterine incision,** and, relatively, with rupture of membranes (ROM), oligohydramnios, known uterine or fetal anomaly, unexplained uterine bleeding, or active phase of labor.

- **ECV reduces the incidences of non-cephalic birth and cesarean delivery.** Because ECV is associated with a very low incidence of adverse events and with a significant decrease in cesarean delivery, **all women at or near term with non-vertex presentations should be offered an ECV attempt. Success rates** roughly average **about 50–70%.** Success is increased with **higher parity,** and **transverse or oblique lie.**

- There is **insufficient evidence to assess the best gestational age** at which to perform ECV. It is effective starting at 34 weeks, with the most common gestational age around 36 weeks in trials.

- Tocolysis with **beta-mimetics** prior to attempt at ECV is associated with **fewer failures of ECV,** and **less cesarean deliveries.**

- ECV should be performed in a facility with ready availability for emergency cesarean delivery, after appropriate counseling and consent, with ultrasound available.

- Compared with planned vaginal delivery, **planned cesarean delivery** for the **term** breech fetus is associated with **decrease in perinatal or neonatal death or serious neonatal morbidity,** but no difference in death or neurodevelopmental delay at 2 years after delivery.

- There is **insufficient evidence** to assess if outcomes of the **preterm** fetus presenting breech are affected by mode of delivery.

- There is **insufficient evidence** to assess the best mode of delivery for the **non-vertex second twin.** Vaginal delivery of the second non-vertex twin may be a reasonable management option for an expert operator, possibly by breech extraction.

Definitions

- Malpresentation: fetus presenting with the fetal head not in the lower uterine segment.
- Presentation: fetal body part which is in the lower uterine segment (lowest in the uterus, and closest to the cervix).
- Malposition: fetal position that is not anterior.
- Position: relationship of presenting part (usually occiput for head) to pelvic outlet.

Symptoms

The maternal impression of fetal presentation based on fetal movement is suggestive but, overall, is unreliable for predicting fetal presentation.

Epidemiology/incidence

Breech presentation complicates 3–4% of all pregnancies at term (≥ 37 weeks).[1] Its incidence is inversely proportional to gestational age, with an incidence of about 25% at 28 weeks, 11% at 32 weeks, and 5% at 34 weeks.[2] In 1990, 90% of these presentations resulted in cesarean delivery (compared with 11.6% in 1970), accounting for 15% of all sections, and adding US$1.4 billion to US obstetric costs.[3]

Classifications

Breech

The fetus presents in longitudinal lie, with the head not in the lower uterine segment. Fetal breech presentation is further classified as:

- complete – flexion of the fetal hips and knees
- incomplete – extension of one or both hips (includes footling)
- frank – flexion of the hips and extension of the knees.

Transverse

The fetal longitudinal axis is perpendicular to the long axis of the uterus. The fetus can either present 'back up' (fetal small parts present to cervix) or 'back down' (fetal spine or shoulder present to cervix).

Oblique

The fetal longitudinal axis is diagonal to the long axis of the uterus.

Risk factors/associations

Both maternal and fetal factors can lead to malpresentation, including **uterine anomalies, fibroids, placenta previa, grandmultiparity, contracted maternal pelvis, pelvic tumors, prematurity** (the earlier the gestational age, the higher the incidence of malpresentation), **multiple gestation, polyhydramnios, short umbilical cord, fetal anomalies** (e.g. anencephaly, hydrocephalus), **abnormal fetal motor ability, and prior breech delivery.** Prior breech delivery is associated with a 9% risk of recurrence in subsequent pregnancies.

Complications

The incidences of **congenital anomalies** (up to 6%), **preterm birth, birth trauma, low Apgar scores, and lower pH** are higher with a breech presentation compared with a vertex presentation, **mostly regardless of mode of delivery.**

Breech presentation may be a sign and a consequence of fetal compromise, again regardless of delivery mode. The incidence of **cord prolapse** is about the same with frank breech as with vertex presentations (<1%), 5% with complete breech, up to 15% with footling, and is inversely proportional to gestational age. **Head hyperextension** (associated with spinal cord injury), and **head or arm entrapment** are all associated with breech presentation, and especially with vaginal delivery. Presentation at birth does not seem to affect adult intellectual performance. Cesarean or vaginal delivery for breech presentation does not seem to differ in terms of long-term adult intellectual performance.[4]

Management (Figure 20.1)

Work-up

Fetal presentation should be assessed by Leopold's maneuvers at each visit, starting at ≥ 34 weeks of gestation. If the clinician is unsure, a vaginal examination, or even better an ultrasound if still unclear, is indicated to assess fetal presentation.

Prevention (interventions to prevent malpresentation at delivery)

External cephalic version

Definition: External cephalic version (ECV) is a procedure performed by application of pressure and maneuvers to the maternal abdomen with the goal of turning the fetus to a cephalic presentation, thus increasing the likelihood of vaginal delivery.[1]

Complications: Whereas the rate of short-term fetal bradycardia is ≥ 20%, the need for **urgent cesarean delivery** for non-reassuring fetal heart rate (NRFHR) testing after an ECV is about 1/600.[5] Placental **abruption** (<1%) and **onset of labor** are uncommon complications. Rare fetal deaths following attempts at version are not considered to have been a result of the procedure.[1] Femur fracture has been reported.

Contraindications: Contraindications are generally considered as **any contraindications to vaginal delivery,** such as placenta **previa** or **prior classical uterine incision.** There are no trials on ECV in **multiple gestations,** so the safety and efficacy of this procedure cannot be assessed. Relative contraindications are rupture of membranes (ROM), **oligohydramnios, known uterine or fetal anomaly, unexplained**

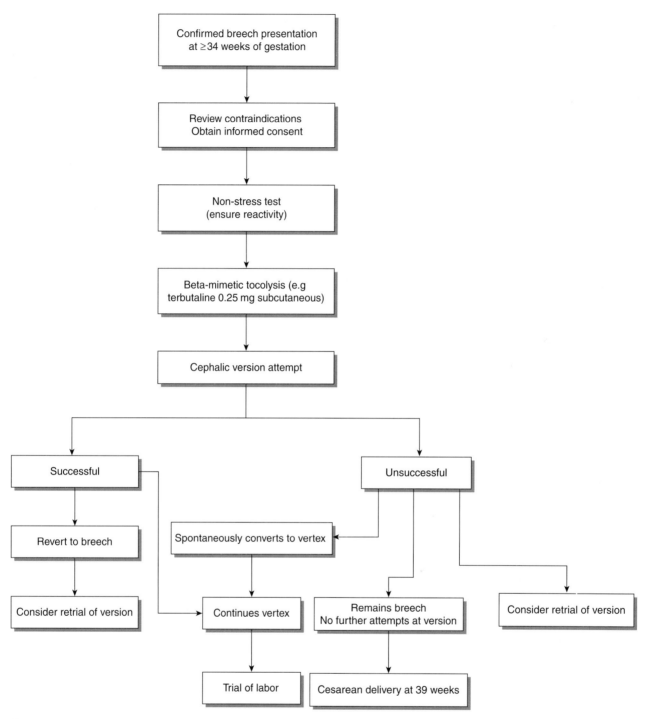

Figure 20.1
Suggested management of breech presentation. (Adapted from ACOG[1])

uterine bleeding, or active phase of labor.[1,6] ECV in women with prior cesarean deliveries is associated with a comparable success rate to that in women without prior cesarean deliveries, but there are insufficient data to assess the safety of this management.[7]

Efficacy: Compared with no ECV, **ECV** at term is associated with a statistically significant and clinically meaningful 62% **reduction in non-cephalic birth** and a 45% **decrease in cesarean delivery**.[8] Because ECV is associated with a very low incidence of adverse events and with a significant decrease in cesarean delivery, **all women at or near term with non-vertex presentations should be offered an ECV attempt.**

Success rates average about **58%**, with a range of 25–80%.[1] Success is increased with **higher parity**, and **transverse or oblique lie** (vs breech). Lower amniotic fluid volume (AFV), anterior placenta, and high maternal body mass index (BMI) might decrease the success rate.[1] There is no scoring system to accurately predict the probability of success of ECV.

Timing of version: Compared with no ECV attempt, **ECV before term reduces non-cephalic births.** There is **insufficient evidence to assess the best gestational age** at which to perform ECV. In general, the later is the gestational age, the lower is the success rate, but there are some occasional reports of successful ECV in women in term labor. 36 weeks is generally considered to be the optimal time for attempted version, and is mostly used in trials. At this gestational age there is felt to be adequate room to turn the fetus while minimizing the risk of reversion to breech after a successful version. At the same time if delivery becomes necessary, a 36-week infant has a low rate of respiratory distress syndrome (RDS) or other complications of prematurity. Compared with ECV at 37 0/7 to 38 0/7 weeks, ECV at **34 0/7 to 36 0/7 weeks** is associated with a non-significant trend for slightly lower (57% vs 66%) non-cephalic presentation at birth and slightly lower (65% vs 72%) cesarean delivery.[9–12]

Tocolysis: Tocolysis with **beta-mimetics** prior to an attempt at ECV is associated with 26% **fewer failures of ECV**, a non-significant reduction in non-cephalic presentations at birth, and 15% **less cesarean deliveries**.[13] Different beta-mimetics have been used, with no evidence as to the best one or its dosage/timing.[13] Tocolysis can be used with success also in a second ECV attempt after a first ECV attempt has failed.[14]

Nitroglycerin has been studied as an agent to improve version success rates. In four small trials, sublingual nitroglycerin was associated with significant side effects, and was **not** found to be **effective**.[13] The terbutaline 0.25 mg subcutaneous 5 minutes prior group was found to have a significantly higher ECV success rate than the nitroglycerin group in one trial.[15]

Fetal acoustic stimulation: Stimulation to the fetal head for 1–3 seconds in midline fetal spine positions is associated with fewer failures of ECV at term in a very small study.[13,16] 11 of 12 versions were successful following stimulation.[16] The crossover arm (patients who failed version without stimulation) were then stimulated, and 8 of 10 patients were successfully verted, for a total of 19/22 successful versions (86%).[16] The initial success rate in the control group of this study was much lower than expected (8%).[16]

Anesthesia: There is insufficient convincing evidence that regional anesthesia affects ECV success. ECV failure,

non-cephalic births, and cesarean sections were reduced in two trials with epidural but not in three with spinal analgesia.[13] ECV success rates increased from 33% to 59% with epidural in one study and from 32% to 69% in another.[3,17] Potential bias in both studies lies in that the care provider was not blinded to placement of epidural.[3,17] It is important to note that **the controls groups had lower success rates than expected**, as, as shown above, the average success rate in the literature, which is mostly without anesthesia, is about 58%. All patients in both studies received terbutaline prior to attempt at version. Some clinicians have postulated that large-volume preloading with epidural may have increased the amniotic fluid volume.[13] The use of spinal anesthesia has not been associated with any benefit in the success of ECV.[6,13]

Other: There are no trials to evaluate the potential effects of hydration or transabdominal amnioinfusion on the success rate of spontaneous version or ECV.

ECV procedure: Given the possible complications, it is prudent to perform ECV in a **facility** with ready availability for emergency cesarean delivery. **Consent** should be obtained after **counseling** regarding possible complications, other options (cesarean delivery), prognosis, and some explanation of the actual procedure. A non-stress test (**NST**) should be performed before and after the procedure. Anesthesia is usually not necessary, and has not been absolutely proven to benefit outcomes. **Beta-mimetic** prophylactic tocolysis should be given (e.g. terbutaline 0.25 mg subcutaneously 5–10 minutes prior to procedure). There is no trial to compare other technical aspects of ECV. The technique using two or one operators can be used. Frequent if not continuous **ultrasound** guidance to assess for fetal well-being and presentation is suggested. Rh-negative women can receive anti-D immunoglobulin. There is no evidence to support immediate induction after successful ECV.

Moxibustion and/or acupuncture

Moxibustion is a form of traditional Chinese medicine that uses heat generated by burning herbs, most often *Artemisia vulgaris* (magwort), to stimulate the acupuncture point BL 67 (Zhiyin in Chinese).[18–22] There is **insufficient evidence** to assess if the use of moxibustion significantly converts a breech to a cephalic presentation. There are differences in interventions (e.g. moxibustion alone or with acupuncture), making it inappropriate to perform a satisfactory meta-analysis. Moxibustion may reduce the need for ECV by 53%, the incidence of non-vertex presentation at term by 35–70%, but mainly in the Chinese trials.[19,20] In the two trials performed in Italy, moxibustion was either not well tolerated by 22% of women and (therefore?) not effective[21] or effective when used with acupuncture.[22] Moxibustion may decrease the use of oxytocin before or during labor for women who had vaginal deliveries.[18] It might be that acupuncture and not moxibustion (especially not at home) is beneficial.[22]

Maternal change in posture

Maternal positioning has been suggested as a means to correct breech presentation in pregnancy. There is insufficient evidence from the small trials reported so far to support the use of postural management for breech presentation.[23] Meta-analysis of these data could not be done, as study designs and outcomes measured were different.[24] Postural management is not associated with a significant effect on the rate of non-cephalic births, either for the subgroup in which no ECV was attempted or for the group overall. No differences were detected for cesarean sections. As such, there is no solid evidence to this practice.[23,24]

Delivery outcomes

It is important to note that the rate of cesarean delivery after ECV is still about double that of pregnancies presenting with spontaneous cephalic presentation because of higher incidences of dystocia and NRFHT after successful ECV.[25]

Mode of delivery – singleton

Term breech

At 4–6 weeks after delivery, compared with planned vaginal delivery, **planned cesarean delivery** is associated with a 67% **decrease in perinatal or neonatal death** (excluding fatal anomalies) **or serious neonatal morbidity.**[26] This reduction is (surprisingly) less for countries with high national perinatal mortality rates.[27] Planned cesarean delivery is associated with a 71% reduction (from 1.15% to 0.26%) in perinatal or neonatal death (excluding fatal anomalies);[26] this was similar for countries with low and high national perinatal mortality rates. One death would be prevented for every 112 cesarean sections planned.[26] A secondary analysis[28] of the short-term outcomes of the Term Breech Trial[27] looked at factors associated with adverse outcomes. The lowest morbidity was found in patients with a planned section prior to the onset of labor. If vaginal birth is the desired route, labor augmentation and a second stage > 60 minutes are associated with poorer outcomes.[28] Factors not shown to affect outcome include induction, parity, use of continuous electronic fetal monitoring, or epidural.[28] A skilled clinician at the delivery was associated with lower adverse outcome: 'skilled clinician' was described by clinicians themselves rather than by years of experience or licensed obstetrician.[28]

At 3 months after delivery, women allocated to the planned cesarean section group reported 38% **less urinary incontinence,** 89% more abdominal pain; and 68% less perineal pain.[29]

At 2 years after delivery, there was **no difference in the combined outcome 'death or neurodevelopmental delay'.** Of 463 vaginal delivery patients followed up at 2 years, there were only 6 deaths and 7 neurodevelopmental delays (2.8%), compared with 2 and 12 patients of 457 patients (3.1%) in the section group.[30] The disappearance at 2 years of age of the difference seen at neonatal follow-up is because most children with serious neonatal morbidity survive and develop normally. Moreover, there might still not be a sample size big enough to detect small differences for the 2 years' data.[30] **Maternal outcomes at 2 years** were also very **similar,** with only **constipation** significantly more **common** in the **cesarean** delivery group (27% vs 20%), while self-reported incontinence was non-significantly different (18% vs 22%).[31] Incontinence was different (16% vs 25%) if comparing women who actually planned and had a cesarean vs those who planned and had a vaginal delivery.[31]

These results are mostly from the Term Breech Trial[27] and its secondary analyses and follow-up.[28–31] Also important to note is that these outcomes are based on deliveries done by 'clinicians who were regarded as experienced at vaginal breech delivery'.[27–31] As the number of breech vaginal deliveries decreases, physician skill to perform this procedure will continue to diminish, with the potential of making vaginal delivery less safe. While it is estimated that > 90% of babies presenting non-vertex are currently delivered by cesarean, there might still be a small role for vaginal delivery for the woman who declines scheduled cesarean or presents in advanced labor. Still, **all women with breech presentation with a large fetus (> 3500 g estimate), unfavorable pelvis, hyperextended head, incomplete or footling breech presentation, NRFHT, severe fetal growth restriction (FGR), or lack of experienced obstetric and anesthesiological operators should absolutely have a cesarean delivery.**

Technical aspects

Cesarean breech delivery: There are no trials to assess the technical aspects of breech (or other malpresentation) cesarean delivery. There is insufficient evidence to assess if intra-abdominal version during cesarean delivery before uterine incision affects outcomes.

Vaginal breech delivery: There are several technical suggestions for assisting a vaginal breech delivery. None is based on trials. There is insufficient evidence to assess if clinical/radiological pelvimetry affects outcomes in the management of breech presentation. Usually a double set up is suggested, so that an attempt at vaginal delivery should be organized in the operating room, ready for possible cesarean delivery.

Some other suggestions are:

- minimal intervention, at least until the abdomen up to the umbilical cord is delivered
- prevention of head extension (with prophylactic Mauriceau maneuver)
- proper use of Pipers forceps (if necessary).

Term transverse or oblique

The same management options exist for transverse/oblique lie as for breech. Fetal version or cesarean delivery are the standards of care, with lack of trial evidence.

Preterm breech

There is **insufficient evidence** to assess if outcomes of the preterm fetus presenting breech are affected by mode of delivery. Very little prospective data, mostly non-randomized, exist regarding vaginal vs cesarean delivery of the premature breech infant.[1] Two trials aimed at assessing this question failed to randomize the planned sample sizes. After 17 months of patient recruiting at 26 different hospitals, only 13 women had been randomized, making it impossible to confer any conclusions in one study.[32] The Iowa Premature Breech Trial was somewhat more successful, recruiting 38 patients over 5 years, with insufficient data for meaningful conclusions.[33] Outcomes in premature breech infants are mainly related to prematurity and/or fetal anomaly, with unclear effect of mode of delivery.[34]

Mode of delivery – twins

Breech second twin

(See also Chapter 38 of *Maternal–Fetal Evidence Based Guidelines*.) Pregnancies at 35–43 weeks with vertex/breech presentation in twin gestations < 7 cm dilated have similar Apgar scores or incidence of neonatal morbidity in the second twin if delivered by vaginal or cesarean birth in a very small trial.[35] There was no incidence of birth trauma or intraventricular hemorrhage (IVH) in any of the 27 breech deliveries.[35] Maternal febrile morbidity and length of stay was increased in the cesarean group.[35] As such, **vaginal delivery of the second non-vertex twin is a reasonable management option**. Attempt at vaginal twin delivery has been supported, especially for twins with estimated fetal weight (EFW) of >1500 g, and can only be performed with adequate experience of the obstetrician, and continuous availability of expert anesthesia, usually in or very close to an operating room. **Total breech extraction** is associated with shorter maternal stay and lower neonatal pulmonary disease, infection, and intensive care nursery (ICN) stay compared with cephalic version in retrospective studies.[35,36] There are no trials for twins presenting with **first twin non-vertex** (about 26%), with recommendation for cesarean delivery made based mostly on data from singleton gestations. Because vaginal delivery of **triplets** is usually associated with an increased risk for fetal, neonatal and infant deaths compared with cesarean delivery, **cesarean section is the route of choice**, even if some small series have recently reported similar outcomes for trial of labor or cesarean delivery for triplets.

Malposition

There is insufficient evidence for assessing the effect of **hands and knees posture** to correct malposition. There are two trials on the effect of hands and knees posture before labor.[37] Compared with a sitting position, 10 minutes in the hands and knees position is associated with a lower likelihood of malposition of the presenting part of the fetus in a small trial, but advice to assume the hands and knees posture for 10 minutes twice daily in the last weeks of pregnancy had no effect on the baby's position at delivery or any of the other pregnancy outcomes measured in a larger trial.[37] No trials of hands and knees posture during labor have been reported.

Anesthesia

For vaginal breech delivery, an anesthesiologist skilled at the pharmacology of uterine relaxation (e.g. nitric oxide) should be present.

Postpartum/breastfeeding

There are no specific recommendations.

References

1. American College of Obstetricians and Gynecologists. External cephalic version. ACOG Clinical Management Guidelines for Obstetrician-Gynecologists, No. 13, February 2000.[review]
2. Hill LM. Prevalence of breech presentation by gestational age. Am J Perinatol 1990; 7: 92–3. [II–3]
3. Mancuso KM, Yancey MK, Murphy JA, Markenson GR. Epidural analgesia for cephalic version: a randomized trial. Obstet Gynecol 2000; 95(5): 648–51. [RCT, n = 108]

4. Eide MG, Oyen N, Skjaerven R et al. Breech delivery and intelligence: a population-based study of 8,738 breech infants. Obstet Gynecol 2005; 105: 4–11. [II–2]

5. Dyson DC, Ferguson JE, Hensleigh P. Antepartum external cephalic version under tocolysis. Obstet Gynecol 1986; 67: 63–8. [II–2]

6. Dugoff L, Stamm CA, Jones OW, Mohling SI, Hawkins JL. The effect of spinal anesthesia on the success rate of external cephalic version: a randomized trial. Obstet Gynecol 1999; 93: 345–9. [RCT, n = 102]

7. Flamm BL, Fried MW, Lonky NM, Giles WS. External cephalic version after previous cesarean section. Am J Obstet Gynecol 1991; 165: 370–2. [II–2]

8. Hofmeyr GJ, Kulier R. External cephalic version for breech presentation at term. Cochrane Database Syst Rev 2007; 1. [5 RCTs, n = 533]

9. Hutton EK, Hofmeyr GJ. External cephalic version for breech presentation before term. Cochrane Database Syst Rev 2007; 1. [meta-analysis: 3 RCTs, n = 515]

10. Hutton EK, Kaufman K, Hodnett E et al. External cephalic version beginning at 34 weeks' gestation versus 37 weeks' gestation: a randomized multicenter trial. Am J Obstet Gynecol 2003; 189(1): 245–54. [RCT, n = 233]

11. Mensink WFA, Huisjes HJ. Is external version useful in breech presentation? Nederlands Tijdschrift voor Geneeskunde 1980; 124: 1828–31. [RCT, n = 102]

12. Van Veelen AJ, Van Cappellen AW, Flu PK, Straub MJ, Wallenburg HC. Effect of external cephalic version in late pregnancy on presentation at delivery: a randomized controlled trial. Br J Obstet Gynaecol 1989; 96(8): 916–21. [RCT, n = 180]

13. Hofmeyr GJ, Gyte G. Interventions to help external cephalic version for breech presentation at term. Cochrane Database Syst Rev 2007; 1. [6 RCTs beta-mimetic tocolysis, n = 617; 4 RCTs nitric oxide donors, n = >100; 1 acoustic stimulation, n = 26]

14. Impey L, Pandit M. Tocolysis for repeat external cephalic version in breech presentation at term: a randomised, double-blinded, placebo-controlled trial. Br J Obstet Gynaecol 2005; 112; 627–31. [RCT, n = 124]

15. El-Sayed YY, Pullen K, Riley ET et al. Randomized comparison of intravenous nitroglycerin and subcutaneous terbutaline for external cephalic version under tocolysis. Am J Obstet Gynecol 2004; 191: 2051–5. [RCT, n = 59]

16. Johnson RL, Strong TH, Radin TG, Elliot JP. Fetal acoustic stimulation as an adjunct to external cephalic version. J Reprod Med 1995; 40(10): 696–8. [II–3]

17. Schorr SJ, Speights SE, Ross EL et al. A randomized trial of epidural anesthesia to improve external cephalic version success. Am J Obstet Gynecol 1997; 177(5): 1133–7. [RCT, n = 69]

18. Coyle ME, Smith CA, Peat B. Cephalic version by moxibustion for breech presentation. Cochrane Database of Syst Rev 2007; 1. [meta-analysis: 3 RCTs, n = 597]

19. Cardini F, Weixin H. Moxibustion for correction of breech presentation. JAMA 1998; 280(18): 1580–4. [RCT, n = 260, in China]

20. Li Q, Wang L. Clinical observation on correcting malposition of fetus by electro-acupuncture. J Trad Chinese Med 1996; 16(4): 260–2. [RCT, n = 111]

21. Cardini F, Lombardo P, Regalia AL et al. A randomized controlled trial of oxybustion for breech presentation. Br J Obstet Gynaecol 2005; 112: 743–7. [RCT, n = 123, in Italy]

22. Neri I, Airola G, Contu G et al. Acupuncture plus moxibustion to resolve breech presentation: a randomized controlled study. J Matern Fetal Neonatal Med 2004; 15: 247–52. [RCT, n = 240, in Italy]

23. Hofmeyr GJ, Kulier R. Cephalic version by postural management for breech presentation. Cochrane Database Syst Rev 2007; 1. [meta-analysis: 5 RCTs, n = 392]

24. Founds S. Maternal posture for cephalic version of breech presentation: a review of the evidence. Birth 2005; 32(2): 137–44. [meta-analysis: 4 RCTs, n = 346, but could not be performed because of flaws in RCTs]

25. Vezina Y, Bujold E, Varin J, Marquette GP, Boucher M. Cesarean delivery after successful external cephalic version of breech presentation at term: a comparative study. Am J Obstet Gynecol 2004; 190(3): 763–8. [II–2, n = 602]

26. Hofmeyr GJ, Hannah ME. Planned caesarean section for term breech delivery. Cochrane Database Syst Rev 2007; 1. [meta-analysis: 3 RCTs, n = 2,396]

27. Hannah ME, Hannah WJ, Hewson SA et al. The Term Breech Collaborative Group Planned caesarean section versus planned vaginal birth for the breech presentation at term: a randomized multicenter trial. Lancet 2000; 356(9239): 1375–83. [RCT, n = 2088]

28. Su M, McLeod L, Ross S et al; Term Breech Trial Collaborative Group. Factors associated with adverse perinatal outcome in the Term Breech Trial. Am J Obstet and Gynecol 2003; 189(3): 740–5. [secondary analysis of RCT, n = 2083]

29. Hannah ME, Hannah WJ, Hodnett ED et al; Outcomes at 3 months after planned cesarean vs planned vaginal delivery for breech presentation at term. JAMA 2002; 287: 1822–31. [RCT analysis of 3-Month questionnaire follow-up, n = 1596]

30. Whyte H, Hannah ME, Saigal S et al; Term Breech Trial Collaborative Group. Outcomes of children at 2 years after planned cesarean birth versus planned vaginal birth for breech presentation at term: The International Randomized Term Breech Trial. Am J Obstet Gynecol 2004; 191: 864–71. [RCT analysis of 2-year children follow-up, n = 923]

31. Hannah ME, Whyte H, Hannah WJ et al; Term Breech Trial Collaborative Group. Maternal outcomes at 2-years after planned cesarean section versus planned vaginal birth for breech presentation at term: the international randomized Term Breech Trial. Am J Obstet Gynecol 2004; 191: 917–27. [2-year maternal follow-up of RCT, n = 917]

32. Penn ZJ, Steer PJ, Grant A. A multicoated randomized control trial comparing elective and selective caesarean section for the delivery of the preterm breech infant. Br J Obstet Gynecol 1996; 103(7): 684–9. [RCT, n = 13; stopped recruitment]

33. Zlatnik FJ. The Iowa premature breech trial. Am J Gerontol 1993; 10(1): 60–3. [RCT, n = 38]

34. Cibils LA, Karrison T, Brown L. Factors influencing neonatal outcomes in the very-low-birth-weight fetus (< 1500 grams) with breech presentation. Am J Obstet Gynecol 1994; 171(1): 35–42. [II–2]

35. Rabinovici J, Barkai G, Reichman B, Serr DM, Mashiach S. Randomized management of the second nonvertex twin: vaginal delivery or cesarean section. Am J Obstet Gynecol 1987; 156(1): 52–6. [RCT, n = 60]

36. Mauldin JG, Newman RB, Mauldin PD. Cost-effective management of the vertex and non-vertex twin gestation. Am J Obstet Gynecol 1998; 179: 864–9. [II–2]

37. Hofmeyr GJ, Kulier R. Hands and knees posture in late pregnancy or labour for fetal malposition (lateral or posterior). Cochrane Database Syst Rev 2007; 1. [meta-analysis: 2 RCTs, n = 2647]

21

Shoulder dystocia

Vincenzo Berghella

KEY POINTS

- Approximately 50% of cases of brachial plexus injury do not occur in association with shoulder dystocia, and 4% occur after cesarean delivery.
- **Risk factors** for shoulder dystocia include **prior shoulder dystocia** (recurrence risk about 15%); **macrosomia, previous macrosomia, diabetes mellitus, obesity, post-term, induction, epidural anesthesia, prolonged second stage,** and **operative (forceps/vacuum) vaginal delivery.**
- **Complications** of shoulder dystocia include **brachial plexus injury, fractures, hypoxic-ischemic encephalopathy, long term neurologic disability,** and even **death** for the baby; severe (third and fourth degree) **perineal lacerations** and **postpartum hemorrhage** for the mother.
- Since shoulder dystocia is **not easily predictable by risk factors,** obstetricians must **be prepared for the condition at every delivery.**
- **Prevention strategies** include cesarean for estimated fetal weight (EFW) > 5000 g in non-diabetic women and EFW > 4500 g in diabetic women; avoid operative vaginal delivery in presence of significant risk factors.

Table 21.1 *Management of shoulder dystocia*
- Ask for help (anesthesia, neonatology, colleagues, nursing, etc.)
- McRobert's maneuver (> 60–80% success)
- Suprapubic pressure
- Shoulder rotation:
- Rubin's maneuver
- Wood's corkscrew maneuver
- Delivery of posterior arm
- Episiotomy
- 'All-fours'
- Clavicle fracture
- Cephalic replacement (Zavanelli maneuver)
- Symphisiotomy

(McRobert's, suprapubic pressure, shoulder rotation, and delivery of posterior arm are the initial maneuvers, usually successful in > 90% of cases).

- **Management of shoulder dystocia involves asking for help** (anesthesia, neonatology, colleagues, nursing, etc.) **and different maneuvers, as shown in detail in Table 21.1**

Diagnosis/definition

The definition of shoulder dystocia is difficult delivery of the baby's shoulders requiring additional maneuvers to gentle downward traction of the fetal head.[1] Shoulder dystocia pertains only to a vertex presentation. Unfortunately, there are no accepted objective diagnostic criteria, making diagnosis subjective.

Signs

Retraction of the delivered fetal head against the maternal perineum ('turtle sign').

Epidemiology/incidence

The incidence is about **1%** (range 0.1–2%, also depending on definition) of vertex vaginal deliveries.

Etiology/basic pathophysiology

Shoulder dystocia is related, most commonly, to the impaction of the anterior fetal shoulder behind the maternal pubis symphysis, or, less commonly, to the impaction of the posterior shoulder on the sacral promontory.[1] **Approximately 50% of cases of brachial plexus injury do not occur in association with shoulder dystocia, and 4% occur after cesarean delivery,** so that external maneuvers and forces at vaginal delivery may not be responsible for injury from shoulder dystocia.[2] In fact, the estimated pressures from endogenous forces are 4–9 times greater than those calculated for clinician-applied forces.[3]

Risk factors/associations

Risk factors (and warning/predictive signs) are **prior shoulder dystocia (recurrence risk about 15%); macrosomia, previous macrosomia, diabetes mellitus, obesity, post-term, induction, epidural anesthesia, prolonged second stage, and operative (forceps/vacuum) vaginal delivery.**

Complications

Perinatal

Perinatal complications are brachial plexus injury (transient, 4–40%; persistent, < 10%), **fractures** (clavicle, humerus – up to 15%); **hypoxic-ischemic encephalopathy; long term neurologic disability** (up to 5–10%); and even **death** (usually < 5–10%).

Maternal

Maternal complications are severe (third and fourth degree) **perineal lacerations** and **postpartum hemorrhage.** Zavanelli maneuver and symphysiotomy may be associated with significant morbidity.

Management

Principles

Shoulder dystocia is one of the most common severe complications in pregnancy. **Since it is not easily predictable by risk factors, obstetricians must be prepared for this condition at every delivery.**

Prevention

Shoulder dystocia is most often unpredictable and unpreventable.[1] There is no accepted effective algorithm for prevention of shoulder dystocia. Risk factors should be reviewed, as in some cases prevention is possible. **Risk of shoulder dystocia should be discussed with any woman with a risk factor, including risk factors that occur in labor. Prevention strategies include cesarean for estimated fetal weight (EFW) > 5000 g in non-diabetic women and EFW > 4500 g in diabetic women and avoidance of operative vaginal delivery in the presence of significant risk factors.** There is insufficient evidence to support labor induction in the non-diabetic woman suspected of having macrosomia (see Chapter 40 of *Maternal–Fetal Evidence Based Guidelines*). EFW (either clinical or by ultrasound) **should be documented before every labor.**

Preconception counseling

Women with prior shoulder dystocia have about a 15% risk of recurrence. Counseling should include discussion of risk factors of prior shoulder dystocia, review of which risk factors are present in the current pregnancy, and also possible complications. If several significant risk factors are still present, the woman may opt for cesarean delivery. If risk factors are not present (except for prior shoulder dystocia), the woman may decide after counseling for either trial of labor or cesarean delivery.

Therapy

There are no specific trials to guide management. Level II-3 and III evidence suggests the interventions shown in Table 21.1. These interventions go from most successful/least invasive to most invasive, but there are insufficient data to assess the most safe and effective sequence of interventions for shoulder dystocia.

Ask for help

Help could come from anesthesia, neonatology, colleagues, nursing, etc.

External maneuvers

McRobert's maneuver

McRobert's maneuver is a reasonable initial maneuver as it is easy, safe, and effective. It involves hyperflexion and abduction of the hips, causing cephalad rotation of the symphysis pubis and flattening of the lumbar lordosis, which frees the impacted shoulder.[1] Use of this maneuver doubles the intrauterine pressure developed by contractions alone.[4] By bringing the uterus closer to the diaphragm, the maneuver possibly increases the efficiency of pushing. McRobert's maneuver is effective in resolving shoulder dystocia in about 60–80% of cases.

Suprapubic pressure

Pressure, usually with the fist, is exerted on the symphysis pubis to dislodge the impacted anterior shoulder.

Internal maneuvers

Shoulder rotation

Rubin's maneuver (Figure 21.1):[5] Adduction of either the anterior (usually) or posterior shoulder can achieve manual 'disimpaction' of the anterior shoulder from under the

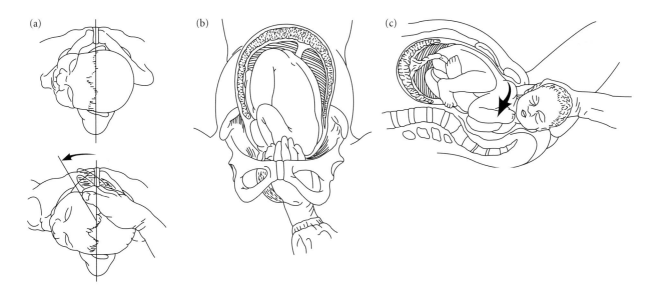

Figure 21.1
Rubin's maneuver. (a) and (b) Pressure is exerted on the posterior surface of the most accessible part of the shoulder to facilitate abduction and disimpaction of the anterior shoulder. (c) Further rotation and adduction toward the fetal chest reduces the bisacromial diameter and results in the movement of the shoulders in a transverse position, facilitating passage of the anterior side of the shoulder beneath the pubic arch. (Reproduced from Ramsey et al,[5] with permission)

symphysis pubis, if space permits the insertion of the hand/fingers.

Wood's corkscrew maneuver (Figure 21.2):[5] Abduction of fetal shoulders through pressure exerted on the anterior surface of the posterior shoulder can facilitate rotation of the impacted anterior shoulder to an oblique position and subsequently into the posterior pelvis, while the posterior shoulder comes into the anterior pelvis.

Delivery of posterior arm

The posterior arm is (internally) flexed at the elbow and gently extracted from hand to shoulder.

Episiotomy

Episiotomy is not absolutely necessary, but might be helpful, especially to perform the internal maneuvers just described.

'All fours'

In one study, placing the patient in an 'all-fours' position resolved 83% of cases of shoulder dystocia.[6]

Clavicle fracture

Intentional fracture of the fetal clavicle, preferably performed 'in-to-out' (e.g. trying to avoid fetal vessel or lung injury).

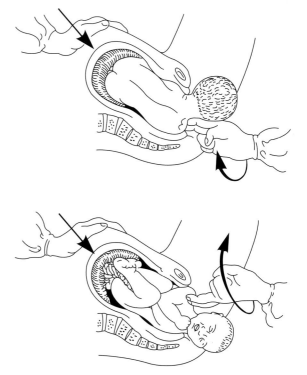

Figure 21.2
Wood's corkscrew maneuver. Initial pressure exerted on the anterior surface of the posterior shoulder facilitates rotation of the posterior shoulder anteriorly (upper). With concurrent synchronized downward pressure, the shoulder 'screws' though the maternal pelvis, disimpacting the previously impacted shoulder (lower). (Reproduced from Ramsey et al,[5] with permission)

Table 21.2	*Documentation in cases of shoulder dystocia*

- Date and time note
- Time of delivery of head
- Record case as shoulder dystocia
- Which shoulder was anterior (right or left)
- Maneuvers used, in order (see Table 21.1)
- Episiotomy (yes or no, and which type); lacerations
- Time of delivery of shoulders
- Duration of shoulder dystocia (difference between time of head and shoulder deliveries)
- Birth weight
- Apgar score (at 1, 5, and 10 minutes)
- Umbilical artery pH (recommended)
- Movement of neonatal arms in delivery room (which and how much)
- Neonatology personnel present or time of arrival
- Destination nursery (special or not)
- Estimated blood loss (ml)
- Anesthesia (type)
- Who was present at delivery?
- Postpartum counseling to mother/family
- Any other data or comments

Cephalic replacement (Zavanelli maneuver)[7]

If all above maneuvers have failed, an attempt can be made at gently pushing the head back into the uterus, and delivering by cesarean section.

Symphisiotomy[8]

If all above maneuvers have failed, a scalpel can be used to separate the cartilage of the pubis symphysis to enlarge the pelvis and facilitate vaginal delivery.

Fundal pressure should be **avoided**, as it may worsen shoulder dystocia (impaction of shoulder).

Anesthesia

An anesthesiologist should be present to ensure adequate analgesia, and prompt preparation for cesarean delivery if needed.

Postpartum

It is important to **document all maneuvers** used in detail, and time from delivery of head to delivery of shoulders (most prognostic variable for neonatal outcome) (Table 21.2). Open and honest communication with the mother and family after delivery is recommended.

Neonatal/infant follow-up

Table 21.3 describes the most common palsies associated with shoulder dystocia. Erb's palsy is by far the most common, and the one with the best prognosis. Erb's palsy is caused by excessive widening of the head–shoulder angle. Occasionally, an Erb's palsy can occur on the posterior shoulder, via impaction on the sacral promontory. Prolonged intrauterine maladaptation can result even in total brachial plexus palsy. The lower plexus nerves can instead be injured by the force applied to the arm in abduction or posterior rotation, but not by more violent traction than that which can produce an Erb's palsy.[9] In fact **in only about 50% of cases of neonatal brachial plexus palsies is shoulder dystocia present**, since the stretching of the nerves occurs because of internal disproportional descent of the head and body of the fetus while the anterior (sometimes posterior) shoulder does not move.[2,10] Over 90% of neonates with Erb's palsy with shoulder dystocia recover within 1 year, with most recovery already evident at 3–6 months. Erb's palsy without shoulder dystocia has only a 60% recovery rate, and in about 68% of cases involves the posterior shoulder. Only about 40% of babies with Klumpke's palsy recover by 1 year. If permanent injury (5–8%) occurs, there is insufficient evidence to assess if surgery is effective.

Table 21.3	*Palsies associated with shoulder dystocia*		
Palsy	Description	Level	Frequency (%)
Erb's palsy (also known as Erb–Duchenne palsy)	Paralysis of flexion, abduction, internal and external rotation of the forearm	C5, C6	>98
Klumpke's palsy	Paralysis of the thumb, fingers, and pronation of the forearm	C8, T1	<1
Complete brachial plexus palsy	Both Erb's palsy and Klumpke's palsy	C5, T1	<1

References

1. American College of Obstetricians and Gynecologists. Shoulder dystocia. ACOG Practice Bulletin No. 40, Obstet Gynecol 2002; 105: 1045–9. [review]

2. Gherman RB, Ouzounian JG, Goodwin TM. Brachial plexus palsy: an in utero injury? Am J Obstet Gynecol 1999; 180: 1303–7. [review]

3. Gonik B, Walker A, Grimm M. Mathematical modeling of forces associated with shoulder dystocia: a comparison of endogenous and exogenous sources. Am J Obstet Gynecol 2000; 182: 689–91. [III]

4. Buhimschi CS, Buhimschi IA, Malinow A, Weiner CP. Use of McRoberts' position during delivery and increase in pushing efficiency. Lancet 2001; 358: 470–1. [II–2]

5. Ramsey PS, Ramin KD, Field CS, Rayburn WF. Shoulder dystocia; rotation maneuvers revisited. J Reprod Med 2000; 45: 85–8. [III]

6. Bruner JP, Drummond SB, Meenan AL, Gaskin IM. All-fours maneuver for reducing shoulder dystocia during labor. J Reprod Med 1998; 43: 439–43. [II–3]

7. Sandberg EC. The Zavanelli maneuver: 12 years of recorded experience. Obstet Gynecol 1999; 93: 312–17. [review]

8. Bjorklund K. Minimally invasive surgery for obstructed labour: a review of symphisiotomy during the twentieth century (including 5000 cases). Br J Obstet Gynaecol 2002; 109: 236–48. [review]

9. Jennett RJ, Tarby TJ, Krauss RL. Erb's palsy contrasted with Klumpke's and total palsy: different mechanisms are involved. Am J Obstet Gynecol 2002; 186: 1216–20. [II–3]

10. Sandmire HF, DeMott RK. Erb's palsy: concepts of causation. Obstet Gynecol 2000; 95: 940–2. [III]

22

Abnormal third stage of labor*

Julie T Crawford, and Jorge E Tolosa

KEY POINTS

- Adequate physical examination, intravenous access, anesthesia and nursing support are important for third-stage complications.
- Misoprostol, in particular rectally, is helpful even as first agent for treatment of primary postpartum hemorrhage (PPH).
- Oxytocin IV can be used as a uterotonic for PPH.
- There is insufficient evidence to assess all other interventions for PPH.
- Umbilical vein injection of oxytocin, or prostaglandin $F_{2\alpha}$, or sulprostone IV increase delivery of placenta in cases of retained placenta.
- There is insufficient evidence to assess interventions for uterine inversion.

POSTPARTUM HEMORRHAGE (PPH)

Definitions

Primary postpartum hemorrhage

Blood loss at delivery within 24 hours exceeding:
- Vaginal delivery: >500 ml (≤500 ml is considered physiological)
- Cesarean delivery: >1000 ml (≤1000 ml is considered physiological).

Secondary postpartum hemorrhage

Excessive blood loss >24 hours and <12 weeks postpartum.

Incidence

About 3% of all births. About 500 000 women die annually across the world from causes related to pregnancy and childbirth, of which one-quarter are caused by one complication of the third stage of labor, i.e. primary PPH.[1] In the developing world, the risk of maternal death from PPH is approximately 1 in 1000 deliveries, while in developed countries it is about 1 in 100 000 deliveries. In developed countries, <2% of postnatal women are admitted to hospital with secondary PPH, half of them undergoing uterine surgical evacuation; in developing countries, PPH is a significant contributor to maternal death.

Etiology

- Lack of efficient uterine contraction (uterine atony) – commonest cause of primary PPH.
- Retained parts of the placenta.
- Vaginal or cervical lacerations.
- Uterine rupture – rare.
- Clotting disorders, uterine inversion, or rupture – extremely rare.

Risk factors

Risk factors for primary PPH include first pregnancy, maternal obesity, a large baby, twin pregnancy, prolonged or augmented labor, and antepartum hemorrhage. High multiparity does not appear to be a strong risk factor, either in high- or low-income countries, even after controlling for maternal age. Despite the identification of risk factors, primary PPH often occurs unpredictably in low-risk women.

Complications

Hypovolemic shock, disseminated intravascular coagulation (DIC), renal failure, hepatic failure, adult respiratory distress syndrome, and death.

*Comprises postpartum hemorrhage, retained placenta, and uterine inversion (see also Chapter 8).

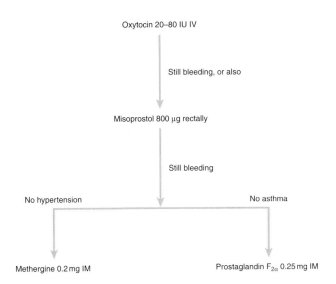

Oxytocin 20–80 IU IV

Still bleeding, or also

Misoprostol 800 µg rectally

Still bleeding

No hypertension   No asthma

Methergine 0.2 mg IM   Prostaglandin F$_{2\alpha}$ 0.25 mg IM

Figure 22.1
Suggested management of uterotonic agents for primary postpartum hemorrhage.

Management

Primary postpartum hemorrhage

- Obtain help (multidisciplinary approach).
- Vigorous **uterine massage** until firm.
- Identify and **repair** any vaginal and cervical **lacerations**. Place initial suture above the apex. Ensure adequate exposure; if necessary, transfer patient to surgical suite.
- **Manually explore the uterus**; ensure adequate intravenous (IV) access.
- Laboratory tests: complete blood count with platelet concentration, blood type, antibody screen, fibrinogen, fibrin split products, prothrombin time, and partial prothrombin time.
- Administer **uterotonic drugs** (Figure 22.1):
  1. Oxytocin 20–80 IU in 1000 ml of normal saline (NS), fast IV drip, and/or
  2. Misoprostol 800–1000 µg rectally
  3. Methergine 0.2 mg intramuscular (IM) (if evidence of hypertension do not administer) every 2–4 hours, and/or
  4. Carboprost tromethamine (Hemabate; prostaglandin F$_{2\alpha}$ [PGF$_{2\alpha}$]) 0.25 mg IM every 15–90 minutes. Maximum dose is 2 mg (do not administer if asthma).

Rectal misoprostol is a useful 'first-line' drug for the treatment of **PPH**. Compared with a combination of IM syntometrine injection and oxytocin infusion, **rectal misoprostol 800 µg** is associated with a statistically significant **reduction in the number of women who continued to bleed after the intervention and those who required medical co-interventions to control the bleeding**.[2] There is no significant difference between the two groups regarding surgical interventions to control intractable hemorrhage, including hysterectomy, internal iliac artery ligation, and/or uterine packing. There no specific trials on oxytocin, or methergine or PGF$_{2\alpha}$ vs placebo or vs each other for treatment of PPH. There is insufficient evidence to identify the best drug combinations, route, and dose for the treatment of PPH, or to evaluate the effects of rectal misoprostol on maternal mortality, serious maternal morbidity, or hysterectomy rates in women with PPH.

- Place Foley catheter to monitor urine output.
- If retained placental products are suspected, perform uterine curettage.
- Transfusion of blood and blood products, as necessary.
- There are no randomized controlled trials (RCTs) on the following techniques (either against placebo or against each other):
  - Uterine tamponade: packing, Foley catheter, or Sengstaken-Blakemore tube.
  - If stable: consider selective pelvic arterial embolization or ballooning. Fever, contrast media renal toxicity, and leg ischemia are rare but reported complications of this procedure.
  - If unstable or failed management as above, consider surgical techniques: suture bleeding sites; uterine artery ligation; B-Lynch stitch for uterine compression; or hysterectomy.
  - If intractable bleeding, consider hemostatic drugs: factor VIIa and tranexamic acid.

Secondary postpartum hemorrhage

No information is available from RCTs to inform the management of women with secondary PPH.

RETAINED PLACENTA

Definition

The placenta is undelivered at ≥ 30 minutes after delivery despite active management of the third stage.

Incidence

The incidence of retained placenta is **0.5–1%**.

Etiology

- Preterm birth: incidence is inversely proportional to gestational age.
- Cord avulsion: incidence is 3% with controlled cord traction, especially in inexperienced operators.
- Placenta accreta (be aware of risk factors – see Chapter 24).

Complications

Hemorrhage, infection, or genital tract trauma.

Management

- Provide adequate anesthesia.
- Attempt manual extraction.
- Once placental margin is identified, gently peel the placenta from the uterine wall and remove it. May consider ultrasound to ascertain if placental removal is complete.
- Palpate and massage the fundus until firm.
- **Umbilical vein injection of oxytocin (10 or 20 IU in 1 or 2 ml)** in NS (18–19 ml) is effective in the management of retained placenta at 20–30 minutes by **decreasing the need for manual placental removal** compared with NS alone or expectant management.[3] No discernible difference is detected in length of third stage of labor, blood loss, hemoglobin, change in hemoglobin, blood transfusion, curettage, infection, hospital stay, fever, abdominal pain, and oxytocin augmentation. Umbilical vein injection of NS plus oxytocin compared with umbilical vein injection of plasma expander is associated with higher, but not statistically significant, incidence of manual removal of placenta, and no difference in blood loss in one small trial.[3] Compared with expectant management, **umbilical vein injection of NS alone** does **not** show any significant difference in the incidence of manual removal of the placenta, and should not be used.[3]
- Umbilical vein injection of **$PGF_{2\alpha}$ 20 mg in 20 ml NS is more effective than even 30 IU of oxytocin** in preventing need for manual placental removal, but no difference is observed in blood loss, fever, abdominal pain, and oxytocin augmentation in a small trial.[3] There are no significant differences in manual removal between NS plus prostaglandin and NS plus oxytocin.
- **Sulprostone**, a synthetic prostaglandin E_2, given as 250 µg IV over 30 minutes, **reduces the need for manual removal of the placenta** by 49% (retained placenta expelled in 52% of sulprostone cases vs 18% of placebo controls), and is associated with lower blood loss by avoiding manual removal of placenta.[4]
- There is insufficient data to support or refute prophylactic antibiotics.
- If continued bleeding, see above for management of PPH.
- Consider diagnosis of placenta accreta.

UTERINE INVERSION
Definition

Collapse of the uterine fundus into the endometrial cavity.

Incidence

Incidence varies widely, but is approximately 1 in 2500 deliveries.

Risks

Excess cord traction, fundal pressure, fundal cord insertions, and abnormal placentations.

Management

There are no RCTs to guide management of uterine inversion. Suggested management:

- Summon anesthesia and nursing staff.
- Provide large-bore access and IV fluid therapy.
- Withhold uterotonic agents.
- To decrease bleeding, avoid separating the placenta.
- Consider pharmacological uterine relaxation:
  - magnesium sulfate IV bolus
  - terbutaline IV 0.25 mg subcutaneously × 1
  - nitroglycerin 50–500 µg orally or by anesthesia.
- Manual manipulation of the uterus: reposition the portion of the uterus that inverted last. Grasp the uterus with palm with fingers posteriorly and the thumb anteriorly.
- Rare – surgical intervention (laparotomy) if cannot correct by vaginal manipulation alone:
  - Huntington procedure – clamps are placed on the round ligaments 2 cm deep in the inversion and gentle upward traction applied. Repeat clamping as necessary.
  - Haultain procedure – an incision is made in the posterior portion of the inversion ring to increase its size and to reposition the uterus.
- Uterotonic agents when uterus repositioned:
  - Oxytocin 20–40 IU/L NS IV, Methergine 0.2 mg IM every 6 hours as needed, or Hemabate 0.25 mg IM repeated every 25–60 minutes as needed.
- Treat PPH or retained placenta as mentioned above.

References

1. American College of Obstetricians and Gynecologists. Postpartum hemorrhage. ACOG Educational Bulletin No. 243. American College of Obstetricians and Gynecologists; Washington, DC: 1998. [review]
2. Lokugamage AU, Sullivan KR, Niculescu I et al. A randomized study comparing rectally administered misoprostol versus syntometrine combined with an oxytocin infusion for the cessation of primary post partum hemorrhage. Acta Obstet Gynecol Scand 2001; 80(9): 835–9. [RCT, n = 64 women with PPH > 500 ml. Syntometrine IM + syntocinon IV + 4 placebo tablets per rectum vs 800 µg (4 tablets) misoprostol per rectum + a placebo NS 2 ml IM + placebo crystalloid IV infusion]
3. Carroli G, Bergel E. Umbilical vein injection for management of retained placenta. Cochrane Database Syst Rev 2007; 1. [12 RCTs, n => 1000]
4. van Beekhuizen HJ, de Groot AN, DeBoo T et al. Sulprostone reduces the need for manual removal of the placenta in patients with retained placenta: a randomized controlled trial. Am J Obstet Gynecol 2006; 194: 446–50. [RCT, n = 103]

23

Post-term pregnancy

Vincenzo Berghella

KEY POINTS

- Post-term pregnancy is defined as a **singleton** pregnancy that has lasted until **≥ 42weeks or ≥ 294 days.**
- **Complications** include, for the baby, increased incidences of **meconium aspiration, intrauterine infection, oligo hydramnios, macrosomia, non-reassuring fetal heart testing (NRFHT), low umbilical artery pH, low 5-minute Apgar score, dysmaturity syndrome,** and **perinatal mortality;** for the mother, increased risk of **labor dystocia, perineal injury,** and **cesarean delivery.**
- **Pregnancies with risk factors** such as maternal (e.g. hypertension, diabetes, etc.) and fetal (growth restriction, etc.) diseases necessitate special management, as described in the **pertinent guidelines.**
- **Prevention** of post-term pregnancy can be effectively achieved with **routine early pregnancy (< 20 weeks) ultrasound** and with **stripping of membranes** starting at 38 or 41 weeks.
- There is insufficient evidence to assess the efficacy of antepartum testing for pregnancies after their due date, but twice-weekly fetal testing starting at 41 weeks with the non-stress test (NST), or NST and amniotic fluid volume (AFV), or biophysical profile (BPP) have been proposed.
- At ≥ 41 weeks, even if the cervix is still unfavorable, **routine induction of labor reduces perinatal mortality,** mainly as a result of the **decrease in fetal deaths.** Routine induction of labor is associated with a **decrease in the incidence of cesarean delivery** in women who are nulliparous, ≥ 41 weeks, induced with prostaglandins, or delivered in a center with a cesarean delivery rate >10%.
- In women with a prior cesarean delivery, induction of labor is associated with an increase in uterine rupture.

Diagnosis/definition

Post-term pregnancy is defined as a pregnancy that has lasted until ≥ 42 weeks, or ≥ 294 days, or ≥ 14 days after the due date (estimated date of confinement or EDC).[1]

Prolonged pregnancy can be defined as a pregnancy that has lasted until ≥ 41 weeks, or ≥ 287 days, or ≥ 7 days after the EDC.[2] The term postdates can signify a pregnancy that lasted until ≥ 40 weeks, or ≥ 280 days, but is often defined differently in the literature and should be probably avoided.[1] All these definitions may have been differently described in the literature, but it is important to be clear when using these terms that everyone involved understands their meaning. These definitions and this chapter's guideline pertain to **singleton gestations.** For multiple gestations, please refer to Chapter 38 in *Maternal–Fetal Evidence Based Guidelines.*

Epidemiology/incidence

The incidence of post-term pregnancy is about 7%.[1]

Etiology/basic pathophysiology

The most frequent cause of post-term pregnancy is an error in dating.[1] See Chapter 3 for accurate dating criteria and ultrasound benefits, as well as below.

Risk factors/associations

Poor (wrong) dating; prior post-term pregnancy; nulliparity; long (> 28 days) cycles without early ultrasound; placental sulfatase deficiency; anencephaly; male fetus.

Complications

Perinatal

Meconium aspiration, intrauterine infection, oligohydramnios, macrosomia, non-reassuring fetal heart testing (NRFHT), low umbilical artery pH, and **low 5-minute Apgar score** have all been associated with post-term pregnancy. **Perinatal mortality** (fetal and neonatal deaths) is twice as high at ≥ 42 weeks and 6 times as high at ≥ 43 weeks compared with 39–40 weeks.[1] **Dysmaturity syndrome** is present in about 20% of neonates born post-term, and has some of the characteristics above, as well as possibly hypoglycemia, seizures, from uteroplacental insufficiency, and unclear long-term outcome but increased risk of infant death.[1]

Maternal

Women giving birth post-term are at increased risk of **labor dystocia, perineal injury,** and **cesarean delivery** with their complications.[1]

Pregnancy considerations

Every woman should be counseled early in pregnancy that up to 50% of gestations, especially in nulliparous women, last until past the due date (EDC). This is physiological, and natural for humans. The incidence of fetal death is significantly higher than that of neonatal death at ≥ 283 days (≥ 40 weeks and 3 days).[3] In large series, delivery at 38 weeks is associated with the lowest risk of perinatal death, but the risk of perinatal death is < 1–2/1000 up to 41 weeks and 6 days.[4] **It is important to identify risk factors such as maternal (e.g. hypertension, diabetes, etc.) and fetal (growth restriction, etc.) diseases that necessitate special management,** as described in the pertinent guidelines.

Management (Figure 23.1)

Preconception counseling

Women with prior post-term pregnancy are at increased risk for recurrent post-term pregnancy. Prevention strategies should be discussed.

Work-up

Early ultrasound < 20 weeks of gestation can prevent post-term pregnancy, and therefore the need for induction.

Prevention

Routine early ultrasound to reduce post-term pregnancies

Compared with no routine early ultrasound, **routine early pregnancy (< 20 weeks) ultrasound reduces by 32–39% the incidence of post-term pregnancy and of induction**

for post-term pregnancy[5,6] (see also Chapter 3). Accurate assessment of gestational age is extremely important in improving perinatal morbidity and mortality.

Stripping of membranes

Compared with no sweeping (stripping), **sweeping of the membranes,** performed weekly as a general policy in women at term (e.g. weekly starting at 38 weeks), **is associated with reduced duration of pregnancy** and **reduced frequency of pregnancy continuing beyond 41 weeks and 42 weeks.**[2,7] To avoid one formal induction of labor, sweeping of membranes must be performed in 8 women. **Risk of cesarean section and maternal or neonatal infection is similar. Serial sweeping of membranes starting at 41 weeks every 48 hours** also **decreases the risk of post-term pregnancy** from 41% to 23%, with efficacy both in nulliparous and multiparous women.[8] Discomfort during vaginal examination and other adverse effects (bleeding, irregular contractions) are more frequently reported by women allocated to sweeping, but are not associated with complications (see also Chapter 17).

Breast and nipple stimulation to reduce post-term pregnancies

Breast and nipple stimulation daily starting at 39 weeks has not been sufficiently studied to ascertain safety, but it does appear to reduce the incidence of post-term pregnancy by 48%.[9,10]

Antepartum testing

There are insufficient data to assess the best mode of fetal monitoring after the EDC, as there are no trials to assess the effect of antepartum testing on these pregnancies compared with no testing. Since fetal death rates incrementally increase after the EDC, it seems reasonable to test fetuses to assure well-being, especially at ≥ 41 weeks.[1,3,4] The most used options include the non-stress test (NST) (also called cardiography), biophysical profile (BPP), and modified BPP. Modified BPP includes NST and ultrasound measurement of maximum pool depth of amniotic fluid volume (AFV). Other tests have been described, with even less evidence for efficacy. Doppler ultrasound of any vessel, including the umbilical artery, is not effective in the management of post-term pregnancy. Compared with fetal monitoring using **NST and AFV,** computerized cardiotocography, amniotic fluid index, fetal breathing, fetal tone, and fetal body movements were associated with increased incidence of inductions and similar outcomes in a small trial in women ≥ 42 weeks.[11] At ≥ 41 weeks, **twice-weekly testing** is recommended,[1] but is not based on trials (see also Chapter 51 of *Maternal–Fetal Evidence Based Guidelines*).

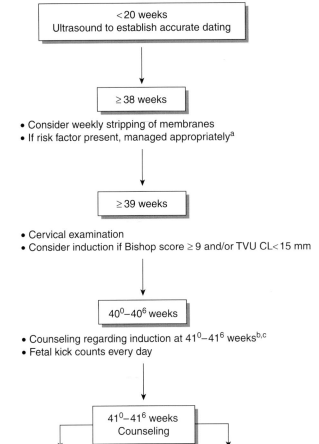

Figure 23.1
Management of post-term pregnancy. TVU, transvaginal ultrasound; CL, cervical length; 2×/wk, twice per week; NST, non-stress test; AFV, amniotic fluid volume assessment; NRFHT, non-reassuring fetal heart testing.

[a]Risk factor examples include hypertension, diabetes mellitus, fetal growth restriction (FGR), multiple gestation, etc. Please see guideline (chapter) pertinent to specific risk factor for management.
[b]Suggest induction for all women between 41⁰ and 41⁶ weeks.
[c]See Chapter 17 for effective induction management.

Interventions

Favorable cervix:≥ 41weeks

There is insufficient evidence to assess any interventions in the woman at ≥41 weeks (or even earlier) with a favorable cervix – Bishop score ≥9 or transvaginal ultrasound cervical length (TVU CL) <15 mm – as no trials have focused on or included these pregnancies in sufficient numbers. As the complications of induction in these women, especially if multiparous, are minimal to absent, it seems reasonable to offer at least, if not recommend, **induction.**[1]

Unfavorable cervix: routine induction of labor at ≥ 41 weeks

Compared with expectant management, **routine induction of labor at ≥41 weeks reduces perinatal mortality** by 80%.[6] This benefit is from the effect of induction of labor after 41 weeks and the **decrease in fetal deaths**. About 500 inductions must be performed to prevent one perinatal death. The use of analgesia, NRFHT, operative vaginal or cesarean delivery rates, and other neonatal outcome measures are similar with induction or expectant management. Routine induction of labor is associated with a **decrease in the incidence of cesarean delivery** in women who are nulliparous, ≥41 weeks, induced with prostaglandins, or delivered in a center with a cesarean delivery rate >10%. Routine induction is more cost-effective than expectant management. Women at ≥41weeks are more satisfied with induction than expectant management[12] (see also Chapter 17 for other induction risks and benefits, as well as management of induction).

In **women with a prior cesarean delivery**, induction is associated with a higher incidence of uterine rupture, especially in the nulliparous woman with an unfavorable cervix. Therefore, if the woman desires vaginal birth after cesarean (VBAC), it seems reasonable to wait until 40–41 weeks for spontaneous labor, but then a repeat cesarean delivery can be offered to avoid the induction risks.[1]

References

1. American College of Obstetricians and Gynecologists. Management of postterm pregnancy. ACOG Practice Bulletin No. 55. Obstet Gynecol 2004; 104: 639–46. [review]
2. Berghella V, Rogers RA, Lescale K. Stripping of membranes as a safe method to reduce prolonged pregnancies. Obstet Gynecol 1996; 87:(6): 927–9. [RCT, n=142]
3. Divon MY, Ferber A, Sanderson M, Nisell H, Westgren M. A functional definition of prolonged pregnancy based on daily fetal and neonatal mortality rates. Ultrasound Obstet Gynecol 2004; 23: 423–6. [II–2, n=656134]
4. Smith GCS. Life-table analysis of the risk of perinatal death at term and post term in singleton pregnancies. Am J Obstet Gynecol 2001; 184: 489–96. [II–2, n=700878]
5. Neilson JP. Ultrasound for fetal assessment in early pregnancy. Cochrane Database Syst Rev; 2007; 1.[meta-analysis: 9 RCTs, n=>24000]
6. Crowley P. Interventions for preventing or improving the outcome of delivery at or beyond term. Cochrane Database Syst Rev 2007; 1. [meta-analysis: 26 RCTs (variable quality), n=>25000; early ultrasound: 4 RCTs, n=21776; induction at ≥41weeks: 19 RCTs, n=7925]

7. Boulvain M, Stan C, Irion O. Membrane sweeping for induction of labour. Cochrane Database Syst Rev 2007; 1. [meta-analysis: 22 RCTs, n=2797]

8. de Miranda E, van der Bom JG, Bonsel GJ, Rosendaal FR. Membrane sweeping and prevention of post-term pregnancy in low-risk pregnancies: a randomized controlled trial. Br J Obstet Gynaecol 2006; 113: 402–8. [RCT, n=742]

9. Elliott JP, Flaherty JF. The use of breast stimulation to prevent post-date pregnancy. Am J Obstet Gynecol 1984; 149: 628–32. [RCT]

10. Kadar N, Tapp A, Wong A. The influence of nipple stimulation at term on the duration of pregnancy. J Perinatol 1990; 10: 164–6. [RCT]

11. Alfirevic Z, Walkinshaw SA. A randomised controlled trial of simple compared with complex antenatal fetal monitoring after 42 weeks of gestation. Br J Obstet Gynaecol 1995; 102: 638–43. [RCT]

12. Hannah ME, Hannah WJ, Hellman J et al; Canadian Multicenter Post-Term Pregnancy Trial Group. Induction of labour as compared with serial antenatal monitoring in post-term pregnancy. A randomized controlled trial. N Engl J Med 1992; 326: 1587–92. [RCT, n=3407]

24

Placenta previa, placenta accreta, and vasa previa[*]

Vincenzo Berghella

KEY POINTS

- Total (complete) placenta previa is defined as a placenta that covers the internal os. **Marginal (incomplete) placenta previa** is defined as a placenta that comes within 0.1–2.0 cm of the internal os but does not cover it. **Low-lying placenta** is defined as a placenta that comes between 2.1–3.5 cm from internal os.
- **Placental location should be assessed any time an ultrasound is performed.** If placenta previa is suspected, a transvaginal ultrasound (TVU) should be performed.
- The risk of previa at delivery depends on several factors, especially gestational age (GA) at detection, how many millimeters the placenta overlaps the internal os or its distance from it, prior cesarean delivery, etc. **Most previa diagnosed before the third trimester resolve.**
- Women who have the inferior edge of the placenta ≥ 1 cm from the internal os at around 20 weeks do not require further ultrasounds for placental location.
- All patients with suspected placenta previa (i.e. inferior placental edge < 1 cm from the internal os or overlying the os by < 2.5 cm at around 20 weeks) should be **rescanned at least once** between 32 and 35 weeks' gestation to assess for persistence of true placenta previa. **Measuring distance from placental edge to internal os in the third trimester can help estimate the risk of bleeding with trial of labor.**
- For patients with low-lying placenta or marginal previa, velamentous cord insertion, succenturiate lobed or bilobed placenta, **vasa previa should be excluded by TVU.**
- All patients with **prior cesarean delivery and placenta previa** need at least some comment on signs (see Table 24.4) on ultrasound regarding the degree of concern for **placenta accreta.**
- Women with placenta previa and either **hemodynamic instability; other causes of bleeding; ≥ 3 episodes of** bleeding; other obstetric complications; serious maternal medical disorders; lack of telephone at home; or lack of immediate transport from home are usually managed in the hospital.
- The best GA for delivery of a woman with placenta previa is unknown, but most authors recommend around **36–38 weeks.**
- Women with a **complete placenta previa** should be delivered by **cesarean.** If the placenta is **within 1–2 cm of the internal os, a cesarean delivery should be offered.** In women with the **placenta ≥ 2 cm from the internal os, a trial of labor** should be encouraged.
- **Risk factors for placenta accreta** include **prior cesarean delivery, placenta previa, prior uterine surgery, prior myomectomy, prior dilatation and evacuation (D&E), Asherman's syndrome, submucosal leiomyomata, maternal age ≥ 35 years old, multiparity, and smoking.**
- **Complications** of placenta accreta include **hysterectomy, injury to other organs, blood transfusion, disseminated intravascular coagulation (DIC), infection, death,** as well as **preterm birth (PTB) and small for gestational age (SGA).**
- There are **no trials** to assess any interventions in the management of placenta accreta. There are benefits and risks for all three main approaches, which are **attempts at spontaneous placental delivery, planned hysterectomy,** and **expectant/medical management.** Although an attempt at placental delivery is a common approach, planned hysterectomy is associated with the least complications and should be offered if the diagnosis is highly suspected and the woman does not desire further fertility. Expectant/medical management has been insufficiently studied, and should be considered only when the woman wants to preserve her fertility and no active uterine bleeding is present.

---

[*]For normal or abnormal third stage, including postpartum hemorrhage, retained placenta, and uterine inversion, see Chapters 8 and 22.

PLACENTA PREVIA

Diagnoses/definitions (established by transvaginal ultrasound – TVU)

- Total (complete) placenta previa – placenta covers the internal os.
- Marginal (incomplete) placenta previa – placenta edge comes within 0.1–2.0 cm of the internal os but does not cover it.
- Low-lying placenta – placenta comes between 2.1 and 3.5 cm from internal os.

The use of the term **partial placenta previa** should be discontinued. Total placenta previa can cover the internal os symmetrically or asymmetrically. Asymmetric placenta previa may resolve in the third trimester and evolve into a marginal previa. Many studies have differing definitions for all of these terms.

Symptoms

About two-thirds of complete placenta previas at delivery have antepartum vaginal bleeding. Therefore about 33% do not have any symptoms before possibly catastrophic complications at delivery if not previously identified by ultrasound.

Epidemiology/incidence

The incidence of placenta previa at term is **0.5–2%**. The incidence of placenta previa is much higher earlier in gestation, but most of these cases resolve, especially when detected in the first or second trimester (Table 24.1).

Risk factors/associations

Prior cesarean delivery, any other uterine surgery (e.g. dilatation and evacuation [D&E], dilatation and curettage [D&C], hysteroscopy, etc.), multiparity, cocaine abuse.

Complications (Table 24.2)

Preterm birth (PTB) < 37 weeks, neonatal death (1%), antepartum and/or postpartum hemorrhage.[1]

Management

Principles

Placental location should be assessed any time an ultrasound is performed. If placenta previa is suspected, a **TVU should be performed.** A change in the relative position of the placenta in respect to the internal os (**placental migration**) is observed in all cases, with some estimating this

Table 24.1 *Prediction of previa persistence until delivery according to gestational age at ultrasound detection, type of previa, and prior cesarean delivery* [2, 4–8]

	GA at detection					
	11–14 weeks	15–19 weeks	20–23 weeks	24–27 weeks	28–31 weeks	32–35 weeks
Incidence (%)	42	10	4	3	2	1
Incomplete previa,[a] no prior cesarean (%)	NA	6	11	12	35	39
Incomplete previa, prior cesarean (%)	NA	7	50	40	38	63
Complete previa, no prior cesarean (%)	NA	20	45	56	89	90
Complete previa, prior cesarean (%)	NA	41	73	84	88	89
Overall	<1	3–12	14–34	49	62	73
Degree of overlap (mm) and persistence of previa (%)	≥15–25 mm: 5	≥25 mm: 40	≥25 mm: 90–100	≥20 mm: 90–100	NA	NA

[a]Incomplete previa defined[4] as placental inferior edge partially covering or reaching the margins of the internal os. GA, gestational age; NA, not available.

Table 24.2	*Complications of placenta previa*[1]			
Placenta	PTB < 37 weeks (%)	Antepartum hemorrhage (%)	Cesarean delivery (%)	Postpartum hemorrhage (%)
Complete previa	33	57	100	12
Marginal previa	23	48	90	5
Low-lying placenta	8	28	37	8

PTB, preterm birth.

migration at an average of 0.5 cm/week in marginal and low-lying placentas.[2] The placenta does not in fact migrate. The apparent upward movement is due to the growth and development of the lower uterine segment. Another concurrent explanation may be that in some cases part of the placenta overlying the internal os undergoes atrophy. This may also lead to vasa previa and/or a succenturiate lobe.

Work-up
Pelvic examination

Because of the reliability of ultrasound for diagnosis of previa, the technique of double set-up examination is unnecessary in most cases. However, if employed, double set-up examination should be performed in the operating room (OR) with the patient prepped and draped for cesarean delivery.

Ultrasound

Transvaginal ultrasound is the gold standard test for the diagnosis of placenta previa. It is very safe in these women.[3] The risk of previa at delivery depends on several factors (see above), especially gestational age (GA) at detection, how many millimeters the placenta overlaps the internal os or its distance from it, prior cesarean delivery, etc. **Most previa diagnosed before the third trimester resolve** (see Table 24.1).[2,4–8] Interestingly, pregnancies with 'resolved' placenta previa or even low-lying placenta are still at increased risk for third trimester bleeding, uterine atony, hemorrhage, cesarean delivery, and prolonged hospitalization.[9]

Women who have the inferior edge of the placenta ≥ 1 cm **from the internal os at around 20 weeks do not require further ultrasounds for placental location** as they are exceedingly unlikely to have placenta previa at delivery if the ultrasound was done accurately. Women who have the inferior placental edge **overlapping the internal os by ≥ 25 mm at around 20 weeks** have been reported to almost **always have persistence of previa even by term**[10] (see Table 24.1), and therefore may also not benefit from ultrasound follow-up, as they require cesarean delivery in all cases.[2]

All **patients with suspected placenta previa (i.e. inferior placental edge < 1 cm from the internal os or overlying the os by < 2.5 cm at around 20 weeks) should be rescanned at least once** between **32 and 35 weeks'** gestation to assess for persistence of true placenta previa. **Measuring the distance from the placental edge to internal os in the third trimester can help to estimate the risk of bleeding with trial of labor.**

For **all patients** (especially those with previa), the **placental cord insertion** (PCI) site should be identified. If there is a velamentous cord insertion, serial scans for fetal growth should be ordered.

For patients with succenturiate placental lobes or marginal previa in which the PCI is low or cannot be easily identified, **vasa previa** should be excluded by TVU (see below).

All patients with **prior cesarean delivery and placenta previa** need at least some comment on ultrasound regarding the degree of concern for **placenta accreta** (see below).

Prenatal care

All patients with **total placenta previa** should be on **pelvic rest** (no vaginal penetration). Activity recommendations in women with **marginal previa** should be **individualized** and based on GA, prior bleeding, and the distance between the placenta and the internal os. There is no evidence to support the use of autologous blood donation/transfusion for placenta previa.[11]

Therapy/interventions
Management at home vs hospitalization

Women with **hemodynamic instability, other cause of bleeding, ≥ 3 episodes of bleeding, other obstetric complications, serious maternal medical disorders, lack of telephone at home, and lack of immediate transport from home** have not been studied in a trial in regards to home management, as they are **usually managed in the hospital.**

Home vs hospitalization is obviously associated with about 18.5 reduced days of length of stay in hospital antenatally in a small trial.[12] There is little evidence of any clear advantage or disadvantage to a policy of home vs hospital care, with **similar maternal and fetal outcomes**. The one woman who had a hemorrhage severe enough to require immediate transfusion and delivery was in the home care group. Women with hemodynamic instability, other cause of bleeding, ≥ 3 episodes of bleeding, other obstetric complications, serious maternal medical disorders, lack of telephone at home, and lack of immediate transport from home were excluded from this study.[12]

So after an antenatal bleeding episode related to placenta previa, women may be allowed to go home if they do not have fresh bleeding for a period of 4–7 days after admission, in the absence of the above criteria.

Cervical cerclage

Cervical cerclage does not appear to be an effective intervention for women with placenta previa. Cervical cerclage vs no cerclage is associated with a 4.8 days reduced length of stay in hospital antenatally, reduced risk of PTB < 34 weeks by 55%, of the birth of a baby weighing < 2 kg by 66%, or of having a low 5-minute Apgar score by 81% in two small trials.[13–15] In general, these possible benefits were more evident in the trial of lower methodological quality.

Tocolysis

There is insufficient evidence (no trials) to assess the effect of tocolysis in the management of placenta previa.

Antepartum testing

There are insufficient data to assess the effect of antenatal testing on outcomes.

Delivery

There is insufficient evidence to assess the best timing and mode of delivery for women with different types of placenta previa, with no trials available. Suggestions are based on retrospective cohort studies of limited quality, and should be interpreted cautiously.

Timing: Selected women with placenta previa and vaginal bleeding of < 3 episodes can be managed as outpatients between 24 and 36 weeks. The best GA for delivery of a woman with placenta previa is unknown, but most authors recommend **36–38 weeks** and some consideration for possible fetal lung maturity (FLM) amniocentesis.

Mode: Women with a **complete** (covering the internal os) **placenta previa** should be delivered by **cesarean**.

If the placenta is **within 1 cm of the internal os**, a **cesarean delivery should be offered.**

There are insufficient data to make a firm recommendation if the placenta is **1.1–2.0 cm from the internal os.** A **cesarean delivery can also be offered,** as few women who attempt a vaginal delivery are successful, and may have complications (see Table 24.2).[2] Patients may labor only as long as they have been informed of the increased risks and that the facilities and personnel are available for emergent operative delivery if necessary.

In women with the **placenta ≥ 2 cm from the internal os**, a **trial of labor** should be encouraged. In *low-lying* placenta, when the placenta is at least **2 cm** from the internal os, patients should be encouraged to undergo trial of labor, but need to be informed of the slight increased risks of bleeding and cesarean delivery (see Table 24.2), and should deliver where facilities and personnel are available for emergent operative delivery if necessary.[16] When the distance from the placental edge to the internal os is ≥ 3 cm, there appears to be no increased risk of bleeding, and attempted vaginal delivery should be encouraged.

PLACENTA ACCRETA
Diagnosis/definition

Placenta accreta is defined as a placenta which is abnormally adherent and sometimes invasive to the uterus, due to total or partial **lack of the decidua basalis layer**. The Nitabuch membrane, a fibrinoid layer that separates the deciduas basalis from the placental villi, is imperfectly developed. Unfortunately, the diagnosis is controversial. Postpartum histological examination would require both placenta and uterus, and sampling of the whole interface, conditions that are almost never present. If only the placenta is examined histologically, the specimen is usually in pieces, only a few placental surfaces are sampled, and small areas that might contain myometrial tissue may be missed. So, in cases of clinically suspected placenta accreta, failure to demonstrate adherence of myometrial tissue to the maternal surface of the placenta cannot always be used to exclude this diagnosis.[17] Moreover, incidental finding of placenta accreta at histological examination is not uncommon.[17] The diagnosis of placenta accreta may be suspected by history (especially prior cesarean delivery) or by ultrasound, but it is not 100% accurate by these methods (see below).

Epidemiology/incidence

1/2500 deliveries (and increasing, as cesarean delivery rates increase).

Classification

- Placenta accreta (vera): chorionic villi are attached directly but do not invade the myometrium.
- Placenta increta: placental villi invade the myometrium.
- Placenta percreta: placental villi invade beyond the whole myometrium, into the uterine serosa and possibly into adjacent organs (especially the bladder).

Risk factors/associations

Prior cesarean delivery (Table 24.3).[18] Most morbidity from repeat cesarean delivery derives from accreta and hysterectomy. **Risk factors include placenta previa, prior uterine surgery, prior myomectomy, prior D&Es, Asherman's syndrome, submucosal leiomyomata, maternal age ≥ 35 years old, multiparity, and smoking.**

Complications

- Maternal: **hysterectomy, injury to other organs, blood transfusion, DIC, infection, and death** (<1–7%) (see Table 24.3).
- Perinatal: **PTB and small for gestational age (SGA)**.[19]

Management

There are **no trials** to assess any interventions in the management of placenta accreta.

Work-up

Ultrasonography is the gold standard for antenatal diagnosis of placenta accreta. Ultrasonographic signs of placenta accreta are shown in Table 24.4.[20] It is important to know that even the combinations of all these signs is not 100%

Table 24.3 *Risk of placenta previa and/or accreta (and other complications) according to number of prior cesarean delieveries*[18]

	1st CD	2nd CD	3rd CD	4th CD	5th CD	$\geq$ 6th CD
Previa (%)	6.4	1.3	1.1	2.3	2.3	3.4
Accreta (no previa) (%)	0.03	0.2	0.1	0.8	0.8	4.7
Accreta (previa) (%)	3.3	11	40	61	67	67
Hysterectomy (%)	0.7	0.4	0.9	2.4	3.5	9.0
Blood transfusion (%)	4.0	1.5	2.3	3.7	4.3	15.7
Cystotomy (%)	0.1	0.1	0.3	1.2	1.9	4.5
Ureteral injury (%)	0.03	0.01	0.02	0.07	0.4	1.1
Bowel injury (%)	0.1	0.1	0.1	0.3	0	1.1

CD, cesarean delivery.

Table 24.4 *Ultrasonographic signs of placenta accreta*

Gray-scale signs	Color Doppler signs
Loss of retroplacental hypoechoic zone	Dilated vascular channels with diffuse lacunar flow
Progressive thinning of the retroplacental hypoechoic zone (myometrium) <2 mm	Irregular vascular lakes with focal lacunar flow
Multiple placental lakes	Hypervascularity linking placenta to bladder
Thinning of the uterine serosa–bladder wall complex (percreta)	Dilated vascular channels with pulsatile venous flow over cervix
Elevation of tissue beyond the uterine serosa – extension of the placenta beyond the myometrium (percreta)	Poor vascularity at sites of loss of hypoechoic zone

sensitive and/or specific for the diagnosis for accreta. Most studies report sensitivity, specificity, and positive and negative predictive values of about 80–90%.[20] Three-dimensional and power Doppler ultrasound have been insufficiently studied to be assessed adequately.

Further evaluation of possible placenta accreta includes **magnetic resonance imaging (MRI)** (especially T_2 and short tau inversion recovery [STIR] images), which may be informative, especially for posterior previas and to assess possible bladder involvement.[21] Cystoscopy can be considered in cases where bladder invasion is highly suspected by radiologic studies.

Preparations and plans for delivery

If placenta accreta is suspected, appropriate counseling and preparations should be made. **Multidisciplinary management** is important. Labor and delivery staff should be notified regarding delivery plans and location, as well as **nursing, surgery, anesthesia**, and **neonatology** staff. Interventions have not been tested in any trial, and so each intervention should be discussed with patients, making sure they understand that the interventions have **not** been clearly shown to improve outcomes and their utilization is not considered a 'standard of care.' Complications should be reviewed, as well as approach to management, with consideration of different options: attempt at placental delivery, planned hysterectomy, or expectant management. Additional preventive or therapeutic interventions as described below should be discussed, allowing patient input into management given the lack of trials guiding care.

Preoperative laboratory tests include at least type and crossmatch. Notify **blood bank**: blood products should be available in the OR at the time of the procedure. Consider reserving **cell saver** for the OR. Consider bowel prep: clear liquids day before procedure; Fleets Phospho-soda or Fleets enema are options.

Notification of back-up consultants

Anesthesia: Notify of possible need for massive transfusion, and for central monitoring.

Urology: Notify for possible cystoscopy, with possible placement of ureteral stents in OR pre-procedure, with standby for possible back-up.

CVIR: CardioVascular and Interventional Radiology may be notified for placement of uterine artery catheters and/or balloons or coils/plugs pre-procedure vs standby. This intervention has not been studied in a trial, and even case-control studies do not confirm its efficacy.[22]

Gyn/Oncology: A gyn/oncologist or other experienced pelvic surgeon should be notified as possible back-up.

Delivery

It is advisable to perform the delivery in the **main** OR rather than in Labor and Delivery (L&D) OR. **These cases should be the first scheduled operations of the day**. If done in the L&D OR, expect a long operating time and therefore reserve at least two cesarean delivery slots. The best GA for delivery of a woman with placenta accreta is unknown, but most authors recommend **36–38 weeks** and some consideration for possible FLM amniocentesis. Consider a course of steroids for elective cesarean delivery before 39 weeks. If patient accepts, arrange for two doses to be given 24 hours apart, with the second dose to be administered at least 24 hours before delivery. There are three main approaches to managing placenta accreta after cesarean delivery.

Attempt at delivery of placenta: In many cases, as accreta cannot be confirmed with 100% accuracy by radiological studies, an attempt at spontaneous placental delivery is made. A bladder flap may be beneficial in case a hysterectomy is later necessary. A uterine incision should be made, if possible, away from the placenta, which therefore should be 'mapped' by ultrasound beforehand. If spontaneous placental delivery fails, the operator must decide if either manual placental removal in pieces or hysterectomy is the next intervention, based on several factors, including the degree of invasiveness and amount of bleeding. Areas of the placental bed which will bleed can be oversewn with **sutures**, but usually these are in the very low uterine segment and cervix, and often continue to bleed despite suturing or **uterotonics**. **Ligation** of blood supply is often not beneficial, given the high number of collateral vessels. **Packing** has been used as a temporary measure to control bleeding. **Hysterectomy** may be necessary if uterine bleeding cannot be controlled, hopefully *before* massive blood loss and cardiovascular instability. Given most bleeding is from the lower part of the uterus, total hysterectomy including the cervix is usually necessary. Gravid hysterectomy is associated with an incidence of maternal mortality of up to 7%, with a 90% incidence of transfusion, 28% incidence of postoperative transfusion, and a 5% incidence of ureteral injuries or fistula formation.[23]

Planned hysterectomy: If the **diagnosis is highly suspected** by history and radiological studies (e.g. multiple prior cesarean deliveries, placenta previa, and several ultrasonographic findings of placenta accreta), and the **woman does not desire further fertility** (e.g. had requested tubal ligation), it might be prudent to deliver the neonate and proceed with hysterectomy while the placenta remains attached.[24] In these controlled situations, maternal morbidity of gravid hysterectomy may be decreased, but fertility is lost.

Expectant or medical management: There are over a dozen reports of expectant or medical management of placenta accreta. The placenta is left in situ, with either no therapy or, most commonly, **methotrexate** therapy. Medical management should be **considered only when the woman wants to preserve her fertility** and **no active uterine bleeding is present**. The cord is ligated, and the uterus closed with the placenta in situ. Antibiotic prophylaxis is suggested given the risk of infection, and short-term uterotonics for postpartum hemorrhage prevention, but there are no trials on these interventions. Follow-up is carried out with serial ultrasounds to monitor involution and decrease in placental vascularity. Quantitative human chorionic gonadotropin (HCG) should be monitored serially. If HCG levels plateau, or uterine size or placental vascularity do not decrease by 72 hours, methotrexate is usually given as 1 mg/kg on alternate days for a total of 4–6 doses, or according to HCG levels and ultrasonographic findings.[25] Women on methotrexate should be monitored with liver function tests (LFTs), platelet counts, and creatinine levels. Over 90% of the reports state successful outcomes, with future pregnancies and avoidance of gravid hysterectomy. In some cases, hysterectomy may be needed for late-occurring hemorrhage.

Postpartum

Consider reservation of an intensive care unit bed.

VASA PREVIA
Diagnosis/definition

Umbilical vessels, unsupported by placenta or cord, run through the membranes below the presenting part, going over, or in close proximity to, the internal os.

Symptoms

Usually asymptomatic.

Epidemiology/incidence

< 1/2500 deliveries.

Classification

- Type 1: vasa previa result from velamentous cord insertion.
- Type 2: vasa previa result from vessels running between placental lobes.

Risk factors/associations

Low-lying placenta or marginal previa, velamentous cord insertion, succenturiate lobed or bilobed placenta, multiple gestations, and in vitro fertilization (IVF).

Complications

Low Apgar scores, neonatal anemia with need for transfusion, and perinatal mortality (36%).[26]

Management
Principles

Timing of bleeding with antenatally diagnosed vasa previa is variable, and impossible to predict.

Work-up

Women with risk factors (see above) should have a TVU, possibly using color Doppler, for evidence of vessels overlying or in close proximity to the internal os. Not all vasa previa can be detected, even by very careful experienced operators using color Doppler. Prenatal diagnosis of vasa previa is associated with a 3% perinatal mortality, compared with a 56% mortality in cases not diagnosed prenatally.[26]

Therapy

Data to support the management of antenatally diagnosed vasa previa are currently lacking. Hospitalization after viability may be reasonable, but is not supported by trial data. Cesarean delivery is recommended for all women at 35 weeks, or earlier if preterm premature rupture of membranes (PPROM), preterm labor (PTL), or significant bleeding occur.[26]

References

1. Bhide A, Prefumo F, Moore J, Hollis B, Thilaganathan B. Placental edge to internal os distance in the late trimester and mode of delivery in placenta praevia. Br J Obstet Gynaecol 2003; 110: 860–4. [II–2, n = 82 previas]
2. Oppenheimer L, Simpson P, Holmes N, Dabrowski A. Diagnosis of low-lying placenta: can migration in the third trimester predict outcome? Ultrasound Obstet Gynecol 2001; 18: 100–2. [II–2]
3. Sherman SJ, Carlson DE, Platt LD, Mediaris AL. Transvaginal ultrasound: does it help in the diagnosis of placenta praevia? Ultrasound Obstet Gynecol 1992; 2: 256 60. [RCT, n = 38]
4. Dashe JS, McIntire DD, Ramus RM, Santos-Ramos R, Twickler DM. Persistence of placenta previa according to gestational age at ultrasound detection. Obstet Gynecol 2002; 99: 692–7. [II–2, n = 714]

5. Mustafa SA, Brizot ML, Carvalho MH et al. Transvaginal ultrasonography in predicting placenta previa at delivery: a longitudinal study. Ultrasound Obstet Gynecol 2002; 20: 356–9. [II–2]

6. Taipale P, Hiilesmaa V, Ylostalo P. Diagnosis of placenta previa by transvaginal sonographic screening at 12–16 weeks in a nonselected population. Obstet Gynecol 1997; 89: 364–7. [II–2]

7. Becker RH, Vonk R, Mende BC, Ragosh V, Entezami M. The relevance of placental location at 20–23 gestational weeks for prediction of placenta previa at delivery: evaluation of 8650 cases. Ultrasound Obstet Gynecol 2001; 17: 496–501. [II–2]

8. Taipale P, Hiilesmaa V, Ylostalo P. Transvaginal ultrasonography at 18–23 weeks in predicting placenta previa at delivery. Ultrasound Obstet Gynecol 1998; 12: 422–5. [II–2]

9. Newton ER, Barss V, Cetrulo CL. The epidemiology and clinical history of asymptomatic midtrimester placenta previa. Am J Obstet Gynecol 1984; 148: 743–8. [II–2]

10. Oyalese Y. Placenta previa and vasa previa: time to leave the Dark Ages. Ultrasound Obstet Gynecol 2001; 18: 96–9. [review]

11. Dinsmoor MJ, Hogg BB. Autologous blood donation with placenta previa: is it feasible? Am J Perinatol 1995; 12: 382–4. [II–2]

12. Wing DA, Paul RH, Millar LK. Management of the symptomatic placenta previa: a randomized, controlled trial of inpatient versus outpatient expectant management. Am J Obstet Gynecol 1996; 175: 806–11. [RCT, n = 53 women with ultrasound diagnosis of placenta previa after antepartum hemorrhage, with singleton pregnancy; gestation 24–36 weeks; intact membranes; normal fetal anatomy. Outpatient care (discharged home after around 72 hours; weekly ultrasound scans; readmitted to hospital (and subsequently discharged) if they had a second bleed; hospitalized if they had a third bleed) vs inpatient care in bed except for use of bathroom. Women in both groups received weekly corticosteroids until 32 weeks and underwent amniocentesis for assessment of fetal lung maturation at 36 weeks with caesarean section thereafter unless the placenta had risen]

13. Neilson JP. Interventions for suspected placenta praevia. Cochrane Database Syst Rev 2007; 1. [meta-analysis: 3 RCTs, n = 117 (53 for home, 64 for cerclage)]

14. Cobo E, Conde-Agudelo Delgado J, Canaval H, Congote A. Cervical cerclage: an alternative for the management of placenta previa? Am J Obstet Gynecol 1998; 179: 122–5. [RCT, n = 39]

15. Arias F. Cervical cerclage for the temporary treatment of patients with placenta previa. Obstet Gynecol 1988; 71: 545–8. [RCT, n = 25]

16. The Royal College of obstetricians and Gynaecologist. Placenta praevia: diagnosis and management. Clinical green-top guideline No. 27. the Royal College of Obstetricians and Gynaecologists, London: January 2001. [guideline]

17. Jacques SM, Qureshi F, Trent VS, Ramirez NC. Placenta accreta: mild cases diagnoses by placental examination. Int J Gynecol Pathol 1996; 15: 28–33. [II–2]

18. Silver RM, Landon MB, Rouse DJ et al. Maternal morbidity associated with multiple repeat cesarean deliveries. Obstet Gynecol 2006; 107: 1226–32. [II–2]

19. Gielchinsky Y, Mankuta D, Rojansky N et al. Perinatal outcome of pregnancies complicated by placenta accreta. Obstet Gynecol 2004; 104: 527–30. [II–2]

20. Chou MM, Ho ES, Lee YH. Prenatal diagnosis of placenta previa accreta by transabdominal color Doppler ultrasound. Ultrasound Obstet Gynecol 2000; 15: 28–35. [II–3]

21. Palacios Jaraquemada JM, Bruno CH. Magnetic resonance imaging in 300 cases of placenta accreta: surgical correlation of new findings. Acta Obstet Gynecol Scand 2005; 84: 716–24. [II–2]

22. Levine AB, Kuhlman K, Bonn J. Placenta accreta: comparison of cases managed with and without pelvic artery balloon catheters. J Matern Fetal Med 1999; 8: 173–6. [II–2]

23. O'Brien JM, Barton JR, Donaldson ES. The management of placenta percreta: conservative and operative strategies. Am J Obstet Gynecol 1996; 175: 1632–8. [II–2]

24. American College of Obstetricians and Gynecologists. Placenta accreta. ACOG Committee Opinion No. 266, January 2002 [review]

25. Hundley AF, Lee-Parrotz A. Managing placenta accreta. OBG Management 2002; 8: 18–33. [review]

26. Oyelese Y, Catanzarite V, Prefumo F et al. Vasa previa: the impact of prenatal diagnosis on outcomes. Obstet Gynecol 2004; 103: 937–42. [II–2]

25

Abruptio placentae

John F Visintine

KEY POINTS

- Approximately 0.5–1% of all pregnancies are complicated by placental abruption.
- Nearly 50% of women with placental abruption have no identifiable risk factors. Risk factors include **abruption in a prior pregnancy,** maternal **hypertensive disorders, advanced maternal age, smoking, cocaine, polyhydramnios, multiple gestation, (preterm) premature rupture of membranes, chorioamnionitis, elevated maternal serum alpha-fetoprotein,** and **abdominal trauma.** Association with thrombophilias has not been confirmed by prospective studies.
- **Complications** include **antepartum and postpartum hemorrhage, disseminated intravascular coagulation (DIC),** and **acute renal failure,** as well as **perinatal mortality, preterm delivery, fetal hypoxia** and/or **exanguination,** and **growth restriction.**
- The diagnosis of placental abruption is primarily a clinical one. **History, physical examination, laboratory** and **ultrasonographic** studies guide management. Ultrasound is primarily useful in ruling out other causes of third trimester bleeding.
- There are no trials to assess any intervention for prevention of abruption or its complications.
- Prompt **delivery** is indicated **if the pregnancy is near term.** However, if < 34 weeks, expectant management for mild (grade 1) abruptions may allow time for glucocorticoid administration. Maternal or fetal compromise necessitates delivery. A decision to delivery interval of ≤ 20 minutes is associated with a substantial reduction in neonatal morbidity and mortality in cases of fetal bradycardia.
- The mode of delivery is dependent primarily on the condition of the mother and fetus:
  - in most cases, for mild abruption (grade 1, no evidence of maternal or fetal compromise) – **vaginal delivery** is indicated
  - moderate abruption (grade 2, evidence of fetal non-reassuring testing) – rapid delivery typically by **cesarean** is indicated
  - severe abruption (grade 3, fetal demise, often with DIC) – **vaginal delivery** is indicated.

Definition

Placental abruption (also known as abruptio placentae) is defined as a premature separation of a normally implanted placenta.

Signs and symptoms

Signs and symptoms of placental abruption are shown in Table 25.1.[1] About 10% of abruption present with only concealed (occult) bleeding. Occasionally the presenting sign is fetal death.

Epidemiology/incidence

Approximately **0.5–1%** of all pregnancies are complicated by placental abruption.[2] This incidence in the USA has recently increased, mainly in the African-American population, the ethnic group at highest risk, especially for severe (or grade 3) abruption.[2] About 60% of abruptions occur preterm, and 50% occur prior to labor.

Table 25.1 *Clinical findings in women with placental abruption[1]*	
Clinical finding	Percent
Vaginal bleeding	78
Fetal non-reassuring testing	60
Uterine–abdominal tenderness/back pain	66
Uterine contractions (> 5/10 minutes)	17
Uterine hypertonus	17

Genetics

The association of placental abruption with thrombophilia has not been confirmed in prospective studies, with insufficient evidence so far (see Risk factors section).

Etiology/basic pathophysiology

The etiology of placental abruption is not completely understood. Premature separation of the placenta and the resultant decidual hemorrhage are thought to result from **rupture of small arterial vessels in the basal layer of the decidua**. Gross findings associated with placental abruption include adherent retroplacental clot with depression or disruption of the underlying placental tissue. Placental bed biopsies in cases of placental abruption show an absence of physiological trophoblastic invasion, dilated vessels, and recent thrombosis.[3] Microscopic changes associated with abruption resulting in perinatal mortality include thrombosed arteries and necrosis of the deciduas basalis, and large recent infarcts and stromal fibrosis in the terminal villi of the placental parenchyma.[4] Couvelaire first reported a severe form of placental abruption characterized by hemorrhagic infiltration between myometrial fibers that extends to the serosal surface.[5] As fetal growth restriction (FGR) is seen in about 80% of cases of abruption, the condition probably represents the **final expression** of a long-standing pregnancy disorder.

Classification (Table 25.2)

A uniformly accepted classification system for placental abruption does not exist. The clinical classification system originally published by Page in 1954 has been used by subsequent authors as a means of grouping placental abruptions in those that can be potentially managed conservatively (grade 1) and those that require more aggressive management (grades 2 and 3).[6]

Table 25.3	*Risk factors for placental abruption*
Prior abruption	
Chronic hypertension	
Severe pre-eclampsia	
Smoking	
Cocaine	
Chorioamnionitis	
Unexplained elevated MS-AFP	
(P)PROM	
Advanced maternal age	
Polyhydramnios	
Multiple gestation	
Trauma	
Thrombophilia?	

MS-AFP, maternal serum alpha-fetoprotein;
(P) PROM, (preterm) premature rupture of membranes.

Risk factors/associations (Table 25.3)

Nearly 50% of women with placental abruption have no identifiable risk factors.[7]

- History of an **abruption in a prior pregnancy**: the risk of recurrence is about 5–17%.[8] After two abruptions, the risk of recurrence is about 25%.
- Maternal **hypertensive disorders**: associated with up to almost 50% of grade 3 abruption cases. In particular, chronic hypertension (incidence 1.5–2.5%, odds ratio [OR] = 2.8), superimposed pre-eclampsia (about 3%), and severe pre-eclampsia (OR = 4.1), but not mild pre-eclampsia (OR = 0.9), are associated with placental abruption.[9,10] The underlying maternal vascular disease is the etiology of both hypertension and abruption.
- **Advanced maternal age** is associated with placental abruption (OR = 1.6).[11]

Table 25.2	*Clinical classification of placental abruption*				
Grade[a]	Clinically evident bleeding	Uterine tenderness/tetany	Maternal hypotension	Maternal coagulopathy	NRFHR testing
1	Yes	Yes or no	No	No	No
2	Yes or no	Yes	No	Rare	Yes
3	Yes or no	Yes	Yes	Often	Death

[a]Grade 0: diagnosis based on examination of the placenta. NRFHR, non-reassuring fetal heart rate.

Adapted from Sholl[6]

- **Smoking:** a 90% increase in abruption in women who smoke compared with controls. Smoking is responsible for 15–25% of episodes of abruption.[9]
- **Cocaine:** 1.9% rate of abruption.[12]
- **Polyhydramnios** has been associated with placental abruption in patients > 37 weeks' gestation.[13]
- **Multiple gestation:** 1.2% risk of abruption in twins, 1.5% in triplets.[14]
- **Preterm premature rupture of membranes** (PPROM): OR = 3.5.[15] Evidence of old decidual hemorrhage can be found in nearly 40% of placentas from patients with PPROM.[16]
- **Chorioamnionitis:** OR = 9.[15] Neutrophil infiltration of the fetal membranes and cervix as seen with PROM and chorioamnionitis is associated with placental abruption.[17]
- Unexplained **elevated maternal serum alpha-fetoprotein (MS-AFP)** in the second trimester: OR = 6–10 for placental abruption.[18,19]
- Acquired and inherited **thrombophilia** have been associated with abruption only in case-control studies:[20] factor V Leiden homozygote (OR = 17), factor V Leiden heterozygote (OR = 6), prothrombin (G20210A) gene mutation (OR = 29), methylenetetrahydrofolate deficiency (OR = 2), homocysteinemia (OR = 3), activated protein C resistance (OR = 6), and anticardiolipin immunoglobulin G (IgG) antibodies (OR = 20).[21] The first prospective study of women who were heterozygous for **factor V Leiden** found **no increased risk of adverse pregnancy outcomes, including placental abruption.**[22]
- **Abdominal trauma** is a recognized cause of placental abruption, but is responsible for only 1% of cases.[23] See also Chapter 25 in *Maternal–Fetal Evidence Based Guidelines.*

Complications

Maternal

- **Antepartum hemorrhage** remains a leading cause of maternal mortality. For pregnancies ending in stillbirth, hemorrhage related to abruptio placentae is the leading cause of maternal mortality.[24]
- **Disseminated intravascular coagulation** (DIC) was first reported to occur in association with placental abruption by De Lee in 1901.[25] The development of DIC is thought to be due to a release of thromboplastins, as well as consumption of coagulation factors secondary to an enlarging hematoma. Nearly 30% of patients who present with a severe (grade 3) abruption develop DIC.
- **Acute renal failure** is a potential maternal complication associated with abruption. Fortunately the incidence of acute renal failure appears to be decreasing, possibly due to improved medical management.
- **Postpartum hemorrhage secondary to uterine atony** is associated with abruption, as are postpartum **anemia** and **infection.**

Perinatal

Perinatal mortality (both fetal and neonatal deaths) varies from 4 to 12/1000.[26] This high perinatal mortality with abruption is attributable, in part, to its association with **preterm delivery.** Of the excess perinatal deaths, about 55% can be attributed to prematurity. The remaining perinatal mortality is associated with **fetal hypoxia, exanguination, and FGR.**

Management (Figure 25.1)

Unfortunately there are **no trials to assess any intervention for prevention of abruption or its complications.** Recommendations for management are primarily based on expert opinion or at best retrospective case-control studies.

Prevention

Smoking cessation counseling, avoidance of cocaine, and, if possible, avoidance of other risk factors can prevent abruptio placentae.

Preconception counseling

Women with risk factors should be counseled regarding the risk and complications of placental abruption, as well as interventions for its prevention.

Work-up

- The **diagnosis** of abruption is usually made **clinically,** and confirmed by gross or histological examination of the placenta. Placental abruptions may, however, be occult, at times presenting as preterm labor, and going undiagnosed until after delivery. Using the clinical criteria listed in Table 25.1, as well as ultrasound evaluation, the diagnosis of placental abruption is made prior to delivery in only 62% of cases,[1] so that >30% of cases of abruption may go undiagnosed until examination of the placenta after delivery.
- **History and physical examination,** as well as appropriate laboratory and ultrasonographic studies, guide management. Routine assessment should be conducted, including **vital signs, oxygenation status, and urine output. Laboratory** assessment may include a **hematocrit, platelet count, coagulation studies** (prothrombin time [PT], partial thromboplastin time [PTT], fibrinogen), **blood type and screen, or cross-match, serum creatinine, and a drug screen.** Other causes of third trimester bleeding must be excluded. The **differential diagnosis** includes placenta previa, vasa previa, cervical lesions (e.g. malignancy), and vaginal lesions.

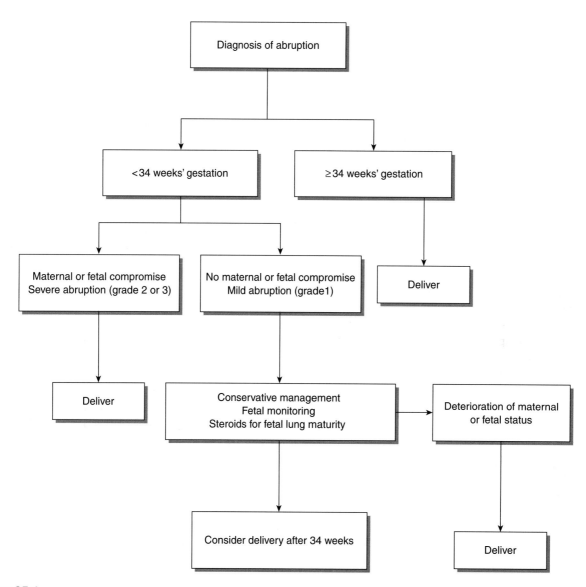

Figure 25.1
Management of abruptio placentae.

- An **ultrasound examination** is useful primarily in the exclusion of placenta previa or vasa previa. The sensitivity and specificity of ultrasound in the diagnosis of placental abruption were 24% and 96%, respectively, in one study.[27] So, while ultrasound is very helpful in ruling out other causes of third trimester bleeding, it lacks the sensitivity needed to reliably detect placental abruption.[27] The echogenicity of the collection of blood of an abruption depends on the time the ultrasound is performed relative to the onset of symptoms.[28] Acute hemorrhage is hyperechoic to isoechoic compared with the placenta. Resolving hematomas become hypoechoic within 1 week and sonolucent within 2 weeks.
- A **vaginal speculum examination** should be performed to rule out cervical or vaginal sources of bleeding.

- **Laboratory findings** (Table 25.4) associated with placental abruption such as prolonged PT, prolonged PTT, hypofibrinogenemia, and thrombocytopenia are markers of DIC or a consumptive coagulopathy, and are typically not present until later in the course of disease. D-dimer, a fibrin degradation product, had a sensitivity and specificity for placental abruption of 66% and 93%, respectively, in one study.[29]

General principles

Once the diagnosis of placental abruption has been made, attention should be focused on ensuring maternal and fetal well-being. **Maternal status** should be addressed, with attention paid to signs or symptoms of hemorrhage, hypovolemic

Table 25.4	Laboratory results in women with abruption
Test	Percent positive
D-dimer	66
Thrombocytopenia (<100 000/mm³)	13
Prolonged prothrombin time	20
Prolonged thromboplastin time	7
Hypofibrinogenemia	7

Adapted from Nolan et al[29]

shock, and DIC. The frequency of repeated evaluations is dependent primarily on the acuity and severity of the abruption. Preparations should be made in anticipation of potential maternal complications. This should include **intravenous access; two large-bore peripheral lines** will allow for rapid fluid or blood component replacement. The **availability of blood** or blood components may be lifesaving; therefore, close cooperation with blood banking services is essential.

Fetal status is typically assessed with **continuous electronic fetal monitoring,** at least in the acute setting. For women with a chronic abruption, once clinically stable, intermittent monitoring may be a consideration.

Timing of delivery (see Figure 25.1)

Near-term abruption: ≥ 34 weeks

Prompt delivery is indicated if the pregnancy is near term.[30–32] Fortunately, rapid labor often ensues as a result of the abruption.

Preterm abruption: < 34 weeks

Maternal or fetal compromise necessitates delivery. In selected patients with mild (grade 1) abruption, with no evidence of maternal or fetal compromise, expectant management may allow time for glucocorticoid administration, and appears to be a safe option.[1,6,32] Antepartum testing should be frequent, and at least initially continuous. There does not appear to be any increased morbidity or mortality associated with tocolytic use in selected patients.[6,33] In this setting, magnesium sulfate is the tocolytic agent used most frequently in the USA due to its cardiovascular side-effect profile, but its effectiveness has not been sufficiently studied.[33]

Mode of delivery

Deciding on the method of delivery is dependent primarily on the condition of the mother and fetus.

Mild abruption (grade 1): no evidence of maternal or fetal compromise

With close monitoring of the mother and fetus, **vaginal delivery** may be accomplished. In studies of women with mild (or grade 1) abruptions, mothers who delivered vaginally had a similar perinatal mortality rate to mothers who had a cesarean delivery.[30]

Moderate abruption (grade 2): evidence of fetal compromise

Rapid delivery, typically **cesarean delivery,** is indicated. In a recent study of placental abruption complicated by fetal bradycardia, a decision to delivery interval of ≤ 20 minutes was associated with substantially reduced neonatal morbidity and mortality.[34]

Severe abruption (grade 3): fetal death, often with DIC

Vaginal delivery is preferred in this group, as a cesarean delivery may exacerbate maternal hemorrhage. If present, DIC will typically resolve with evacuation of the uterus, with possible improvement in clotting parameters even prior to delivery.[35,36]

Anesthesia

No specific suggestions. Anesthesia support is particularly important with DIC, hemorrhagic shock, and massive transfusion cases.

Postpartum

Attention should be paid to hemodynamic state and possible late hemorrhage from uterine atony after abruption.

References

1. Hurd WW, Miodovnik M, Hertzberg V, Lavin JP. Selective management of abruptio placentae: a prospective study. Obstet Gynecol 1983; 61(4): 467–73. [II–2]
2. Ananth CV, Oyelese Y, Yeo L, Pradhan A, Vintzileos AM. Placental abruption in the United States, 1979 through 2001: temporal trends and potential determinants. Am J Obstet Gynecol 2005; 192(1): 191–8. [epidemiological review]
3. Dommisse J, Tiltman AJ. Placental bed biopsies in placental abruption. Br J Obstet Gynaecol 1992; 99(8): 651–4. [II–3]
4. Naeye RL, Harkness WL, Utts J. Abruptio placentae and perinatal death: a prospective study. Am J Obstet Gynecol 1977; 128(7): 740–6. [II–3]
5. Couvelaire A. Classic pages in obstetrics and gynecology: Alexandre Couvelaire. Am J Obstet Gynecol 1973; 116(6): 875. [II–3]

6. Sholl JS. Abruptio placentae: clinical management in non acute cases. Am J Obstet Gynecol 1987; 156(1): 40–51. [II–3]

7. Toivonen S, Heinonen S, Anttila M, Kosma VM, Saarikoski S. Reproductive risk factors, Doppler findings, and outcome of affected births in placental abruption: a population-based analysis. Am J Perinatol 2002; 19(8): 451–60. [II–2]

8. Rasmussen S, Irgens LM, Dalaker K. The effect on the likelihood of further pregnancy of placental abruption and the rate of its recurrence. Br J Obstet Gynaecol 1997; 104(11): 1292–5. [II–2]

9. Ananth CV, Smulian JC, Vintzileos AM. Incidence of placental abruption in relation to cigarette smoking and hypertensive disorders during pregnancy: a meta-analysis of observational studies. Obstet Gynecol 1999; 93(4): 622–8. [meta-analysis: 13 studies, n = 1,358,083]

10. Sibai BM, Lindheimer M, Hauth J et al. Risk factors for preeclampsia, abruptio placentae, and adverse neonatal outcomes among women with chronic hypertension. N Engl J Med 1998; 339(10): 667–71.[II–2]

11. Kramer MS, Usher RH, Pollack R, Boyd M, Usher S. Etiologic determinants of abruptio placentae. Obstet Gynecol 1997; 89(2): 221–6. [II–2]

12. Dombrowski MP, Wolfe HM, Welch RA, Evans MI. Cocaine abuse is associated with abruptio placentae and decreased birth weight, but not shorter labor. Obstet Gynecol 1991; 77(1): 139–41. [II–2]

13. Sheiner E, Shoham-Vardi I, Hallak M et al. Placental abruption in term pregnancies: clinical significance and obstetric risk factors. J Matern Fetal Neonatal Med 2003; 13(1): 45–9. [II–2]

14. Salihu HM, Bekan B, Aliyu MH et al. Perinatal mortality associated with abruptio placenta in singletons and multiples. Am J Obstet Gynecol 2005; 193(1): 198–203. [II–2, n = 1.6 million births]

15. Ananth CV, Oyelese Y, Srinivas N, Yeo L, Vintzileos AM. Preterm premature rupture of membranes, intrauterine infection, and oligohydramnios: risk factors for placental abruption. Obstet Gynecol 2004; 104(1): 71–7. [II–2, n = 11 777]

16. Salafia CM, Lopez-Zeno JA, Sherer DM et al. Histologic evidence of old intrauterine bleeding is more frequent in prematurity. Am J Obstet Gynecol 1995; 173(4): 1065–70. [II–2]

17. Lockwood CJ, Toti P, Arcuri F et al. Mechanisms of abruption-induced premature rupture of the fetal membranes: thrombin-enhanced interleukin-8 expression in term decidua. Am J Pathol 2005; 167(5): 1443–9. [II–2]

18. Katz VL, Chescheir NC, Cefalo RC. Unexplained elevations of maternal serum alpha-fetoprotein. Obstet Gynecol Surv 1990; 45(11): 719–26. [II–2]

19. Chandra S, Scott H, Dodds L et al. Unexplained elevated maternal serum alpha-fetoprotein and/or human chorionic gonadotropin and the risk of adverse outcomes. Am J Obstet Gynecol 2003; 189(3): 775–81. [II–2]

20. Kupferminc MJ, Eldor A, Steinman N et al. Increased frequency of genetic thrombophilia in women with complications of pregnancy. N Engl J Med 1999; 340(1): 9–13. [II–2]

21. Alfirevic Z, Roberts D, Martlew V. How strong is the association between maternal thrombophilia and adverse pregnancy outcome? A systematic review. Eur J Obstet Gynecol Reprod Biol 2002; 101(1): 6–14. [II–2]

22. Dizon-Townson D, Miller C, Sibai B et al. The relationship of the factor V Leiden mutation and pregnancy outcomes for mother and fetus. Obstet Gynecol 2005; 106(3): 517–24. [II–2]

23. Higgins SD, Garite TJ. Late abruptio placenta in trauma patients: implications for monitoring. Obstet Gynecol 1984; 63(3 Suppl): 10S–12S. [II–2]

24. Chang J, Elam-Evans LD, Berg CJ et al. Pregnancy-related mortality surveillance – United States, 1991–1999. MMWR Surveill Summ 2003; 52(2): 1–8. [epidemiological review]

25. Page EW, King EB, Merrill JA. Abruptio placentae; dangers of delay in delivery. Obstet Gynecol 1954; 3(4): 385–93. [II–2]

26. Ananth CV, Wilcox AJ. Placental abruption and perinatal mortality in the United States. Am J Epidemiol 2001; 153(4): 332–7. [II–2, n = 53 371]

27. Glantz C, Purnell L. Clinical utility of sonography in the diagnosis and treatment of placental abruption. J Ultrasound Med 2002; 21(8): 837–40. [II–2]

28. Nyberg DA, Cyr DR, Mack LA, Wilson DA, Shuman WP. Sonographic spectrum of placental abruption. Am J Roentgenol 1987; 148(1): 161–4. [II–2]

29. Nolan TE, Smith RP, Devoe LD. A rapid test for abruptio placentae: evaluation of a D-dimer latex agglutination slide test. Am J Obstet Gynecol 1993; 169(2 Pt 1): 265–8; discussion 8–9. [II–2]

30. Knab DR. Abruptio placentae. An assessment of the time and method of delivery. Obstet Gynecol 1978; 52(5): 625–9. [II–2]

31. Combs CA, Nyberg DA, Mack LA, Smith JR, Benedetti TJ. Expectant management after sonographic diagnosis of placental abruption. Am J Perinatol 1992; 9(3): 170–4. [II–2]

32. Bond AL, Edersheim TG, Curry L, Druzin ML, Hutson JM. Expectant management of abruptio placentae before 35 weeks gestation. Am J Perinatol 1989; 6(2): 121–3. [II–2]

33. Towers CV, Pircon RA, Heppard M. Is tocolysis safe in the management of third-trimester bleeding? Am J Obstet Gynecol 1999; 180 (6 Pt 1): 1572–8. [II–2]

34. Kayani SI, Walkinshaw SA, Preston C. Pregnancy outcome in severe placental abruption. Br J Obstet Gynecol 2003; 110(7): 679–83. [II–2]

35. Twaalfhoven FC, van Roosmalen J, Briet E, Gravenhorst JB. Conservative management of placental abruption complicated by severe clotting disorders. Eur J Obstet Gynecol Reprod Biol 1992; 46(1): 25–30. [II–2]

36. Sher G, Statland BE. Abruptio placentae with coagulopathy: a rational basis for management. Clin Obstet Gynecol 1985; 28(1): 15–23. [II–2]

26

Postpartum infections

Juan Carlos Sabogal

Postpartum endometritis

KEY POINTS

- The **diagnosis** of postpartum endometritis is based on the presence of ≥2 of the following: fever > 100.3° F at least twice, ≥6 hours apart; fundal tenderness; tachycardia (heart rate >100 beats/min); and foul-smelling lochia. Endometrial cultures are usually not necessary.
- As postpartum endometritis is most often associated with cesarean delivery, **prevention** is effective by **administration of prophylactic antibiotics** (either ampicillin or a first-generation cephalosporin for just one dose), **spontaneous placental removal, non-closure of both visceral and parietal peritoneum**, and **suture closure or drainage of the subcutaneous tissue when thickness is ≥2 cm.**
- **Gentamicin** and **clindamycin** intravenously, preferably **once-daily dosing**, are most effective for the **treatment** of postpartum endometritis.
- Once uncomplicated endometritis has clinically improved with intravenous therapy (usually 24–48 hours afebrile), oral therapy is not needed.

Diagnosis/definition

The diagnosis is based on clinical criteria. Table 26.1 describes criteria for diagnosis.

Symptoms/signs

Symptoms and signs are described in Table 26.1, plus abdominal pain, malaise, and elevated white blood cell count.

Epidemiology/incidence

Endometritis complicates about 1% of vaginal and about 5–27% of cesarean deliveries.[1] The lower incidence in certain cesarean delivery populations is due to infection precautions

Table 26.1 *Diagnosis of postpartum endometritis*

≥2 of the following:
- Fever >100.3° F, at least twice, ≥6 hours apart
- Fundal tenderness
- Tachycardia (heart rate > 100 beats/min)
- Foul-smelling lochia

at delivery and antibiotic prophylaxis. In specific populations, such as diabetic patients, the risk might be higher.[2]

Etiology/basic pathophysiology

Postpartum endometritis is an inflammatory process that involves both the endometrium and decidual tissue, secondary to infection. Other factors different than colonization itself play a role in pathogenesis, since 94% of postpartum patients have positive cultures from endometrial samples, but only a small fraction actually develop the infection. Bacteria usually ascend from the vagina, and colonize the innermost layer of the endometrial cavity at first. If this is not treated, it might spread locally and through the bloodstream, giving rise to complications that may be life threatening. The use of prophylactic antibiotics has impacted the occurence of such complications dramatically but has not eliminated the risk.

Microbiology

The bacteria are usually either Gram-positive cocci, Gram-negatives, or anaerobes that might be present in the normal female genital tract and reach the endometrium ascending from the vagina (Table 26.2).[3] The infection is usually polymicrobial, as in the vast majority of cases more than one bacterium is found. The presence of these microorganisms and the colonization of the decidua generates multiple microabscesses that trigger the invasion of inflammatory

Table 26.2 *Microorganisms most frequently associated with postpartum endometritis*[3]

Facultative Gram-positive (~50%)
Group B streptococci
Enterococci
Staphylococcus epidermidis
Lactobacillus
Diphtheroids
Staphylococcus aureus
Others

Facultative Gram-negative (~30%)
Gardnerella vaginalis
Escherichia coli
Enterobacter sp.
Proteus mirabilis
Others

Anaerobic (~50%)
Peptococcus asaccharolyticus
Bacteroides sp.
Peptostreptococcus sp
Bacteroides fragilis
Veillonella sp.
Others

Table 26.3 *Risk factors for postpartum endometritis*[4]

Cesarean delivery (directly correlated to its duration)
Labor (directly correlated to its duration)
Rupture of membranes (directly correlated to its duration)
Socioeconomic status
Number of vaginal examinations
Internal fetal monitoring
Manual extraction of placenta
Episiotomy
Forceps delivery
Young age (< 17 years old)[5]
Obesity (BMI > 30)[6]
Operative time
Blood loss[7]
Bacterial vaginosis[8]
GBS colonization[9,10]
Diabetes[2]

BMI, body mass index; GBS, group B streptococcus.

cells, which release chemical mediators responsible for the different manifestations of endometritis.

Risk factors/associations

'Classic' risk factors for postpartum endometriosis are shown in Table 26.3.[2,4–10] The longer is the labor, rupture of membranes, or also time of cesarean delivery, the higher is the risk of infection. Human immunodeficiency virus (HIV)-positive women with CD4 count ≤500 cells/µL have similar risks of postpartum endometritis and wound infection as HIV-negative women if they receive prophylactic antibiotics.[11,12]

Complications

Sepsis is a rare complication.

Management
Work-up

Endometrial cultures are not necessary, as the antibiotic regimens used are so successful, that, whichever microorganism is identified, it is usually susceptible.[13] Although not a current standard of care,[13] some authors recommend the use of endometrial cultures at the time of diagnosis, advocating the need for specific antibiotic coverage,[14] but

no trials are available to assess their efficacy. Elevation of temperature may be the only sign found in patients with endometritis. Since one single episode of temperature ≥100.4° F (38° C) is commonly present in postpartum patients and most of them will not develop any infection, it is recommended that two episodes of temperature elevation are identified in order to consider the diagnosis.[15] Physical examination is the cornerstone for adequate assessment.[16] Although laboratory studies are not criteria for diagnosis, an increased neutrophil count, as well as elevated proportion of bands, may suggest the presence of an infectious disease.[17] On the other hand, **urine analysis and culture** should be obtained, and **blood cultures** at the time of temperature spikes should be taken, particularly in immunocompromised patients or in those at increased risk for bacterial endocarditis. In selected patients, chest X-rays can be taken. Differential diagnosis includes at least atelectasis, pneumonia, viral syndrome, pyelonephritis, and appendicitis.

Prevention

Prophylactic antibiotics (either ampicillin or a first-generation cephalosporin for just one dose), spontaneous placental removal, non-closure of both visceral and parietal peritoneum, and **suture closure or drainage of the subcutaneous tissue when thickness is ≥2 cm** should routinely be performed in cesarean delivery (see Chapter 12). Each of these interventions decreases the incidence of postpartum endometritis and/or fever. In particular, both ampicillin and first-generation cephalosporins have similar efficacy in reducing postoperative endometritis from about 18% to 12% (a 61% decrease), with no added benefit found in using more broad-spectrum agents.[18,19] In urban, indigenous, mainly Afro-American women with incidence of postpartum endometritis over 24% despite first-generation cephalosporin prophylaxis, the addition of doxycycline 100 mg together with the cephalosporin and azithromycin 1 g orally 6–12 hours postoperatively can decrease the incidence of endometritis to 17%, possibly by targeting *Ureaplasma urealyticum.*[20] The number of vaginal examinations, nulliparity, early gestational age, and cefazolin use were predictors of prophylaxis failure in one study.[21]

Therapy

Since more than one microorganism is usually involved, a combination of antibiotics is used to assure proper coverage and prevent resistance. Parenteral, broad-spectrum antibiotics should be initiated and continued until the patient is afebrile. The combination of **gentamicin and clindamycin is appropriate** for the treatment of endometritis.[13] Compared with other regimens, clindamycin and an aminoglycoside are associated with 44% less treatment failures than with the other regimen.[22] Regimens with **activity against penicillin-resistant anaerobic bacteria** are better than those without, as failures of those regimens with poor activity against penicillin-resistant anaerobic bacteria are 94% more likely. Compared with other regimens, either clindamycin/gentamicin or piperacillin/tazobactam, a regimen with an aminoglycoside and penicillin or ampicillin is associated with about twice as many treatment failures. There is no evidence of difference in incidence of allergic reactions. Cephalosporins are associated with less diarrhea. There is no evidence that any one regimen is associated with fewer side effects.[22]

In four studies comparing once-daily with thrice-daily dosing of **gentamicin,** there were fewer failures with **once-daily dosing.** Once-daily gentamicin can be given 5 mg/kg, and once-daily clindamycin phosphate 2700 mg, both intravenously (IV).[23] Thrice-daily dosing consists of clindamycin 900 mg and gentamicin 1.5 mg/kg every 8 hours. It is recommended that levels (peak/trough) of gentamicin be taken after the third dose, to make sure therapeutic regimens are achieved.

Once uncomplicated endometritis has clinically improved with IV therapy (usually 24–48 hours afebrile), antibiotics can be discontinued. Oral therapy is not needed, as, compared with continued oral antibiotic therapy after IV therapy, **no oral therapy** is associated with similar recurrent endometritis or other outcomes in 4 trials.[22]

Response is usually prompt. If fever persists > 48 hours (< 10% of women), the addition of ampicillin for refractory cases can be considered. If fever still persists, pelvic abscess, wound infection, pelvic septic thrombophlebitis, inadequate antibiotic coverage, and retained placental tissue should be ruled out. Also, the likelihood of a resistant organism, a non-genital source of infection (pyelonephritis, pneumonia, IV catheter phlebitis), or non-infectious fever are part of the entities to rule out.[14] There is insufficient evidence to assess the effect of anti-coagulant therapy in refractory cases.

Because of the neonatal implications, information on the mother's condition should be provided to the neonate's healthcare provider.

Breastfeeding

Safe with clindamycin, gentamicin, or penicillin, as well as with most regimens.[24]

Wound infection
KEY POINTS

- **Risk factors** for post-cesarean wound infection are **chorioamnionitis, maternal preoperative condition or infection, pre-eclampsia, higher body mass index (BMI), nulliparity, increased surgical blood loss,** and **diabetes.**
- **Prophylactic antibiotics** (either ampicillin or a first-generation cephalosporin for just one dose) and **suture closure or drainage of subcutaneous fat in women with ≥ 2 cm thickness** prevents post-cesarean wound infection.
- **Penicillin** is the drug of choice. Wound **drainage and debridement of necrotic tissue** may be necessary.
- Compared with healing by secondary intention, **reclosure of the disrupted laparotomy wound** after the infection has resolved **is associated with success in > 80% of women, faster healing times, and fewer office visits.**

Diagnosis/definition

The Center for Disease Control defines and classifies surgical site infection (SSI) as either superficial, deep, or organ/space, as shown in Table 26.4. These criteria should be addressed at the time of diagnosis.[25] The vast majority of significant wound infections in obstetrics are postpartum following cesarean delivery.

Symptoms

Pain, redness, swelling or heat, fever.

Epidemiology/incidence

The incidence of wound infection after cesarean delivery ranges from 2.8 %[26] to 3.5% (in obese patients),[6] to 9.8%.[27]

Etiology/basic pathophysiology

The most common microorganisms identified by cultures from wound infections after cesarean delivery include

Table 26.4 *Classification of surgical site infection (SSI)*[25]

(A) **Superficial:** Infection occurs within 30 days after surgical procedure, involves skin and subcutaneous tissue only, and *at least one* of the following:
1. Purulent drainage from incision
2. Organism isolated from culture of fluid or tissue from SSI
3. At least one of the following – pain, redness, swelling, or heat – and superficial incision is deliberately opened by the surgeon
4. Diagnosis of superficial SSI by surgeon or attending physician

(B) **Deep:** Infection occurs within 30 days from surgical procedure and involves deep soft tissues (fascia, muscle) of the incision, and at least one of the following:
1. Purulent drainage from incision
2. Spontaneous dehiscence or deliberately opened by a surgeon when the patient presents at least one of the following: fever, pain, tenderness
3. An abscess involving the deep incision is found on direct examination during reoperation, or by histopathological or radiological examination
4. Diagnosis of deep SSI by surgeon or attending physician

(C) **Organ/space:** Infection occurs within 30 days from surgical procedure and appears to be related to the operation. Infection involves any part of the anatomy (organs, spaces) other than the incision, which was opened or manipulated during an operation, and at least one of the following:
1. Purulent drainage from a drain placed in the organ/space
2. Organisms isolated from a culture of fluid or tissue in the organ/space
3. An abscess involving the organ/space found on direct examination during reoperation, or by histopathological or radiological examination
4. Diagnosis of an organ/space SSI by surgeon or attending physician

Staphylococcus epidermidis, Enterococcus faecalis, Staphylococcus aureus, Escherichia coli, and *Proteus mirabilis.* The pathophysiology involves either seeding of bacteria from the uterine cavity or from the skin.[26]

Classification

For classification, see Table 26.4.

Risk factors/associations

Risk factors described are **preoperative remote infection, chorioamnionitis, maternal preoperative condition, preeclampsia, higher BMI, nulliparity,** and **increased surgical blood loss.**[6,27,28] Also, **diabetes** has long been considered a classic risk factor, with five times the risk of wound infection as for non-diabetics.[29]

Work-up

In early-onset wound infection (< 48 hours after the procedure), the microorganisms are likely to be either group A streptococcus, or *Clostridium.* A **wound culture** can be taken and a Gram stain will show either Gram-positive cocci, or Gram-positive rods, respectively. There are no trials to confirm the efficacy of obtaining a wound culture.

Prevention

See also Chapter 12.

Prophylactic antibiotics (either ampicillin or a first-generation cephalosporin for just one dose) are associated with a 59% decrease in the incidence of wound infection compared with no antibiotics.[19] The timing for prophylaxis before and after cord clamp is not associated with significant change in neonatal outcomes.[30] **Suture closure or drainage of subcutaneous fat in women with ≥ 2 cm thickness** is associated with a significant decrease in wound disruptions, including infections.[31,32]

Therapy

The onset of the infection defines the need for **antibiotics.** For infection arising < 48 hours after the cesarean delivery, **penicillin** is the drug of choice, with second options being cephalosporins, ampicillin, or erythromycin. Wound **drainage and debridement of necrotic tissue** may be necessary.

In late-onset wound infection (4–8 days postoperatively), the management consists purely of drainage. Antibiotics are not considered indicated in this setting, unless extensive cellulitis is present, or if the patient does not improve after drainage (necrotizing fasciitis should be considered).[14]

Disrupted (open) laparotomy wound, after infection has resolved

There are different ways to manage the open wound.[33]

Compared with healing by secondary intention, **reclosure of the disrupted laparotomy wound is associated with success in > 80% of women, faster healing times** (16–23 days vs 61–72 days), **and fewer office visits.**[34] No serious morbidity or mortality is associated with either method. There is insufficient evidence to assess optimal timing (probably 4–6 days after disruption if non-infected) and technique (superficial vertical mattress or 'en bloc' reclosure of entire wound thickness with absorbable sutures, or adhesive tape) of reclosure, as well as utility of antibiotics. After the wound is free of infection and is granulating properly, local anesthesia can be applied at the bedside and polypropylene mattress stitches can be used to close the skin.

Compared with reclosure using sutures, reclosure using permeable, adhesive tape (Cover-Roll; Biersdorf, Norwalk, CT) is associated with a faster procedure, less pain scores, and similar healing times in a small trial.[35]

Secondary intention closure with negative pressure wound therapy (NPWT), also called vacuum-assisted closure, has not been studied in any trials after cesarean section, but this technique seems to shorten the time needed for closure in non-pregnant adults.[36]

References

1. Brown CE, Stettler RW, Twickler D, Cunningham FG. Puerperal septic pelvic thrombophlebitis: incidence and response to heparin therapy. Am J Obstet Gynecol 1999; 181(1): 143–8. [II–2]

2. Diamond MP, Entman SS, Salyer SL, Vaughn WK, Boehm FH. Increased risk of endometritis and wound infection after cesarean section in insulin-dependent diabetic women. Am J Obstet Gynecol 1986; 155(2): 297–300. [II–2]

3. Rosene K, Eschenbach DA, Tompkins LS, Kenny GE, Watkins H. Polymicrobial early postpartum endometritis with facultative and anaerobic bacteria, genital mycoplasmas, and Chlamydia trachomatis: treatment with piperacillin or cefoxitin. J Infect Dis 1986; 153(6): 1028–37. [RCT]

4. Gibbs RS. Clinical risk factors for puerperal infection. Obstet Gynecol 1980; 55(5 Suppl): 178–84S. [II–2]

5. Magee KP, Blanco JD, Graham JM, Rayburn C, Prien S. Endometritis after cesarean: the effect of age. Am J Perinatol 1994; 11(1): 24–6. [II–2]

6. Myles TD, Gooch J, Santolaya J. Obesity as an independent risk factor for infectious morbidity in patients who undergo cesarean delivery. Obstet Gynecol 2002; 100(5 Pt 1): 959–64. [II–2]

7. Wolfe HM, Gross TL, Sokol RJ, Bottoms SF, Thompson KL. Determinants of morbidity in obese women delivered by cesarean. Obstet Gynecol 1988; 71(5): 691–6. [II–3]

8. Watts DH, Krohn MA, Hillier SL, Eschenbach DA. Bacterial vaginosis as a risk factor for post-cesarean endometritis. Obstet Gynecol 1990; 75(1): 52–8. [II–2]

9. Minkoff HL, Sierra MF, Pringle GF, Schwarz RH. Vaginal colonization with group B beta-hemolytic streptococcus as a risk factor for post-cesarean section febrile morbidity. Am J Obstet Gynecol 1982; 142(8): 992–5. [II–2]

10. Krohn MA, Hillier SL, Baker CJ. Maternal peripartum complications associated with vaginal group B streptococci colonization. J Infect Dis 1999; 179(6): 1410–15. [II–2]

11. Watts DH, Lambert JS, Stiehm ER et al. Complications according to mode of delivery among human immunodeficiency virus-infected women with CD4 lymphocyte counts of < or = 500/microL. Am J Obstet Gynecol 2000; 183(1): 100–7. [II–3]

12. Ferrero S, Bentivoglio G. Post-operative complications after caesarean section in HIV-infected women. Arch Gynecol Obstet 2003; 268(4): 268–73. [II–2]

13. American College of Obstetricians and Gynecologists. Guidelines for Perinatal Care, 2nd edn. ACOG; Washington, DC: 2002. [review]

14. Sweet RL, Gibbs RS. Infectious Diseases of the Female Genital Tract, 4th edn. Lippincott Williams & Wilkins; Philadelphia, PA: 2002. [review]

15. Monif GR, Baker DA. Infectious Diseases in Obstetrics and Gynecology, 5th edn. Parthenon Publishing; New York: 2004. [review]

16. Gabbe SG, Nyebyl JR, Simpson JL. Obstetrics: Normal and Problem Pregnancy, 4th edn. Churchill Livingstone; New York: 2002. [review]

17. Chen KT. Acute and chronic endometritis: < www.uptodate.com >. Accessed 01/02/2006: 2005 up to date, Waltham, MA. [review]

18. Hopkins L, Smaill F. Antibiotic prophylaxis regimens and drugs for cesarean section. Cochrane Database Syst Rev 2007; (1). [meta-analysis: 53 RCTs, n = > 2000]

19. Smaill F, Hofmeyr GJ. Antibiotic prophylaxis for cesarean section. Cochrane Database Syst Rev 2007; 1. [meta-analysis: 81 RCTs, n = > 2000]

20. Andrews WW, Hauth JC, Cliver SP, Savage K, Goldenberg RL. Randomized clinical trial of extended spectrum antibiotic prophylaxis with coverage for Ureaplasma urealyticum to reduce post-cesarean delivery endometritis. Obstet Gynecol 2003; 101(6): 1183–9. [RCT, n = 597]

21. Chang PL, Newton ER. Predictors of antibiotic prophylactic failure in post-cesarean endometritis. Obstet Gynecol 1992; 80(1): 117–22. [II–2]

22. French LM, Smaill FM. Antibiotic regimens for endometritis after delivery. Cochrane Database Syst Rev 2007; 1. [meta-analysis: 38 RCTs, n = 3983]

23. Livingston JC, Llata E, Rinehart E et al. Gentamicin and clindamycin therapy in postpartum endometritis: the efficacy of daily dosing versus dosing every 8 hours. Am J Obstet Gynecol 2003; 188(1): 149–52. [RCT, n = 110]

24. Briggs GG, Freeman RK, Yaffe SJ. Drugs in Pregnancy and Lactation, 5th edn. Lippincott Williams & Wilkins; Baltimore, MD: 1998. [review]

25. Mangram AJ, Horan TC, Pearson ML, Silver LC, Jarvis WR. Guideline for prevention of surgical site infection, 1999. Centers for Disease Control and Prevention (CDC) Hospital Infection Control Practices Advisory Committee. Am J Infect Control 1999; 27(2): 97–132; quiz 133–4; discussion 96. [guideline]

26. Martens MG, Kolrud BL, Faro S, Maccato M, Hammill H. Development of wound infection or separation after cesarean delivery. Prospective evaluation of 2,431 cases. J Reprod Med 1995; 40(3): 171–5. [II–1]

27. Tran TS, Jamulitrat S, Chongsuvivatwong V, Geater A. Risk factors for postcesarean surgical site infection. Obstet Gynecol 2000; 95(3): 367–71. [II–2]

28. Vermillion ST, Lamoutte C, Soper DE, Verdeja A. Wound infection after cesarean: effect of subcutaneous tissue thickness. Obstet Gynecol 2000; 95(6 Pt 1): 923–6. [II–2]

29. Cruse PJ, Foord R. A five-year prospective study of 23,649 surgical wounds. Arch Surg 1973; 107(2): 206–10. [II–1]

30. Wax JR, Hersey K, Philput C et al. Single dose cefazolin prophylaxis for postcesarean infections: before vs. after cord clamping. J Matern Fetal Med 1997; 6(1): 61–5. [RCT]

31. Anderson ER, Gates S. Techniques and materials for closure of the abdominal wall in caesarean section. Cochrane Database Syst Rev 2007; 1. [meta-analysis]

32. Chelmow D, Rodriguez EJ, Sabatini MM. Suture closure of subcutaneous fat and wound disruption after cesarean delivery: a meta-analysis. Obstet Gynecol 2004; 103(5 Pt 1): 974–80. [meta-analysis]

33. Sarsam SE, Elliott JP, Lam GK. Management of wound complications from cesarean delivery. Obstet Gynecol Surv 2005; 60(7): 462–73. [review]

34. Wechter ME, Pearlman MD, Hartmann KE. Reclosure of the disrupted laparotomy wound: a systematic review. Obstet Gynecol 2005; 106(2): 376–83. [meta-analysis: 8 RCTs, n = 324. Includes both CDs, gynecologic and GI laparotomies]

35. Harris RL, Magann EF, Sullivan DL, Meeks GR. Extrafascial wound dehiscence: secondary closure with suture versus noninvasive adhesive bandage. J Pelvic Surg 1995; 1: 88–91. [RCT, n = 27]

36. Eginton MT, Brown KR, Seabrook GR, Towne JB, Cambria RA. A prospective randomized evaluation of negative-pressure wound dressings for diabetic foot wounds. Ann Vasc Surg 2003; 17(6): 645–9. [RCT]

27

The neonate

Gary Emmett and Jay S. Greenspan

KEY POINTS

- **Necessary equipment** for neonatal stabilization must be available.
- **Personnel trained in neonatal resuscitation** should be present at every delivery.
- Neonatal resuscitation begins with **drying, stimulating, and clearing the airway.** If further resuscitation is necessary, it is frequently due to respiratory failure and can be resolved with **support of airway and breathing.**
- A difficult transition may be anticipated by infants at risk and may be due to hypothermia, hypoglycemia, or congenital anomalies.
- Low-risk infants are > 36 weeks' gestation, of birth weight 2500–4200 g, Apgar > 7 at 5 minutes, normal vital signs, and no signs of congenital anomalies or respiratory distress.
- **The preterm infant** is at **greater risk** for complications in the delivery room and thereafter. Additional resuscitation considerations should be the establishment of **intravenous access and airway pressure.** Protocols for stabilization and transfer as needed should be proactively determined.

Delivery room management[1–4]

The minutes around birth are the riskiest time in a person's life. Every newborn has the right to a resuscitation performed at a high level of competence. A competent resuscitation means that the proper equipment and well-trained personnel must be available at each delivery. The **necessary equipment** is shown in Table 27.1.

Initiation of resuscitation

The majority of newborns experiencing apnea and/or bradycardia require **airway clearance, stimulation, and ventilation.** The need for medication is rare. The first steps include:

1. Thermal management (placing the infant under a preheated radiant warmer, dry and stimulate infant, replace wet blankets with warmed and dry ones).

Table 27.1 *Necessary equipment for neonatal resuscitation in the delivery room*

1. Suction equipment

   a. Bulb syringe
   b. Mechanical suction
   c. Suction catheters (various sizes)
   d. Feeding tubes
   e. Meconium aspirator

2. Bag mask equipment

   a. Neonatal resuscitation bag with pressure manometer
   b. Face masks (various sizes)
   c. Oxygen source and tubing (blender preferable)
   d. Oxygen flow meter

3. Intubation equipment

   a. Laryngoscope (with 0 and 1 blades)
   b. Endotracheal tubes (2.5–4.0 mm)
   c. Stylet

4. Other equipment

   a. Alcohol
   b. Stethoscope
   c. Gloves
   d. Scissors
   e. Tape
   f. Stopcocks
   g. Syringes (1–20 ml)
   h. Umbilical artery and vein tray with catheters (3.5F and 5F)
   i. Warmer

2. Airway clearance (suction mouth and gently suction nares – infants are obligate nose breathers).
3. Tactile stimulation (if drying and suctioning fail, rub the infant's back).

On occasion, medications may be necessary and should be available:

1. Epinephrine 1:10 000; 0.1–0.3 ml/kg intravenous (IV) or via endotracheal tube (ET) given rapidly.
2. Volume expanders (whole blood, normal saline, 5% albumin-saline, Ringer's lactate); 10 ml/kg IV over 5 minutes.
3. Sodium bicarbonate 0.5 mEq/ml; 2 mEq/kg IV given over at least 2 minutes.
4. Naloxone hydrochloride 0.4 mg/ml; 0.1 mg/kg ET or IV given rapidly.

Delivery room resuscitation

Each newborn should be assessed for the need to treat using the Apgar score (scored 0–10, with 1 or 2 points scored for each of heart rate, respiratory effort, muscle tone, reflex irritability, color). The algorithm in Figure 27.1 can be used as a guideline for the resuscitation of a term or near-term infant.

The difficult transition

Successful transition to extrauterine life generally occurs over the first hours after birth. Delay in transition can occur for many reasons. Common causes of delayed transition are listed in Table 27.2.

In addition to the resuscitation steps for the newborn, in infants with signs of poor transition (tachypnea, cyanosis, mottled skin or pallor, tremors and/or jitteriness), consideration should be given for measuring their temperature, arterial blood saturation (pulse oximetry or blood gas), and blood glucose.

Hypoglycemia

Infants of diabetics, infants with congenital abnormalities of the pancreas, and large and small for gestational age infants may become hypoglycemic. For blood sugar <45 mg/dl, infants should be treated with early feeds or IV 10% glucose 5–10 ml/kg followed by repeat testing. If a large for gestational age infant does not stabilize its glucose within 5 minutes, an IV line must be placed.

Respiratory distress

Signs and symptoms include tachypnea, retractions, nasal flaring, grunting, cyanosis, and apnea. Differential diagnosis includes abnormalities of lungs (including respiratory distress or aspiration syndromes, infections, pneumothorax, and congenital lung abnormalities), airway (including choanal

Table 27.2 *Causes of delayed transition*
Hypothermia
Hypoglycemia
Retained pulmonary fluid
Preterm infants
Multiple births
Infants who are small or large for gestational age (<2500 g or >4200 g)
Infants ≥42 weeks' gestation
Infants born through meconium
Infants with low Apgar scores (e.g. <7 at 5 minutes)
Infants of diabetics
Infants of mothers on tocolytics
Infants of mothers using licit and illicit drugs
Infants with congenital problems, including chromosomal disorders
Infants with neonatal illnesses such as infection

atresia, tracheal–esophageal fistula, and micrognathia), cardiovascular system (primarily cyanotic, congestive or congenital heart diseases, and pulmonary hypertension), neurological system (such as infection, hypoxic injury, and hydrocephalus), blood (anemia or polycythemia), infections, metabolic problems, or exposure to maternal drugs. Treatment involves ensuring airway patency and intubation if necessary, provision of supplemental oxygen by blow-by, bag, and mask, or via an endotracheal tube, and initiation of a work-up (complete blood count [CBC] with differential, chest radiograph, blood gas, and C-reactive protein [CRP]).

Meconium

Meconium is passed in approximately 10% of fetuses prior to delivery. Small amounts may be of no consequence. The risk of aspiration is greater with large amounts, and 'pea soup'-colored meconium. Suctioning can take place for all infants with meconium when the head is delivered (intrapartum suction) and after delivery for infants who are depressed or with thick, particulate meconium, but this is not confirmed by recent trials (see Chapter 19), in particular for the vigorous infants with thick meconium-stained fluid. If performed, suctioning meconium is best done by applying suction directly to an endotracheal tube. Continuous suction is applied during tube withdrawal with a vacuum set to approximately 100 mmHg (3–5 seconds). Free-flow oxygen

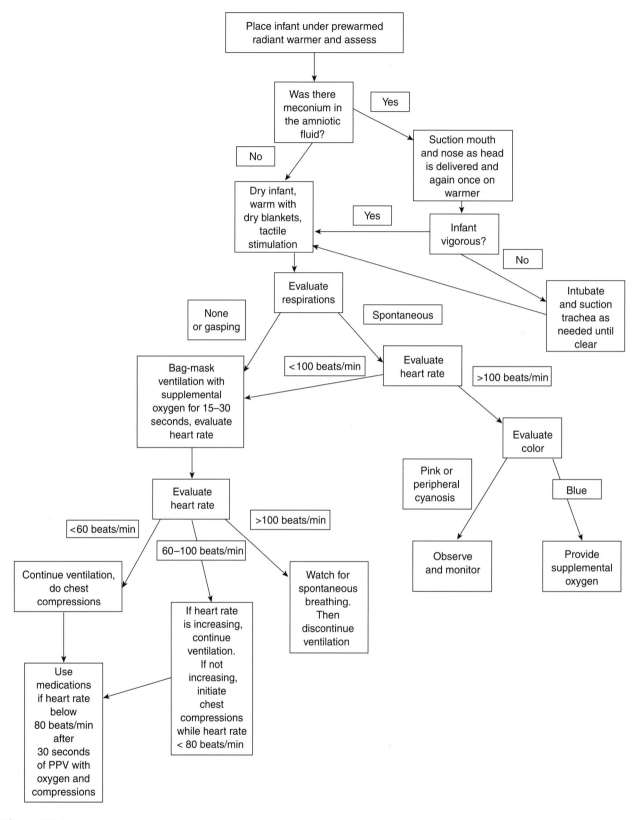

Figure 27.1
Neonatal resuscitation algorithm. PPV, positive pressure ventilation.

should be provided through tubing during this procedure. Reintubation should be repeated until returns are nearly free of meconium. After several passes of the tube, it may be appropriate to leave the tube in place for delivery of positive pressure ventilation (PPV). After tracheal suctioning, consideration should be given to suctioning the stomach contents to prevent aspiration. Wait until the resuscitation is completed to minimize the adverse effects of a potential vagal response.

Common malformations affecting transition

Some congenital abnormalities of the newborn can present as problems in the delivery room. Common malformations and their stabilization before transfer to a tertiary care intensive care nursery include:

1. Choanal atresia – secure an oral airway.
2. Pierre Robin sequence (small chin with potential airway obstruction) – insert oral airway; if not allowing adequate respiration, consider intubation.
3. Congenital diaphragmatic hernia – decompress the stomach with a nasogastric or orogastric (NG/OG) tube and intubate the airway.
4. Abdominal wall defects (omphalocele and gastroschisis) – cover defect with sterile gauze soaked in sterile normal saline and place infant in a sterile bag fastened above defect.
5. Neural tube defects – cover defect with sterile gauze soaked in normal saline and consider placing infant in sterile bag fastened above defect using latex-free gloves and equipment.

Care of the well baby

Little intervention is needed for the infant with no risks and a normal delivery. It is important, therefore, to determine which baby can go to the well nursery and which must be more fully evaluated.

Low risk

(Can be admitted without pediatric specialist consultation.) Criteria include weight > 2.5 kg and gestational age > 36 weeks, Apgar score > 7 at 5 minutes, infants with normal vital signs (i.e. respiratory rate < 60 beats/min and heart rate 100–160 beats/min), and infants without obvious congenital anomalies and showing no signs of distress.

Some risk

(May be admitted after pediatric specialist consultation.) Criteria include infants at risk because of neonatal abstinence,

sepsis, rupture of membranes > 16 hours, exposure to group B streptococcus that is inadequately treated, maternal temperature of > 100.4°F within 24 hours of delivery, infants born to diabetic mothers, infants born outside of the hospital, infants of unclear gestation, and infants > 4200 g.

Initial care of the newborn

The infant must be observed for an adequate transition. This includes the assessment of vital signs every 30 minutes for about 2 hours and a general assessment by a skilled staff member to observe for signs of an abnormal transition.

Newborn screening

There are no trials to assess benefits of neonatal screening. In fact, there is a lot of controversy on which screening tests should be recommended for every newborn. There is a marked state-to-state and country-to-country variation. In 2005 the American College of Medical Genetics (ACMG) released their recommendations for a uniform newborn screening panel (Table 27.3).[5] As 12 of the 29 disorders recommended for screening have an incidence of < 1 in 100 000, and the effectiveness of screening has not been proven for most of the 29 conditions, the debate will continue regarding newborn screening.[6]

Circumcision

There is insufficient evidence to recommend this procedure, which can have serious complications. If desired by the parents, after extensive counseling and consent, the neonate must be first in stable condition. The presence of any of the following conditions requires the review of a pediatrician prior to the procedure:

1. Reason to suspect neonatal infection or illness.
2. Congenital anomalies, ambiguous genitalia, micropenis (< 2.5 cm from pubic bone to tip), family history of excessive bleeding.
3. Hypospadias, epispadias, chordae.

Infants should be > 12 hours old (to allow for normal transition), should have voided first and be fasting for 1 hour prior to procedure. Pain control should be utilized such as a penile dorsal nerve block, topical analgesic creams, or a subcutaneous ring block. Sucrose water or wine may also provide some pain control. Techniques used for circumcision include the PlastiBell, the Mogen, and the Gomco methods. After the procedure, pain control can be provided with acetaminophen (15 mg/kg dose every 6 hours) as well as breastfeeding. A gauze wrap is generally maintained for 24 hours and, thereafter, the wound should be kept clean with plain water and covered with a lubricant such

Table 27.3 *Disorders recommended by the ACMG Task Force for inclusion in newborn screening*[a]

Disorders of organic acid metabolism
Isovaleric acidemia
Glutaric aciduria type 1
3-Hydroxy-3-methylglutaric aciduria
Multiple carboxylase deficiency
Methylmalonic acidemia, mutase deficiency form
3-Methylcrotonyl-CoA carboxylase deficiency
Methylmalonic acidemia, Cb1 A and Cb1 B forms
Propionic acidemia
Beta-ketothiolase deficiency

Disorders of fatty acid metabolism
Medium-chain acyl-CoA dehydrogenase deficiency
Very long-chain acyl-CoA dehydrogenase deficiency
Long-chain L-3-hydroxy acyl-CoA dehydrogenase deficiency
Trifunctional protein deficiency
Carnitine uptake defect

Disorders of amino acid metabolism
Phenylketonuria
Maple syrup urine disease
Homocystinuria
Citrullinemia
Argininosuccinic acidemia
Tyrosinemia type 1

Hemoglobinopathies
Sickle cell anemia
Hemoglobin S-beta-thalassemia
Hemoglobin SC disease

Other disorders
Congenital hypothyroidism
Biotinidase deficiency
Congenital adrenal hyperplasia
Galactosemia
Hearing deficiency
Cystic fibrosis

[a]The American College of Medical Genetics (ACMG) Task Force also recommended reporting an additional 25 disorders ('secondary targets') that can be detected through screening but that do not meet the criteria for primary disorders. At this time, there is state-to-state variation in newborn screening; a list of the disorders that are screened for by each state is available at http://genes-r-us.uthscsa.edu.
CoA, coenzyme A; Cb1 A, cobalamin A; and Cb1 B, cobalamin B.

Adapted from Natowitz.[6]

as Vaseline. The parents can be instructed to expect a white-yellow discharge for 5–7 days.

Care of the preterm infant

The delivery of a preterm infant follows many of the guidelines generated for the term infant. These infants, born at ≤ 36 weeks' gestation, are at high risk for problems immediately following birth and in the subsequent newborn period. Delivery room management includes similar resuscitation steps with accentuated attention to drying and maintaining thermal stability, close observation of blood glucose and volume requirements, and close observation and response to respiratory distress and failure. The prophylactic placement of IV access should be considered and the early institution of positive airway pressure may be necessary to prevent respiratory failure. Preparation and anticipation of the delivery with the availability of the proper equipment and personnel for stabilization and transport will optimize survival.

Neonatal encephalopathy and cerebral palsy[7]

Neonatal encephalopathy

Neonatal encephalopathy is a clinically defined syndrome of disturbed neurological function in the earliest days of life in the term infant, manifested by difficulty initiating and maintaining respiration, depression of tone and reflexes, subnormal level of consciousness, and, often, seizures; it can result from a myriad of conditions and may or may not result in permanent neurological impairment.

Hypoxic-ischemic encephalopathy

Also called postasphyxial encephalopathy, hypoxic-ischemic encephalopathy is a subtype of neonatal encephalopathy for which the etiology is considered to be a limitation of oxygen and blood flow near the time of birth. The usual progression of events is:

Intrapartum hypoxic-ischemic injury

↓

Neonatal encephalopathy

↓

Cerebral palsy

Cerebral palsy

Cerebral palsy (CP) is a chronic static neuromuscular disability characterized by aberrant control of movement or posture, appearing early in life and not the result of a recognized progressive disease:

- CP affects 2–3/1000 live births.
- Prevention is elusive.
- Incidence of neonatal encephalopathy attributed to intrapartum hypoxia in absence of other preconception or antepartum abnormalities is about 1.6 in 10 000 infants.
- spastic quadriplegia is the only type of CP associated with birth asphyxia.
- the majority of cases of CP do *not* result from isolated intrapartum hypoxia with resultant asphyxia and organ damage.

Etiology of cerebral palsy

- prematurity
- developmental malformations
- metabolic defects
- autoimmune and coagulation disorders
- infections
- hypoxia.

Clinical signs

Historically, four non-specific clinical signs were often assumed to be adequate evidence of birth asphyxia and hypoxic-ischemic neonatal encephalopathy in the absence of objective criteria:

1. meconium staining
2. non-reassuring fetal heart rate (FHR) pattern
3. low Apgar score
4. neonatal encephalopathy.

These signs are not sufficient to make any diagnosis since:

- Abnormal FHR patterns to predict subsequent CP have a **99% false-positive rate.**
- Less than one-quarter of infants with neonatal encephalopathy have evidence of hypoxia or ischemia at birth.
- Intrapartum hypoxia is uncommonly the sole cause of neonatal encephalopathy or CP.

Timing of neonatal encephalopathy

- 69%   Only antepartum risk factors.
- 25%   Both antepartum risk factors and evidence for intrapartum hypoxia.
- 4%   Intrapartum hypoxia without antepartum risk factors.
- 2%   No recognized risk factors.

Apgar scores and cerebral palsy

- 0–3 at 5 minutes: 0.3–1% of babies with CP.
- 0–3 at 10 minutes: 10% of babies with CP (but rate drops to 5% if score improves at 15 and 20 minutes).
- < 3 at 15 minutes: 53% mortality, 36% of survivors with CP.
- < 3 at 20 minutes: 60% mortality, 57% of survivors with CP.

75% of children with **CP** had **normal Apgar** scores at birth.

- Criticism of the management of labor should not be confused with CP causation because the two often may not be linked.

Criteria that define an acute intrapartum event sufficient to cause cerebral palsy

Essential criteria (must meet all four):
- metabolic acidosis in fetal umbilical artery: pH < 7.0 and base deficit > 12 mmol/L
- early onset of neonatal encephalopathy born at or > 34 weeks' gestation
- CP of the spastic quadriplegic or dyskinetic type
- exclusion of other identifiable etiologies.

Criteria that collectively suggest intrapartum timing but are non-specific to asphyxial insults

- Sentinel (signal) hypoxic event immediately before or during labor.
- Sudden and sustained fetal bradycardia or absence of FHR variability with persistent late or variable decelerations, when pattern was previously normal.
- Apgar 0–3 beyond 5 minutes.
- Onset of multisystem organ involvement within 72 hours.
- Early neuroimaging with evidence of acute non-focal cerebral abnormality.

References

1. Emmett GA. Field Guide to the Normal Newborn. Lippincott Williams & Wilkins; Philadelphia, PA, 2004. [review]
2. Bloom RS, Cropley C. Textbook of Neonatal Resuscitation. American Heart Association; Dallas, TX 1995. [review]
3. Kattwinkel J (ed.). Textbook of Neonatal Resuscitation, 4th edn. American Academy of Pediatrics; Elk Grove Village, IL: 2000. [review]
4. Fanaroff AA, Martin RJ. Neonatal–Perinatal Medicine: Diseases of the Fetus and Infant, 7th edn. Mosby; St. Louis, MD, 2002. [review]

5. Maternal and Child Health Bureau: Newborn screening: toward a uniform screening panel and system. Maternal and Child Health Bureau; Rockville, MD: March 2005: http://mchb.hrsa.gov/screening [guideline]

6. Natowicz M. Newborn screening – setting evidence-based policy for protection. N Engl J Med 2005; 353: 867–70. [review]

7. Neonatal encephalopathy and cerebral palsy. Defining the pathogenesis and pathophysiology. American College of Obstetricians and Gynecologists and American Academy of Pediatrics; 2003. [review]

Part III

Gynecologic issues related to pregnancy

28

Medical management of first trimester pregnancy loss

Manish Gopal

KEY POINTS

- Diagnose first trimester pregnancy loss by transvaginal ultrasound and/or serial β-human chorionic gonadotropin (β-HCG) levels.
- There are **three main options** for the woman with first trimester spontaneous loss that is still not complete: **expectant, medical, and surgical management. Successful** management means **complete evacuation** of the uterus. The success of each of these approaches depends on several factors, in particular the **type of loss** (with no symptoms, e.g. missed loss, vs with symptoms such as bleeding and cramping, e.g. incomplete loss), and **estimated gestational age.** A loss with symptoms is easier to end, as is one that is < 9 weeks of gestation.
- **Surgical management** is the option with the **highest (>97%) success rate.** Endometritis or hemorrhage rates are ≤1%. Maternal safety is highest with **manual vacuum aspiration,** when regional or general anesthesia can be avoided.
- **Medical management is significantly more effective than expectant management. Misoprostol 800 μg vaginally, with a repeated dose** on day 1–3 if complete evacuation is not confirmed, has **high safety** (endometritis or hemorrhage ≤1%), and success rates of **81% with anembryonic gestation, 88% with embryonic or fetal death, and 93% with incomplete or inevitable abortion** in women at <13 weeks of gestation.
- Mifepristone 200–600 μg orally followed by misoprostol in 24–48 hours, or intramuscular (IM) methotrexate followed by misoprostol in 3–5 days, as well as other regimens, are effective but possibly slightly less safe options.

Definitions

First trimester pregnancy loss (PL)

Spontaneous loss of pregnancy from conception to < 14 weeks. The term spontaneous abortion is equivalent, but

should be avoided since women associate negative feelings with this term. Miscarriage is a lay term for PL. This chapter concerns these types of losses:

- early first trimester PL – loss of pregnancy between conception and 9 6/7 weeks
- late first trimester PL – loss of pregnancy between 10 and 13 6/7 weeks.

Anembryonic pregnancy loss

No embryo identified (e.g. missed abortion, blighted ovum).

Embryonic pregnancy loss

Embryo identified, but then non-viable (e.g. embryonic demise).

This chapter does not discuss voluntary (elective) termination (induced abortion).

Diagnosis of first trimester loss

Transvaginal ultrasound

Missed abortion

Mean gestational sac size of ≥20 mm and no heart beat by transvaginal ultrasound.

Embryonic demise

Crown–rump length (CRL) of ≥5 mm and no heartbeat by transvaginal ultrasound.

With a mean gestational sac size of >10 mm, a yolk sac should be seen to help discriminate a true gestational sac from a pseudosac (associated with abnormal pregnancy).

β-*Human chorionic gonadotropin*

Increase of β-human chorionic gonadotropin (β-HCG) of <15% over ≥48 hours. If the β-HCG is >1500 mlU/mL, a gestational sac should be visualized by transvaginal ultrasound; if the gestational sac is not seen in the uterus, suspect ectopic pregnancy.

Symptoms

Vaginal bleeding, lower abdominal cramping, and premature dilation of cervix.

Epidemiology/incidence

It is estimated that up to 60% of conceptions end up in early losses, most not clinically recognized (e.g. 'late cycle'). About 15–20% of clinically recognized pregnancies end up as first trimester losses.

Etiology

Chromosomal abnormalities are responsible for >50% of all spontaneous abortions, most commonly translocations and aneuploidy. Many spontaneous losses may be secondary to other genetic defects that are impossible to discern by simple karyotype. TORCH (toxoplasmosis, other agents, rubella, cytomegalovirus, herpes simplex) infections, poorly controlled pregestational diabetes or other medical disorders, antiphospholipid antibodies, drug abuse, tobacco use, alcohol use, Müllerian anomalies, and many other factors are also associated with spontaneous losses.

Contraindications

Hemodynamically or medically unstable patients are not candidates for expectant or medical management. Molar pregnancies should be evacuated by dilatation and evacuation (D&E). Ectopic pregnancy is another contraindication to medical management. Bleeding disorder, or severe anxiety may be best managed by D&E.

Complications

Complications are incomplete and septic abortions, need for surgical evacuation, and hemorrhage requiring transfusion. The risk of maternal death from induced voluntary abortion in the USA is about 1/100 000, and varies from 0.1/100 000 at 8 weeks to about 9/100 000 at 21 weeks. The risk of death from infection using mifepristone for medical abortion is <1/100 000. These risks may be similar or even less with medical termination of a first trimester pregnancy loss.

Management

Principles

There are **three main options** for the woman with first trimester spontaneous loss which is still not complete: **expectant, medical,** and **surgical management.** Successful management means complete evacuation of the uterus. For medical management, failure also means the need for surgical evacuation. The success of each of these approaches depends on several factors, in particular the **type of loss** (with no symptoms, e.g. missed loss, vs with symptoms such as bleeding and cramping, e.g. incomplete loss), and **estimated gestational age.** A loss with symptoms is easier to end, as is one that is <9 weeks of gestation. Moreover, there are several types of medical management approaches, and several surgical approaches.

Medical management

Three main drugs have been used:

- Prostaglandins E_1: **misoprostol** (oral, vaginal), and gemeprost (vaginal) are uterotonics that result in cervical softening and contractions that expel the products of conception.
- **Mifepristone** (oral) is an antiprogesterone that results in starvation of the uterine lining. This results in capillary breakdown and synthesis of prostaglandins.
- **Methotrexate** (IM or oral) antagonizes folic acid, a cofactor needed for synthesis of nucleic acids. It is toxic to the rapidly dividing cells of the trophoblast.

Surgical management

Dilatation and evacuation is the historic, more common approach, usually in the operating room. **Manual vacuum aspiration is a safe alternative for gestations of 6–12 weeks with early pregnancy failure.** In women with incomplete abortion <13 weeks, manual vacuum aspiration is associated with a 91.5% success rate, with a 9.8% rate of complications, and a 94.7% acceptability rate, which are similar to misoprostol 600 μg orally (rates of 96.3%, 0.9%, and 94.2%, respectively).[1]

Medical vs expectant management

Medical management is significantly more effective than expectant management. Expectant management of missed abortion may be justified only for the woman who is very committed, or who has difficulty in accepting the diagnosis and moving directly to therapy. Expectant management may be a reasonable option with incomplete loss and intrauterine contents of $< 50\,mm^3$, as the success rate is about 78%.[2]

Medical vs surgical management

Without accounting for the factors mentioned above, **surgical management is about 50% more effective at achieving complete evacuation of the uterus than all medical management** (about 100% vs 60–80% evacuation) in an overall meta-analysis.[2]

Compared with vacuum aspiration, **misoprostol 800 μg vaginally** has **similar safety** (endometritis or hemorrhage ≤1% in each group), and lower but **good efficacy (84% vs 97%** complete expulsion at day 8).[2,3] This approach involves women at < **13 weeks of gestation**, with anembryonic gestation or embryonic or fetal death, of which some have incomplete abortion. If on day 3, transvaginal ultrasonography did not confirm complete evacuation, misoprostol 800 μg vaginally was repeated. With this approach, the **success rate is 81% with anembryonic gestation, 88% with embryonic or fetal death, and 93% with incomplete or inevitable abortion.** The success rate ranged from 65% to 93%, and increased with multiple dose regimens. Patients receiving misoprostol vaginally have decreased gastrointestinal side effects and improved pharmacokinetics.[2,4–7] Side effects of prostaglandins include diarrhea, nausea, and vomiting. These are increased when misoprostol is given orally.

Up to day 63 gestation (< 9 weeks), an alternative is **mifepristone** 200 mg, with misoprostol 800 μg vaginally 1–2 days after. Mifepristone followed by prostaglandin administration leads to 95% effectiveness or complete abortion. Doses of 200 mg and 600 mg have similar success rates followed by misoprostol (400–800 μg) or gemeprost 0.5 or 1 mg administered over 24–48 hours.[2,8–13] Women > 35 years old and smokers, or those with cardiovascular disease, should not receive the mifepristone/sulprostone regimen.

Up to day 49 gestation (< 7 weeks), **methotrexate** 50 mg/m² IM or orally, with misoprostol 800 μg vaginal 3–7 days later has also been shown to have > 80% success rates. One trial compares the oral with the IM route and found no difference in side effects. Prostaglandin administration should follow 3–7 days after methotrexate.[2,14–17] When using methotrexate, renal, liver, and hematological laboratory tests must be evaluated prior to administration of the medication.

Antibiotics

There is not sufficient evidence to recommend prophylactic antibiotics for spontaneous first trimester pregnancy loss.[18]

Follow-up

There are no trials to assess management of follow-up after pregnancy loss in the first trimester. After expectant or medical management, **β-HCG should probably be followed to zero**. Even with apparent complete miscarriage at transvaginal ultrasound after expectant management, about 5.9% of women have an ectopic pregnancy.[19] If chorionic villi are obtained at D&E, there is usually no need for a β-HCG follow-up.

References

1. Weeks A, Alia G, Blum J et al. A randomized trial of misoprostol compared with manual vacuum aspiration for incomplete abortion. Obstet Gynecol 2005; 106: 540–7. [RCT, n = 317]
2. Sotiriadis A, Makrydimas G, Papatheodorous S, Ioannidis JP. Expectant, medical, or surgical management of first trimester miscarriage: a meta-analysis. Obstet Gynecol 2005; 105: 1104–13. [meta-analysis: 27 RCTs, n = >1000]
3. Zhang J, Gilles JM, Barnhart K et al. A comparison of medical management with misoprostol and surgical management for early pregnancy failure. N Engl J Med 2005; 353: 761–9. [RCT, n = 652]
4. Khan RU, El-Refaey H, Sharma S, Sooranna D, Stafford M. Oral, rectal, and vaginal pharmacokinetics of misoprostol. Obstet Gynecol 2004; 103(5 Pt 1): 866–70. [II–3]
5. Muffley PE, Stitely ML, Gherman RB. Early intrauterine pregnancy failure: a randomized trial of medical versus surgical treatment. Am J Obstet Gynecol 2002; 187(2): 321–5; discussion 325–6. [RCT, n = 50]
6. Demetroulis C, Saridogan E, Kunde D, Naftalin AA. A prospective randomized control trial comparing medical and surgical treatment for early pregnancy failure. Hum Reprod 2001; 16(2): 365–9. [RCT, n = 80]
7. Bagratee JS, Khullar V, Regan L, Moodley J, Kagoro H. A randomized controlled trial comparing medical and expectant management of first trimester miscarriage. Hum Reprod 2004; 19(2): 266–71. [RCT, n = 104]
8. El-Refaey H, Templeton A. Early abortion induction by a combination of mifepristone and oral misoprostol: a comparison between two dose regimens of misoprostol and their effect on blood pressure. Br J Obstet Gynaecol 1994; 101: 792–6. [RCT]
9. McKinley C, Thong KJ, Baird DT. The effect of dose of mifepristone and gestation on the efficacy of medical abortion with mifepristone and misoprostol. Hum Reprod 1993; 8(9): 1502–5. [RCT]
10. Rodger MW, Logan AF, Baird DT. Induction of early abortion with mifepristone (RU 486) and two different doses of prostaglandin pessary (gemeprost). Contraception 1989; 39(5): 497–502. [RCT]
11. WHO Task Force on Post-ovulatory Methods of Fertility Regulation. Comparison of two doses of mifepristone in combination with misoprostol for early medical abortion: a randomised trial. Br J Obstet Gynaecol 2000; 107: 524–30. [RCT]
12. WHO Task Force on Post-ovulatory Methods for Fertility Regulation. Lowering the doses of mifepristone and gemeprost for early abortion: a randomised controlled trial. Br J Obstet Gynaecol 2001; 108: 738–42. [RCT]
13. Tang OS, Chan CC, Ng EH, Lee SW, Ho PC. A prospective, randomized, placebo-controlled trial on the use of mifepristone with sublingual or vaginal misoprostol for medical abortions of less than 9 weeks gestation. Hum Reprod 2003; 18(11): 2315–18. [RCT, n = 80]
14. Carbonell JL, Velazco A, Varela L et al. Misoprostol 3, 4, or 5 days after methotrexate for early abortion. Contraception 1997; 56: 169–74. [RCT]

15. Wiebe ER. Oral methotrexate compared with injected methotrexate when used with misoprostol for abortion. Am J Obstet Gynecol 1999; 181: 149–52. [RCT, n = 100]

16. Carbonell JL, Varela L, Velazco A et al. Oral methotrexate and vaginal misoprostol for early abortion. Contraception 1998; 57: 83–8. [RCT]

17. Creinin MD, Vittinghoff E, Galbraith S, Klaisle C. A randomized trial comparing misoprostol three and seven days after methotrexate for early abortion. Am J Obstet Gynecol 1995; 173: 1578–84. [RCT, n = 20]

18. Prieto JA, Eriksen NL, Blanco JD. A randomized trial of prophylactic doxycycline for curettage in incomplete abortion. Obstet Gynecol 1995; 85: 692–6. [RCT, n = 240]

19. Condous G, Okaro E, Khalid A, Bourne T. Do we need to follow up complete miscarriages with serum human chorionic gonadotropin levels? Br J Obstet Gynaecol 2005; 112: 827–9. [II–3]

29

The adnexal mass

Irina D Burd, David F Silver, and Norman G Rosenblum

KEY POINTS

- There are **no trials** on any intervention for adnexal mass in pregnancy.
- Complications related to the adnexal mass in gravid patients may include **severe pain** (5–26%), **ovarian torsion** (7–12%), **cyst rupture** (9%), **pelvic impaction and obstruction of labor** (5–17%), and **ovarian cancer** (< 5%).
- **Ultrasound,** with transvaginal and Doppler capabilities, **is the mainstay of diagnosis and prognosis.**
- For **persistent adnexal mass in pregnancy,** early preoperative **consultation with a gynecologic oncologist, anesthesiologist, and neonatologist** is recommended.
- Management in the **first trimester** is almost uniformly **expectant** when the clinical presentation is not acute.
- Intervention in the **third trimester** is typically **deferred until delivery or the postpartum period.**
- **Surgery** in pregnancy is reserved for adnexal masses that persist in the second trimester, and are either complex, with papillations and/or bilateral and > 5 cm, or increase by > 30% in size, or simple but > 10 cm.
- When necessary and feasible, **surgery should be scheduled in the early second trimester** when organogenesis is complete, most spontaneous pregnancy losses have occurred, and the risk for premature delivery is low.
- **Intervention** should be considered **at any point** in gestation **if a mass is complex or suspicious for malignancy and increases in size.**
- If an **adnexal mass** is **identified incidentally at the time of cesarean section,** it should be **removed** and not simply aspirated.
- If a **malignant neoplasm of the ovary** is found at the time of exploration, the surgeon's first obligation is to properly **stage the disease.**
- For more advanced ovarian cancer, the degree of cytoreductive surgery and the timing of initiation of chemotherapy will depend on fetal viability and maternal choice.

Definition/diagnosis

An adnexal mass is any mass in the ovary or tube or attached to them (adnexa). The vast majority (> 90%) of adnexal masses in pregnancy are ovarian. The diagnosis is most accurately made by ultrasound, even if it is possible to diagnose an adnexal mass by bimanual physical examination. A persistent adnexal mass is one that does not resolve by the second trimester.

Epidemiology/incidence

Approximately 1–4% of women are diagnosed with an adnexal mass in pregnancy, but in only 1 in 200 to 1 in 600 pregnancies does the adnexal mass persist to the second trimester.[1] The majority of adnexal masses are simple cysts such as corpus luteum or other functional cysts. Most of them (> 90%) when identified during pregnancy will spontaneously regress prior to the second trimester. The likelihood of regression is inversely related to size. Only 6% of cysts < 6 cm compared with 39% of cysts > 6 cm are persistent into the second trimester of pregnancy.[2–4] Two adnexal conditions are specifically associated with pregnancy and spontaneously regress in the postpartum period requiring no further treatment – **luteomas of pregnancy** and **theca lutein cysts.** Only 1–5% of persistent adnexal masses in pregnancy are malignant ovarian tumors.[2,5] The incidence of ovarian cancer in pregnancy is rare, 1 in 18 000 to 1 in 47 000 deliveries.[6,7]

Classification

Among persistent adnexal masses diagnosed during pregnancy (age group 18–35 years), mature teratomas are the most common, followed by benign serous or mucinous cystadenomas (Table 29.1). Most of the literature on ovarian cancer in pregnancy is based on case reports and series. In

Table 29.1 *Relative frequency of adnexal masses diagnosed in pregnancy*[8]	
Diagnosis	Percent
Mature teratoma	43.0
Serous or mucinous cystadenoma	18.6
Corpus luteum	12.0
Follicular cyst	9.0
Endometrioma	7.1
Fibroids	6.3
Malignancy	2.4
Other	1.6

the largest case series, the most common ovarian cancers found in pregnancy are serous and mucinous tumors of low malignant potential.[8]

Risk factors/associations

Maternal age is a risk factor for ovarian malignancy, but malignancies can occur at any reproductive age. **Assisted reproductive technologies** increase the incidence of enlarged ovaries, cysts, and therefore adnexal masses.

Complications

Complications related to the adnexal mass in gravid patients include **severe pain** (5–26%), **ovarian torsion** (12%), **cyst rupture** (9%), **pelvic impaction, and obstruction of labor** (5–17%).[9] Ovarian torsion, the most common significant complication in pregnancy, may be more common in pregnancy.[10] The risk of **ovarian cancer** is usually < 5%.[10]

Management
Principles

There are **no trials** available to assess any intervention in the management of adnexal mass in pregnancy. As > 90% of these masses resolve and the risk of malignancy is < 5%, expectant management is generally followed with serial ultrasound. If malignancy is suspected, the best gestational age for surgery is about 16–18 weeks, as the risk of loss is lowest.

Work-up
Ultrasound

Highly skilled ultrasonographers may be able to accurately diagnose these conditions (e.g. cancer, torsion) without surgical intervention. Suspicious characteristics of an adnexal mass include **complex** masses consisting of both **solid and cystic components** with nodularity, thick septations, irregular borders, solid masses containing irregular echoes, and papillary projections.[11] Although cancer can be present in a cyst of any size, adnexal masses of ≤ 5 cm have an incidence of malignancy of probably much less than < 1%.[10] In addition to routine ultrasonography, color **Doppler** studies may be used to distinguish between malignant and benign adnexal masses.[12] A low pulsatility index of < 1.0 and low impedance are associated with ovarian neoplasms. **Transvaginal** ultrasound may also help to better visualize the adnexal mass. The overall sensitivity of high-resolution ultrasound in distinguishing malignant from benign adnexal masses is 96.6%, specificity of 77%, and negative predictive value of 99%.[12] After 20 weeks, adnexal masses are more difficult to see by ultrasound given the larger uterine size. However, the definitive diagnosis will require pathological confirmation at all institutions.

Magnetic resonance imaging

Magnetic resonance imaging (MRI) has been used in addition to ultrasound to characterize the adnexal masses. There are insufficient data to assess the effect of MRI on the management of adnexal mass in pregnancy.

Laboratory

Most tumor markers may be elevated in normal pregnancy and are generally **not helpful** in distinguishing between a benign or malignant ovarian mass in pregnancy. For example, up to 16% of pregnant patients may have an elevated CA-125.[13]

Therapy

Treatment planning is dependent upon the timeliness of detection of an adnexal mass in pregnancy. When an adnexal mass is diagnosed in the first trimester, the likelihood of a functional etiology is high as is the probability of spontaneous resolution. In pregnant women, most simple cysts < 6 cm have been shown to spontaneously resolve.[14–17] Given the high obstetric risk during this period, **the management in the first trimester is almost uniformly expectant when the clinical presentation is not acute.**[10] Similarly, **intervention in the third trimester is**

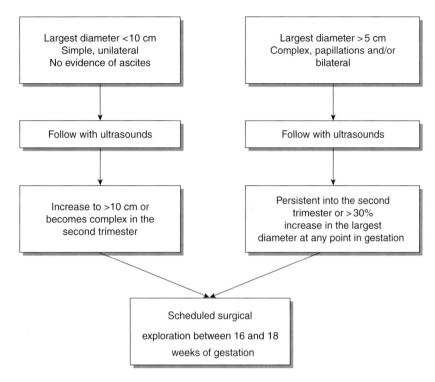

Figure 29.1
Suggested management of the ovarian mass in pregnancy.

typically deferred until delivery or the postpartum period, as the risk of delaying therapy rarely outweighs the risk of surgery to the mother and the fetus. When necessary and feasible, **surgery should be scheduled in the early second trimester** after most functional cysts have resolved, organogenesis is complete, most spontaneous losses have occurred, and the risk for premature delivery is low. **Intervention should be considered at any point in gestation if a mass is complex or highly suspicious for malignancy and increases in size** (Figure 29.1). In addition, **surgical intervention is indicated if torsion, rupture, or hemorrhage is identified.**

Consultations required

For persistent adnexal mass in pregnancy, **early preoperative consultation with a gynecologic oncologist, anesthesiologist, and neonatologist is recommended.**[18] Consultation at < 15 weeks is recommended for better operative planning.

Surgery

When exploration is necessary, all efforts should be made to **avoid unnecessary manipulation of the uterus** to minimize premature uterine contractions. In addition, other

Table 29.2 *Preoperative, intraoperative and postoperative considerations*[19–21]	
Preoperative management	Preoperative hydration – to reduce risk of hypotension, uteroplacental insufficiency, and resultant fetal hypoxemia
Placement	Fifteen percent left lateral tilt if the uterus is greater than 20 weeks to shift off the inferior vena cava/wedge placement under the right hip
Monitoring	All viable fetuses (≥ 24 weeks) can be monitored, either pre- and post–procedure or continuously
Anesthesia	Preoxygenation with 100% oxygen administered by face mask for 3–5 minutes. Halothane, isoflurane, and enflurane decrease uterine tone and may inhibit labor during the operative procedure

intraoperative and postoperative considerations should be kept in mind when operating on a pregnant patient (Table 29.2).[19–21] Whereas, traditionally, a laparotomy was the

Table 29.3	*FIGO staging for ovarian cancer*

Stage I – growth limited to the ovaries

Stage Ia – growth limited to one ovary, no ascites, no tumor on external surface, capsule intact

Stage Ib – growth limited to both ovaries, no ascites, no tumor on external surface, capsule intact

Stage Ic – tumor either stage Ia or Ib but with tumor on surface of one or both ovaries, ruptured capsule, ascites with malignant cells or positive peritoneal washings

Stage II – growth involving one or both ovaries, with pelvic extension

Stage IIa – extension and/or metastases to the uterus or tubes

Stage IIb – extension to other pelvic tissues

Stage IIc – stage IIa or IIb but with tumor on surface of one or both ovaries, ruptured capsule, ascites with malignant cells or positive peritoneal washings

Stage III – tumor involving one or both ovaries, with peritoneal implants outside the pelvis and/or positive retroperitoneal or inguinal nodes; superficial liver metastases

Stage IIIa – tumor grossly limited to pelvis, negative lymph nodes but histological proof of microscopic disease on abdominal peritoneal surfaces

Stage IIIb – confirmed implants outside of pelvis in the abdominal peritoneal surface; no implant exceeds 2 cm in diameter and lymph nodes are negative

Stage IIIc – abdominal implants larger than 2 cm in diameter and/or positive lymph nodes

Stage IV – distant metastases; pleural effusion must have a positive cytology to be classified as stage IV; parenchymal liver metastases

FIGO, Fédération Internationale de Gynécologie et d'Obstétrique (International Federation of Gynecology and Obstetrics).

standard recommendation used to explore the abdomen of a pregnant patient with an adnexal mass, in the 1990s laparoscopy became an acceptable alternative in experienced hands and offers the benefit of a more expeditious recovery.[22–24] However, despite several reports[25,26] suggesting that laparoscopic surgery can be safely performed for ovarian torsion during pregnancy, laparotomy remains the standard of care for surgical management of such patients. Abdominal surgery during pregnancy, in particular laparotomy, has been associated with higher rates of miscarriage and preterm birth compared with no surgery.[10]

If an adnexal mass is identified incidentally at the time of cesarean section, it should be removed and not simply aspirated.[1] With aspiration and cytological evaluation, malignancy could be missed.[27] If a malignant neoplasm of the ovary is found at the time of exploration, the surgeon's first obligation is to properly stage the disease (Table 29.3). Since most present as stage I disease, a unilateral salpingo-oophorectomy, omentectomy, and limited pelvic and para-aortic lymph node dissection is the procedure of choice. If the disease appears to be confined to the pelvis, comprehensive surgical staging is indicated. The staging procedure includes peritoneal cytology, multiple peritoneal biopsies, omentectomy, and pelvic and para-aortic lymph node sampling.

Rarely is a hysterectomy indicated. **For more advanced disease, the degree of cytoreductive surgery and the timing of initiation of chemotherapy will depend on fetal viability and maternal choice, and should be managed by a gynecologic oncologist.**

References

1. Koonings PP, Platt LD, Wallace R. Incidental adnexal neoplasms at cesarean section. Obstet Gynecol 1988; 72: 767–9. [II–3]
2. Hess LW, Peaceman A, O'Brien WF, Winkel CA. Adnexal mass occurring with intrauterine pregnancy: report of fifty-four patients requiring laparotomy for definitive management. Am J Obstet Gynecol 1988; 58: 1029–34. [II–3]
3. Whitecar MP, Turner S, Higby MK. Adnexal masses in pregnancy: a review of 130 cases undergoing surgical management. Am J Obstet Gynecol 1999; 181: 19–24. [II–3]
4. Beischer NA, Buttery BW, Fortune DW, Macafee CA. Growth and malignancy of ovarian tumours in pregnancy. Aust N Z J Obstet Gynaecol 1971; 11: 208–20.[II–3]
5. El Yahia AR, Rahman J, Rahman MS et al. Ovarian tumors in pregnancy. Aust N Z J Obstet Gynecol 1991; 31: 327–30. [II–3]
6. Munnell EW. Primary ovarian cancer associated with pregnancy. Clin Obstet Gynecol 1963; 6: 983–93. [III]
7. Dgani R, Shoham Z, Atar E et al. Ovarian carcinoma during pregnancy: a study of 23 cases in Israel between the years of 1963 and 1984. Gynecol Oncol 1989; 33: 326–31. [II–3]

8. Liu JR, Lilja JF, Johnston C. Adnexal masses in pregnancy. In: Trimble EL, Trimble CL, eds. Cancer Obstetrics and Gynecology. Lippincott, Williams and Wilkins; Baltimore, MD: 1999: 239–48. [III]

9. Struyk AP, Treffers PE. Ovarian tumors in pregnancy. Acta Obstet Gynecol Scand 1984; 63: 421–4. [II–3]

10. Schmeler KM, Mayo-Smith WW, Peipert JF et al. Adnexal masses in pregnancy: surgery compared with observation. Obstet Gynecol 2005; 105: 1098–103. [II–3]

11. Bromley B, Benacerraf B. Adnexal masses during pregnancy: accuracy of sonographic diagnosis and outcome. J Ultrasound Med 1997; 16: 447–54. [II–3]

12. Wheeler TC, Fleischer AC. Complex adnexal mass in pregnancy: predictive value of color Doppler ultrasonography. J Ultrasound Med 1997; 16: 425–8. [II–2, n=34]

13. Niloff JM, Knapp RC, Schaetzi E et al. CA125 antigen levels in obstetric and gynecology patients. Obstet Gynecol 1984; 64: 70–3. [II–3]

14. Hogston P, Lilford RJ. Ultrasound study of ovarian cysts in pregnancy: prevalence and significance. Br J Obstet Gynaecol 1986; 93: 625–8. [II–3]

15. Thornton JG, Wells M. Ovarian cysts in pregnancy: does ultrasound make traditional management inappropriate? Obstet Gynecol 1987; 69: 717–21. [II–3]

16. Bernhard LM, Klebba PK, Gray DL, Mutch DG. Predictors of persistence of adnexal masses in pregnancy. Obstet Gynecol 1999; 93: 585–9. [II–3]

17. Zanetta, G, Mariani, E, Lissoni, A et al. A prospective study of the role of ultrasound in the management of adnexal masses in pregnancy. Br J Obstet Gynecol 2003; 110: 578–83. [II–2, n=79]

18. ACOG Committee Opinion No. 284. Nonobstetric surgery in pregnancy. Obstet Gynecol 2003; 102: 431. [review]

19. Caspi B, Appelman Z, Rabinerson D et al. Pathognomonic echo patterns of benign cystic teratomas of the ovary: classification, incidence and accuracy rate of sonographic diagnosis. Ultrasound Obstet Gynecol 1996; 7: 275–9. [II–2, n=115]

20. Granberg S, Wikland M, Jansson I. Macroscopic characterization of ovarian tumors and the relation to the histological diagnosis: criteria to be used for ultrasound evaluation. Gynecol Oncol 1989; 35: 139–44. [II–3]

21. Hata K, Hata T. Intramural blood flow analysis in ovarian cancer: what does it mean? J Ultrasound Med 1996; 15: 571–5. [II–3]

22. Soriano D, Yefet Y, Seidman DS, Goldenberg M. Laparoscopy versus laparotomy in the management of adnexal masses during pregnancy. Fertil Steril 1999; 71: 955–60. [II–2, n=88]

23. Yuen PM, Ng PS, Leung PL, Rogers MS. Outcome in laparoscopic management of persistent adnexal mass during the second trimester of pregnancy. Surg Endosc 2004; 18(9): 354–7. [II–3]

24. Mathevet P, Nessah K, Dargent D, Mellier G. Laparoscopic management of adnexal masses in pregnancy: a case series. Eur J Obstet Gynecol Reprod Biol 2003; 108(2): 217–22. [II–3]

25. Shalev E, Peleg D. Laparoscopic treatment of adnexal torsion. Surg Gynecol Obstet 1993; 176: 448–50. [II–3]

26. Cohen SB, Oelsner G, Seidman DS et al. Laparoscopic detorsion allows sparing of the twisted ischemic adnexa. J Am Assoc Gynecol Laparosc 1999; 6: 139–43. [II–3]

27. Rodin A, Coltart TM, Chapman MG. Needle aspiration of simple ovarian cysts in pregnancy. Case reports. Br J Obstet Gynaecol 1989; 96: 994–6. [II–3]

30

Cervical cancer screening

Irina D Burd, David F Silver, and Norman G Rosenblum

KEY POINTS

- The only cervical diagnosis that is considered to alter management in pregnancy is invasive cancer.
- Owing to risks of bleeding and premature rupture of membranes, endocervical curettage is generally avoided in pregnancy.
- Diagnostic conization during pregnancy should only be considered when either the biopsy or cytology is suggestive of invasive cancer and the diagnosis of invasion would result in a modification of treatment recommendations, timing, or mode of delivery.
- If the histological diagnosis of invasive cervical cancer is made and a grossly visible lesion is detected, cesarean delivery is indicated and results in better survival outcomes as well as a decreased risk of obstetric bleeding in the intrapartum and postpartum periods.
- If a microinvasive (stage IA1) or a non-visible invasive lesion (stage IA2) is identified, either the abdominal or vaginal route of delivery is acceptable, depending on the obstetric and gynecological circumstances.
- Once the diagnosis of cervical cancer is established, individualized recommendations for the management of the malignancy as well as the pregnancy are formulated with consideration for the stage of disease, gestational age at the time of diagnosis, and the woman's desires regarding the continuation of her pregnancy.

Historic notes

The cytological evaluation of the cervix, known as the Pap smear, was developed in the 1940s by George Papanicolaou MD. The Bethesda System, which standardized terminology for reporting Pap smears in 1988,[1] was subsequently revised in 2001.[2]

Diagnosis/definition

Microinvasive cervical cancer (MCC) is defined as cancer spread to no more than 5 mm into the tissues of the cervix. Invasive cervical cancer (ICC) is defined as cancer spread

from the surface of the cervix to tissue deeper in the cervix, possible spread to part of the vagina, to the lymph nodes, other tissues surrounding the cervix, within the pelvis, or beyond the pelvic areas into nearby organs.

Epidemiology/incidence

The overall rate of an abnormal Pap smear (ASC-US or higher) in the USA from 1995 to 2001 was 6%.[3] The peak age incidence of cervical cancer is in the mid 40s. Cervical cancer is the second most common cancer among women worldwide, the third most common cause of cancer-related death, and the most common cause of mortality from gynecologic malignancy. Although in the majority of developing countries cervical cancer remains the number 1 cause of cancer-related deaths among women, Pap smear screening in developed countries became a preventive medicine issue by accurately detecting preinvasive and early invasive cervical disease. In the USA, the incidence of cervical cancer ranges from 1 to 13 cases in 10 000 pregnancies. About 1% of the women who have cervical cancer are pregnant at the time of diagnosis. The likelihood that a pregnant woman with ASC (atypical squamous cell) pathology has a detectable high-risk human papillomavirus (HPV) is 84%.[4]

Classification

The Pap smear report consists of the following parts:[2]

Specimen type

For example, conventional Pap smear or liquid-based cytology.

Specimen adequacy
Satisfactory for evaluation

- Defined as ≥5000 well-visualized squamous cells on a liquid-based preparation or 8000–12 000 well-visualized squamous cells on a conventional smear.

- The presence of endocervical cells indicates that the area at risk for neoplasia, the transformation zone, has been adequately sampled. In a contrast to the follow-up for an absent endocervical/transformation zone component in non-pregnant population being a repeat Pap in 12 months, pregnant women undergo repeat testing postpartum.[5]

Unsatisfactory for evaluation

- Defined as >75% of the cells being uninterpretable or unlabeled specimen.
- Since women with this result are more likely to have intraepithelial lesions or cancer on follow-up than women with satisfactory Pap smears,[6] the test should always be repeated in 2–4 months.[5] If the Pap smear is repeatedly unsatisfactory, evaluation with colposcopy and/or biopsies is appropriate.[5]

Interpretation/result

Squamous epithelial cell abnormalities

- Atypical squamous cells (ASC) either of:
  - undetermined significance (ASC-US) or
  - suspicious for HSIL (ASC-H).
- Low-grade squamous intraepithelial lesions (LSIL):
  - changes consistent with HPV, mild dysplasia, or CIN 1 (cervical intraepithelial neoplasia grade 1).
- High-grade squamous intraepithelial lesions (HSIL):
  - HSIL includes moderate or severe dysplasia, CIN 2, CIN 3, and carcinoma in situ (CIS), and should indicate if there are features suspicious for invasive disease. When glandular cell abnormalities are present, it should be noted whether there are changes favoring neoplasia.
- Carcinoma.

Glandular cell abnormalities

- Atypical glandular cells (AGC) may be of endocervical, endometrial, or other glandular origin.
- Endocervical adenocarcinoma in situ (AIS).
- Adenocarcinoma.

Ancillary testing done

- human papillomavirus (HPV) testing, which is important in management of ASC-US Pap smear.
- HPV infection is the leading etiological agent in the development of premalignant and malignant lower genital tract disease.
- The most well-studied HPV test is the Hybrid Capture 2 HPV DNA Assay (Digene Corporation), which uses a probe mix for high-risk HPV types 16, 18, 31, 33, 35, 39, 45, 51, 52, 56, 58, 59, and 68. Even though high-risk HPV types 16 and 18 are the viruses most frequently isolated in cervical cancer tissue,[7] the HPV test does not distinguish individual HPV types. The use of the HPV testing was validated in 2001 by a consensus group of the American Society for Colposcopy and Cervical Pathology (see below).[7]

Management
Pregnancy considerations

Pregnancy-induced changes in the cervix include hyperemia, eversion of columnar epithelium, more prominent glands, and increased production and volume of mucus. The decidual changes may exaggerate the colposcopic appearance of CIN. A biopsy during pregnancy may cause substantial bleeding.[8] In pregnancy, the general philosophy for the treatment of intraepithelial neoplasia of the cervix has become expectant management after careful diagnosis.

Screening

The Pap smear is used to screen for cellular abnormalities that are associated with an increased risk for the development of cervical cancer. It selects those women who should have further evaluation, such as HPV DNA testing, colposcopy and/or biopsy, which are then used for treatment decisions. The National Comprehensive Cancer Network (NCCN) panel has adopted a recommendation set forth by the American Cancer Society on initiation and frequency of Pap smear. This recommendation is to start screening within 3 years after the onset of sexual activity or no later than 21 years of age. **Screening** should be recommended to **continue yearly for women younger than 30 years**. Women aged ≥ 30 years old who have had three consecutive cervical cytology test results that are negative, are not immunosuppressed, and have no history of diethylstilbestrol exposure in utero or human immunodeficiency virus (HIV) infection may be screened every 2–3 years. Although testing during pregnancy is not addressed in most screening guidelines, a Pap smear is obtained at the first prenatal visit by many providers, or the above guidelines for non-pregnant women can be followed. There is no difference in unsatisfactory rates, cytology classifications, and accuracy between conventional and liquid-based cervical cytology.[9]

Consultations required

Consultation with a gynecologi oncologist is recommended in cases of cervical cancer.[10] Consultation should occur as early as possible after the diagnosis of cervical cancer for better therapeutic planning.

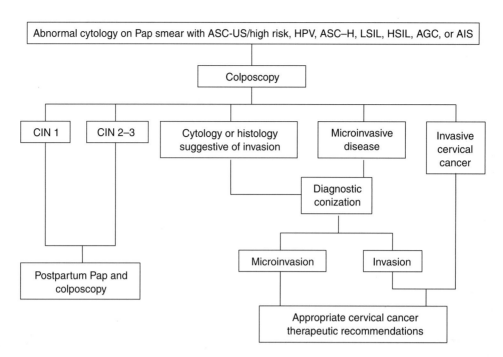

Figure 30.1
Algorithm for the work-up of abnormal cytology in pregnancy. See text for abbreviations.

Natural history/prenatal care/pregnancy course

As in non-pregnant women, women with abnormal Pap smears during pregnancy should undergo colposcopy with directed biopsies of suspicious areas to rule out invasive disease. While necessary colposcopically directed cervical biopsies can be safely performed at any time during pregnancy, many clinicians defer biopsy until the second trimester when the risk of incidental pregnancy loss is minimal. Owing to risks of bleeding and premature rupture of membranes, endocervical curettage is generally not recommended in pregnancy.

Termination issues

Once the diagnosis of cervical cancer is established, individualized recommendations for the management of the malignancy as well as the pregnancy are formulated, with consideration for the stage of disease, gestational age at the time of diagnosis, and the woman's desires regarding the continuation of her pregnancy.

Therapy

There are **no randomized trials** assessing any aspect of management of abnormal Pap smear in pregnancy. Most of the recommendations are based on expert opinion and anecdotal experience.[8] **The only diagnosis that is considered to alter management in pregnancy is invasive cancer.** Management of abnormal Pap smears in pregnancy may follow the recommendations delineated in Figure 30.1.

Colposcopy

Recommendations for **colposcopy** in pregnant patients are similar to those in the non-gravid state, with certain exceptions, as listed in Table 30.1. Colposcopy during pregnancy has as its primary goal to assess for invasive cancer. It is reasonable to follow expectantly cytology results that are not associated with cancer, such as ASC and LSIL, normal Pap but

Table 30.1	*Cervical screening considerations during pregnancy*

- Endocervical brush cytology is safe
- Cervical biopsy is safe
- ECC should be avoided
- For ASC and LSIL, colposcopy can be done during pregnancy or postpartum
- For CIN 2 or CIN 3 in early pregnancy, repeat colposcopy later in pregnancy to rule out invasion
- Delay treatment of any level of CIN until postpartum period
- Cervical conization is recommended if invasion is suspected

ECC, endocervical curettage. For other abbreviations see text.

absence of endocervical cells, or colposcopic impression of CIN 1[11] during pregnancy, with just postpartum follow-up. Colposcopic impression of CIN 2 or CIN 3 can be followed up with colposcopy every 3 months and 6–12 weeks postpartum.

Biopsy

Endocervical sampling is **not performed** in pregnancy.

Cervical biopsy(ies) may be omitted with ASC and LSIL, with colposcopic evaluation either during pregnancy or 6–12 weeks postpartum.[12] Biopsies should be performed for women with colposcopic impression of CIN 3, AIS, or cancer, with the purpose of excluding invasive cancer.

Conization

Cervical conization in pregnancy is primarily used as a diagnostic measure with limited indications (Table 30.2). Unlike standard recommendations for cervical conization in non-obstetric patients with inadequate colposcopies or discordance between Pap smears and colposcopic biopsies, pregnant women with these findings are followed with

Table 30.2 *Indications for conization in pregnancy*

- Histological presence of microinvasive or invasive disease
- Persistent cytological impression of invasive cancer (in absence of histological confirmation)
- Histological presence of adenocarcinoma in situ

serial Pap smears and colposcopies every trimester throughout the remainder of the pregnancy until the postpartum period or the development of histological or cytological evidence of invasive disease. In general, diagnostic conization during pregnancy should only be considered **when either the biopsy or cytology is suggestive of invasive cancer** and the diagnosis of invasion would result in a modification of treatment recommendations, timing, or mode of delivery.

Staging and management

For staging and management please refer to Table 30.3. If a microinvasive (stage IA1) or a non-visible invasive lesion (stage IA2) is identified, either the abdominal or vaginal

Table 30.3 *Staging and management of cervical cancer in pregnancy*			
Stage 0	carcinoma-in-situ		**Preinvasive disease** – not treated in pregnancy
Stage I	the tumor is confined to the cervix		
	IA	microinvasive disease, with the lesion not grossly visible: no deeper than 5 mm and no wider than 7 mm	**Microinvasive cervical cancer** (MCC) – not treated during pregnancy
		IA1 invasion < 3 mm and no wider than 7 mm	
		IA2 invasion > 3 mm but < 5 mm and no wider than 7 mm	
	IB	larger tumor than in IA or grossly visible, confined to cervix	Histologically confirmed, **invasive cervical cancer** (ICC) is the only indication to treat during pregnancy
		IB1 clinical lesion < 4 cm	
		IB2 clinical lesion > 4 cm	
Stage II	extends beyond the cervix, but does not involve the pelvic side wall or lowest third of the vagina		
	IIA	involvement of the upper 2/3 of vagina, without lateral extension into the parametrium	
	IIB	lateral extension into parametrial tissue	
Stage III	involves the lowest third of the vagina or pelvic side wall, or causes hydronephrosis		
	IIIA	involvement of the lowest third of the vagina	
	IIIB	involvement of pelvic side wall or hydronephrosis	
Stage IV	extensive local infiltration or has spread to a distant site		
	IVA	involvement of bladder or rectal mucosa	
	IVB	distant metastases	

route of delivery is acceptable, dependent upon obstetric and gynecological circumstances.

If the histological diagnosis of invasive cervical cancer is made and a grossly visible lesion is detected, cesarean delivery with radical hysterectomy is indicated and results in better survival outcomes as well as a decreased risk of obstetric bleeding in the intrapartum and postpartum periods (see also Chapter 19 of *Maternal–Fetal Evidence Based Guidelines* for additional information on invasive cervical cancer).

Recurrence and follow-up treatment

Seventy-five percent of patients with CIN diagnosed during pregnancy have persistent or progressive disease at postpartum evaluation.[13] A regression rate of only 12% is found in pregnant women with CIN 3, emphasizing the importance of **re-evaluation 6 weeks postpartum.**[14]

Routine surveillance can be resumed if there is no recurrence after the first year. Surveillance consists of Pap smears on a yearly basis for most women, and on a twice-yearly basis for high-risk women (i.e. HIV positive).

Prevention

HPV-16 and -18 vaccine reduces the incidence of both HPV-16 and -18 infection and HPV-16/18-related cervical intraepithelial neoplasia.[15,16] HPV vaccine should be offered routinely to women before 26 years of age, preferably around 12 years of age, or before first intercourse.

References

1. The 1988 Bethesda System for reporting cervical/vaginal cytological diagnoses. National Cancer Institute Workshop. JAMA 1989; 262: 931–4. [review, guideline]
2. Solomon D, Davey D, Kurman R et al. The 2001 Bethesda system: terminology for reporting results of cervical cytology. JAMA 2002; 287: 2114–19. [review, guideline]
3. Benard VB, Eheman CR, Lawson HW et al. Cervical screening in the National Breast and Cervical Cancer Early Detection Program, 1995–2001. Obstet Gynecol 2004; 103: 564–71. [II–3]
4. Lu DW, Pirog EC, Zhu X, Wang HL, Pinto KR. Prevalence and typing of HPV DNA in atypical squamous cells in pregnant women. Acta Cytol 2003; 47(6): 1008–16. [II–3]
5. Davey DD, Austin RM, Birdsong G et al. ASCCP Patient Management Guidelines: Pap Test Specimen Adequacy and Quality Indicators. J Low Genit Tract Dis 2002; 6: 195–9. [guideline]
6. Ransdell JS, Davey DD, Zaleski S. Clinicopathologic correlation of the unsatisfactory Papanicolaou smear. Cancer 1997; 81: 139–43. [II–3]
7. Bosch FX, Manos MM, Munoz N et al. Prevalence of human papillomavirus in cervical cancer: a worldwide perspective. International Biological Study on Cervical Cancer (IBSCC) Study Group. J Natl Cancer Inst 1995; 87: 796–802. [II–3]
8. Massad SL, Wright TC, Cox TJ, Twiggs LB, Wilkinson E. Managing abnormal cytology results in pregnancy. J Low Genit Tract Dis 2005; 9(3): 146–8. [III]
9. Davey E, Barratt A, Irwig L et al. Effect of study design and quality on unsatisfactory rates, cytology classifications, and accuracy in liquid-based versus conventional cervical cytology: a systematic review. Lancet 2006; 367: 122–32. [meta-analysis]
10. ACOG Committee Opinion No. 284. Nonobstetric surgery in pregnancy. Obstet Gynecol 2003; 102: 431. [review]
11. ACOG Practice Bulletin No. 66. Management of abnormal cervical cytology and histology. Obstet Gynecol 2005; 106(3): 645. [review]
12. Wright JD, Pinto AB, Powell MA et al. Atypical squamous cells of undetermined significance in girls and women. Obstet Gynecol 2004; 103: 632–8. [II–3]
13. Palle C, Bangsball S, Andreasson B. Cervical intraepithelial neoplasia in pregnancy. Acta Obstet Gynecol Scand 2000; 79: 306–10. [II–3]
14. Coppola A, Sorosky J, Casper R et al. The clinical course of cervical carcinoma in situ diagnosed during pregnancy. Acta Obstet Gynecol Scand 1997; 67: 162–5. [II–3]
15. Koutsky LA, Ault KA, Wheeler CM et al. A controlled trial of a human papillomavirus type 16 vaccine. N Engl J Med 2002; 347; 1645–51. [RCT, n = 2392]
16. Harper DM, Franco EL, Wheeler C et al. Efficacy of a bivalent L1 virus-like particle vaccine in prevention of infection with human papillomavirus types 16 and 18 in young women: a randomised controlled trial. Lancet 2004; 364: 1757–65.

Index